S0-BJG-451

DISCARD

Humber College Library
3199 Lakeshore Blvd. West
Toronto, ON   M8V 1K8

Better Doctors, Better Patients, Better Decisions

Envisioning Health Care 2020

Strüngmann Forum Reports

Julia Lupp, series editor

The Ernst Strüngmann Forum is made possible through the generous support of the Ernst Strüngmann Foundation, inaugurated by Dr. Andreas and Dr. Thomas Strüngmann.

This Forum was supported by funds from the Deutsche Forschungsgemeinschaft (German Science Foundation)

Better Doctors, Better Patients, Better Decisions

Envisioning Health Care 2020

Edited by

Gerd Gigerenzer and J. A. Muir Gray

Program Advisory Committee:
Gerd Gigerenzer, J. A. Muir Gray, Günter Ollenschläger,
Lisa M. Schwartz, and Steven Woloshin

HUMBER LIBRARIES LAKESHORE CAMPUS
3199 Lakeshore Blvd West
TORONTO, ON.   M8V 1K8

The MIT Press

Cambridge, Massachusetts
London, England

© 2011 Massachusetts Institute of Technology and
the Frankfurt Institute for Advanced Studies

Series Editor: J. Lupp
Assistant Editor: M. Turner
Photographs: U. Dettmar
Typeset by BerlinScienceWorks

All rights reserved. No part of this book may be reproduced in any form
by electronic or mechanical means (including photocopying, recording,
or information storage and retrieval) without permission in writing from
the publisher.

MIT Press books may be purchased at special quantity discounts
for business or sales promotional use. For information, please email
special_sales@mitpress.mit.edu or write to Special Sales Department,
The MIT Press, 55 Hayward Street, Cambridge, MA 02142.

The book was set in TimesNewRoman and Arial.
Printed and bound in the United States of America.

Library of Congress Cataloging-in-Publication Data

Ernst Strüngmann Forum (2009 : Frankfurt am Main, Germany)
Better doctors, better patients, better decisions : envisioning health care
2020 / edited by Gerd Gigerenzer and J. A. Muir Gray.
    p. cm. — (Strüngmann Forum reports)
Forum held in Frankfurt am Main, Germany, Oct. 25–30, 2009.
Includes bibliographical references and index.
ISBN 978-0-262-01603-2 (hardcover : alk. paper)
1. Health education. 2. Medical education. 3. Medicine—Decision
making. 4. Medicine—Forecasting. I. Gigerenzer, Gerd. II. Gray, J. A.
Muir (John Armstrong Muir) III. Title.
RA440.5.E77   2009
362.1—dc22
                                                                2010044699
10 9 8 7 6 5 4 3

Contents

The Ernst Strüngmann Forum

Founded on the tenets of scientific independence and the inquisitive nature of the human mind, the Ernst Strüngmann Forum is dedicated to the continual expansion of knowledge. Through its innovative communication process, the Ernst Strüngmann Forum provides a creative environment within which experts scrutinize high-priority issues from multiple vantage points.

This process begins with the identification of themes. By nature, a theme constitutes a problem area that transcends classic disciplinary boundaries. It is of high-priority interest and requires concentrated, multidisciplinary input to address the issues involved. Proposals are received from leading scientists active in their field and are selected by an independent Scientific Advisory Board. Once approved, a steering committee is convened to refine the scientific parameters of the proposal and select the participants. Approximately one year later, a focal meeting is held to which circa forty experts are invited.

Preliminary discussion on this theme began in 2008, when Gerd Gigerenzer brought the problem of literacy in health care and its impact on the health care system to our attention. In October, 2008, the steering committee—comprised of Gerd Gigerenzer, Muir Gray, Günter Ollenschläger, Lisa Schwartz, and Steven Woloshin—met to identify the key issues for debate and select the participants for the focal meeting, which was held in Frankfurt am Main, Germany, from October 25–30, 2009.

The activities and discourse surrounding a Forum begin well before participants arrive in Frankfurt and conclude with the publication of this volume. Throughout each stage, focused dialog is the means by which issues are examined anew. This often requires relinquishing long-established ideas and overcoming disciplinary idiosyncrasies which might otherwise inhibit joint examination. However, when this is accomplished, a unique synergism results and new insights emerge.

This volume conveys the synergy that arose from a group of diverse experts, each of whom assumed an active role in the process, and is comprised of two types of contributions. The first provides background information on key aspects of the overall theme. These chapters have been extensively reviewed and revised to reflect current understanding. The second (Chapters 8, 12, 13, and 19) summarizes the extensive discussions that transpired. These chapters should not be viewed as consensus documents nor are they proceedings; instead, they transfer the essence of the multifaceted discussions, expose the open questions that remain, and highlight directions for future work.

An endeavor of this kind creates its own unique dynamics and puts demands on everyone who participates. Each invitee contributed not only their time and congenial personality, but a willingness to probe beyond that which is evident, and I wish to extend my sincere gratitude to all. A special word of thanks goes

viii *The Ernst Strüngmann Forum*

to the steering committee, the authors of the background papers, the reviewers of the papers, and the moderators of the individual working groups (Johann Steurer, Ingrid Mühlhauser, Hilda Bastian, and Heather Buchan). To draft a report during the Forum and bring it to its final form in the months thereafter is no simple matter, and for their efforts, we are especially grateful to Gerd Antes, Markus Feufel, Talya Miron-Shatz, Norbert Donner-Banzhoff, and Ralph Hertwig. Most importantly, I wish to extend my appreciation to Gerd Gigerenzer, whose tireless efforts throughout the entire process proved to be invaluable.

A communication process of this nature relies on institutional stability and an environment that encourages free thought. The generous support of the Ernst Strüngmann Foundation, established by Dr. Andreas and Dr. Thomas Strüngmann in honor of their father, enables the Ernst Strüngmann Forum to conduct its work in the service of science. In addition, the following valuable partnerships are gratefully acknowledged: the Scientific Advisory Board, which ensures the scientific independence of the Forum; the Deutsche Forschungsgemeinschaft (German Science Foundation), which provided financial support for this theme; and the Frankfurt Institute for Advanced Studies, which shares its vibrant intellectual setting with the Forum.

Long-held views are never easy to put aside. Yet when this is achieved, when the edges of the unknown begin to appear and gaps in knowledge are able to be identified, the act of formulating strategies to fill these becomes a most invigorating exercise. But this is hardly the end, for if people are to achieve health literacy and if current health care systems are to evolve into patient-centered entities, multiple efforts on many levels are needed. It is our hope that this volume will contribute to these efforts.

Julia Lupp, Program Director
Ernst Strüngmann Forum
Ruth-Moufang-Str. 1
60438 Frankfurt am Main, Germany
http://esforum.de

List of Contributors

Gerd Antes   Deutsches Cochrane Zentrum, Abteilung Medizinische Biometrie und Statistik, Stefan-Meier-Str. 26, 79104 Freiburg, Germany

Hilda Bastian   IQWiG, Institut für Qualität und Wirtschaftlichkeit im Gesundheitswesen, Dillenburger Str. 27, 51105 Köln, Germany

Jean Bousquet   University Hospital and INSERM, Hôpital Arnaud de Villeneuve, Montpellier, France

Bruce Bower   Science News, 1719 N Street N.W., Washington, D.C. 20036, U.S.A.

Henry Brighton   Center for Adaptive Behavior and Cognition, Max Planck Institute for Human Development, Lentzeallee 94, 14195 Berlin, Germany

Heather Buchan   National Institute of Clinical Studies, National Health and Medical Research Council, GPO Box 4530, Melbourne, VIC 3001, Australia

Angela Coulter   Bitterell House, 8 Bitterell, Oxon OX29 4JL, U.K.

David A. Davis   Continuing Healthcare Education and Improvement, Association of American Medical Colleges, 2450 N Street NW, Washington, D.C. 20031, U.S.A.

Michael Diefenbach   Mount Sinai School of Medicine, 5 East 98th Street, New York, NY 10029, U.S.A.

Norbert Donner-Banzhoff   Abteilung für Allgemeinmedizin, Phillips-Universität Marburg, 35032 Marburg, Germany

Glyn Elwyn   Clinical Epidemiology Interdisciplinary Research Group, Cardiff University, Neuadd Meironydd Heath Park, CF 14 4YS, U.K.

Markus A. Feufel   Center for Adaptive Behavior and Cognition, Max Planck Institute for Human Development, Lentzeallee 94, 14195 Berlin, Germany

Wolfgang Gaissmaier   Harding Center for Risk Literacy, Max Planck Institute for Human Development, Lentzeallee 94, 14195 Berlin, Germany

Davina Ghersi   World Health Organisation, Avenue Appia 20, 1211 Geneva 27, Switzerland

Gerd Gigerenzer   Harding Center for Risk Literacy, Max Planck Institute for Human Development, Lentzeallee 94, 14195 Berlin, Germany

Ben Goldacre   Bad Science, 119 Farringdon Road, London EC1R 3ER, U.K.

J. A. Muir Gray   NHS National Knowledge Service, Summertown Pavilion, Middle Way, Oxford OX2 7LG, U.K.

Martin Härter   Universitätsklinikum Hamburg-Eppendorf, Institut und Polyklinik für Medizinische Psychologie, Martinstr. 52, 20246 Hamburg, Germany

Ralph Hertwig   Department of Psychology, University of Basel, Missionsstrasse 64a, 4055 Basel, Switzerland

Günther Jonitz Präsident der Ärztekammer Berlin, Friedrichstr. 16, 10969 Berlin, Germany

David Klemperer University of Applied Sciences, Faculty of Social Science, Seybothstr. 2, 93053 Regensburg, Germany

Kai Kolpatzik Leiter Abteilung Prävention, AOK-Bundesverband, Rosenthaler Str. 31, 10178 Berlin, Germany

Julia Kreis IQWiG, Institut für Qualität und Wirtschaftlichkeit im Gesundheitswesen, Dillenburger Str. 27, 51105 Köln, Germany

France Légaré Research Center, Centre Hospitalier Universitaire de Québec, 10 Rue de L'Espinay, Québec G1L 3L5, Canada

Wolf-Dieter Ludwig Arzneimittelkommission der deutschen Ärzteschaft, Herbert-Lewin-Platz 1, 10623 Berlin, Germany

Marjukka Mäkelä Finnish Office for Health Technology Assessment (Finohta), National Institute for Health and Welfare (THL), Lintulahdenkuja 4, P.O.Box 30, 00271 Helsinki, Finland

Talya Miron-Shatz Ono Academic College, Business School, Marketing Department, 104 Zahal Street, Kiryat Ono, 55000, Israel

Ingrid Mühlhauser Universität Hamburg, Gesundheitswissenschaften, Martin-Luther-King-Platz 6, 20146 Hamburg, Germany

Albert G. Mulley, Jr. Chief, General Medicine, Massachusetts General Hospital, 50 Staniford, St., Suite 900, Boston, MA 02114, U.S.A.

David E. Nelson Cancer Prevention Fellowship Program, National Cancer Institute, Executive Plaza South, Suite 150E, Bethesda, MD 20892–7105, U.S.A.

Norbert Schmacke Arbeits- und Koordinierungstelle, Gesundheits-versorgungsforschung, Universität Bremen, Wilhelm-Herbst-Str.7, 28359 Bremen, Germany

Gisela Schott Drug Commission of the German Medical Association (DCGMA), Berlin, Germany

Jay Schulkin Department of Physiology, Biophysics 1, Neuroscience, Georgetown University, Washington, D.C., U.S.A.

Holger Schünemann McMaster University, Health Science Centre, 1200 Main Street West, Hamilton, Ontario L8N 3Z5, Canada

Lisa M. Schwartz Dartmouth Medical School, HB 7900, Hanover, NH 03755, U.S.A.

Daniela Simon Section of Clinical Epidemiology and Health Services Research, Department of Psychiatry and Psychotherapy, University Medical Centre, Hamburg-Eppendorf, Germany

Richard S. W. Smith Director, UnitedHealth Chronic Disease Initiative, 35 Orlando Road, London SW4 0LD, U.K.

David Spiegelhalter Statistical Laboratory, Centre for Mathematical Sciences, Wilberforce Road, Cambridge CB3 0WB, U.K.

Johann Steurer Horten-Zentrum für Patientenorientierte Forschung, Unispital, 8091 Zürich, Switzerland

Odette Wegwarth   Harding Center for Risk Literacy, Max Planck Institute for Human Development, Lentzeallee 94, 14195 Berlin, Germany

John E. Wennberg   Dartmouth Medical School, 35 Centerra Parkway, Suite 300, Rm. 3018, Lebanon NH 03766, U.S.A.

Claudia Wild   Ludwig Boltzmann Institut für Health Technology Assessment, Garnisonsgasse 7/20, 1090 Vienna, Austria

Steven Woloshin   VA Outcomes Group (111B), Department of Veterans Affairs Medical Center, White River Junction, VT 05009, U.S.A.

Holger Wormer   Institute of Journalism, Universität Dortmund, Emil-Figge-Str. 50, 44227 Dortmund, Germany

Health Literacy:
Is the Patient the Problem?

1

Launching the Century of the Patient

Gerd Gigerenzer and J. A. Muir Gray

Abstract

Efficient health care requires informed doctors *and* patients. The health care system inherited from the 20th century falls short on both counts. Many doctors and most patients do not understand the available medical evidence. Seven "sins" are identified which have contributed to this lack of knowledge: biased funding; biased reporting in medical journals; biased patient pamphlets; biased reporting in the media; conflicts of interest; defensive medicine; and medical curricula that fail to teach doctors how to comprehend health statistics. These flaws have generated a partially inefficient system that wastes taxpayers' money on unnecessary or even potentially harmful tests and treatments as well as on medical research that is of limited relevance to the patient. Raising taxes or rationing care is often seen as the only viable alternative to exploding health care costs. Yet there is a third option: by promoting health literacy, better care is possible for less money. The 21st century should become the century of the patient. Governments and health institutions need to change course and provide honest and transparent information to enable better doctors, better patients, and, ultimately, better health care.

Introduction

Patients appear to be the problem in modern high-tech health care: they are uninformed, anxious, noncompliant folk with unhealthy lifestyles. They demand drugs advertised by celebrities on television, insist on unnecessary but expensive computer tomography (CT) and magnetic resonance imaging (MRI) scans, and may eventually turn into plaintiffs. Patients' lack of health literacy and the resulting costs and harms have received much attention. Consider the following cases.

Almost ten million U.S. women have had unnecessary Pap smears to screen for cervical cancer—unnecessary because, having already undergone complete hysterectomies, these women no longer had a cervix (Sirovich and Welch 2004). Unnecessary Pap tests cause no harm to the patient, but in terms of the health system, they waste millions of dollars which could have been used else-where to better health care.

Every year, one million U.S. children have unnecessary CT scans (Brenner and Hall 2007). An unnecessary CT scan equates to more than a waste of money: an estimated 29,000 cancers result from the approximately 70 million CT scans performed annually in the United States (González et al. 2009); people who have a full-body CT scan can be exposed to radiation levels comparable to some of the atomic-bomb survivors from Hiroshima and Nagasaki (Brenner and Hall 2007). Why don't parents protect their children from unnecessary doses of radiation? They probably would if only they knew. When a random sample of 500 Americans was asked whether they would rather receive one thousand dollars in cash or a free full-body CT, 3 out of 4 wanted the CT (Schwartz et al. 2004).

The uninformed patient is not restricted to the United States. A representa-tive study of 10,228 people from nine European countries revealed that 89% of men and 92% of women overestimated the benefit of PSA and mammography screening tenfold, hundredfold and more, or did not know (Gigerenzer et al. 2007). Why don't people know, or want to know?

Answers that have been proposed range from the perception that patients are not intelligent enough to they just do not want to see numbers, even though most American 12-year-olds already know baseball statistics and their British peers can easily recite the relevant numbers of the Football Association Cup results. Scores of health psychologists and behavioral economists add to the list of suspected cognitive deficits by emphasizing patients' cognitive biases, weakness of will, and wishful thinking. In this view, the problems in health care stem from people who engage in self-harming behavior, focus on short-term gratification rather than long-term harms, suffer from the inability to make forecasts of their emotional states after a treatment, or simply do not want to think but prefer to trust their doctor. The recommended remedies are consequently some form of paternalism that "nudges" the immature patient in the right direction (Thaler and Sunstein 2008). The 20th century has focused the spotlight on the patient who lacks health literacy.

We take a different position. Today's problem is less the patient than the health system we inherited. The patient is only the last element in a chain that actively creates and sustains health illiteracy. In this chapter, we identify seven "sins" of the 20th-century health care system and advocate a change toward a 21st-century system centered around patients—not industries, organizations, or doctors.

Raising taxes or rationing care is often viewed as the only alternative to exploding health care costs. We argue that there is a third option: by promoting health literacy, we can get better care for less money. However, what is ulti-mately at stake is more than just health and money: an educated citizenry is the lifeblood of a modern democracy. We begin with an example that demonstrates how difficult it can be for a patient to make sense out of the barrage of misinformation, so as to be able to make an informed decision.

Misinformed Men: John Q. Public and Otto Normalverbraucher

In his early fifties, John Q. Public intends to make an informed decision about whether to participate in prostate cancer screening with PSA tests. He lives in New York and recalls what Rudi Giuliani, former mayor of New York City, said in a 2007 campaign advertisement (Dobbs 2007):

> I had prostate cancer, 5, 6 years ago. My chance of surviving prostate cancer—and thank God, I was cured of it—in the United States? Eighty-two percent. My chance of surviving prostate cancer in England? Only 44 percent under socialized medicine.

John concludes that he is lucky to live in New York rather than York. He also recalls that back in the late 1990s, Congress initiated a postal stamp featuring "Prostate Cancer Awareness," which promoted "annual checkups and tests." Giuliani and the U.S. Postal Service were obviously of one mind. Yet John looks for further information. He reads that US$3 billion is spent every year on PSA tests and follow-ups, and that the majority of primary care physicians perform routine PSA testing, even in men over 80 years of age. What finally convinces him is that 95% of male urologists and 78% of primary care physicians 50 years and older report that they have undergone PSA screening themselves (Barry 2009). He believes he has enough information and decides that he will take PSA tests because they save lives and lead to little or no harm. Has John Q. Public made an informed decision?

No, but he will likely never know. For one, he may not realize that he was misled by Rudi Giuliani, who presented high 5-year survival rates as suggestive evidence for lower mortality, when in fact differences in survival rates are *uncorrelated* with differences in mortality rates (Welch et al. 2000). In reality, mortality from prostate cancer is about the same in the United States and the United Kingdom, even though most American men take the PSA test and most British men do not. There are two reasons why high survival rates tell us nothing about lower mortality in the context of screening: Screening results in early detection and thus increases 5-year survival rates by setting the time of diagnosis earlier (*lead-time bias*). In addition, it also increases survival rates by including people with non-progressive cancers, which by definition do not lead to mortality (*overdiagnosis bias*; Gigerenzer et al. 2007). Giuliani is not the only one to have misled the public with survival rates; prestigious U.S. cancer centers such as MD Anderson at The University of Texas have done this as well (Gigerenzer et al. 2007). But surely, one might think, John's doctor would provide him with the truth. This, too, is unlikely, because very few doctors know that in screening, survival rates reveal nothing about mortality, just as many do not understand what lead-time bias and overdiagnosis bias are (Wegwarth, Gaissmaier, and Gigerenzer, submitted). This lack of statistical literacy in health may explain why so many urologists themselves take the test. John Q. Public is also unlikely to learn that a U.S. randomized trial found *no* reduction of prostate cancer deaths from combined screening with PSA and digital rectal examination (Andriole et al. 2009), but that one- to two-thirds of men could expect harms such as incontinence and impotence from surgery or radiation.

The American market-driven health care system has no monopoly on producing misinformed patients. In Germany, John Q. Public is known as Otto Normalverbraucher. Otto wants to make an informed decision, too, and—in keeping with the fact that Germans read more health pamphlets than any other European (Gigerenzer et al. 2009)—opens the 114-page pamphlet on prostate cancer published by the Deutsche Krebshilfe (2009), a highly respected nonprofit cancer care organization that receives large amounts of donations from the public. Otto reads that, according to experts, PSA tests are an important method for early detection, and that 10-year survival rates are higher than 80% (Deutsche Krebshilfe 2009:15). He also consults a press release about a recent European randomized trial on prostate cancer screening, which states that PSA screening reduced mortality from prostate cancer by 20%—not as exciting as 80%, but impressive all the same. In the news, Otto reads the unequivocal statement from the president of the German Urology Society: "The study shows without doubt that PSA testing saves lives" (*The Epoch Times*, 26 April 2009). The president is joined by German sport celebrities who recount their personal stories about how early detection saved their lives on TV talk shows and remind Otto to take responsibility for his health—without delay. Just to be sure, Otto consults his urologist, who recommends screening as well. Everything falls into place and he follows suit. Has Otto Normalverbraucher made an informed decision?

No. However, just like John, he will probably never notice. To begin, he may not learn that he has been misled by the 20% figure. What it refers to is a reduction from 3.7 to 3.0 in every 1,000 men who participate in screening, which is an absolute reduction of 0.7 in 1,000, as reported in the original study (Schröder et al. 2009). Framing benefits in terms of *relative risks* (20%) is a common way to mislead the public without actually lying. Second, Otto may not know the subtle distinction between reduced cancer mortality and reduced prostate cancer mortality (multiple cancers exist, which can make it difficult to make correct attributions). The European randomized trial did not report on total cancer mortality, but the U.S. trial did and found no difference in cancer mortality: in the screening group, 23.9 out of 1,000 men died of cancer, compared to 23.8 in the control group. This information is virtually never mentioned in health brochures, which seem more intent on increasing attendance rates than on informing patients. Finally, chances are slim that his urologist knows the scientific evidence and is able to explain to him the pros and cons of PSA screening. Out of a random sample of 20 Berlin urologists, only 2 knew the benefits and harms of PSA screening (Stiftung Warentest 2004). Even when physicians know the evidence, they may practice defensive medicine out of fear of litigation and recommend the test. For instance, only about half of 250 Swiss internists believed that the advantages of regular PSA screening outweigh its harms in men older than 50 years of age, but 75% recommended regular PSA screening to their patients. More than 40% of physicians recommended screening for legal reasons—to protect themselves against potential lawsuits (Steurer et al. 2009).

The scenarios of John Q. Public and Otto Normalverbraucher illustrate some of the ways in which the patient is misled by the health system inherited from the 20th century. In the following sections, we will explain these in more detail. The deluded patient is the victim of a chain of biased information. Such a health care system wastes taxpayers' money, physicians' time, and causes potential harm to patients' health. The main problem is not the patient, but the health care system itself.

The 20th-Century Medical System Produces Health Illiteracy

Why are patients and doctors misinformed about available evidence concerning standard tests and treatments? The problem begins even before medical research starts—with the funding of research. It continues with biased (incomplete or nontransparent) reporting of the results in medical journals and health brochures, and ends with innumerate physicians who misunderstand health statistics. Throughout, seven elements contribute to misinform patients and prevent them from noticing the facts (Table 1.1). It is not an exhaustive list, but constitutes what we believe are some of the most important sources of distortion and confusion.

There are additional factors outside the health care system which cannot be addressed here, such as the remarkably slow pace of educational systems to adjust their curricula to the 21st century so as to include statistical literacy as

Table 1.1   Important sources that contribute to the health illiteracy of patients.

	Biased funding of research
+	Biased reporting in medical journals
+	Biased reporting in health pamphlets
+	Biased reporting in the media
+	Commercial conflicts of interest
+	Defensive medicine
+	Doctors' lack of understanding of health statistics
=	Misinformed patients

a central topic, and the resulting blind spot in teaching health and financial literacy (Gigerenzer et al. 2007). We would like to emphasize that in pointing out the flaws of the 20th-century health system, our aim is not to criticize particular doctors, politicians, or industries but to analyze a system whose primary goal has not always been to provide the best outcome for the patient. Knowledge of the system is essential if we are to change it into a more efficient one that serves the patient.

However, before we continue, let us clarify terms. We use the terms "health literacy" and "statistical literacy" as two overlapping bodies of knowledge, whose intersection is "statistical literacy in health" (Figure 1.1). Statistical literacy in health does not require a degree in statistics. Rather, it means that patients and health care providers have basic competencies in understanding evidence and, most importantly, know which questions to ask. Health literacy, in turn, intersects with "health system literacy" (a basic understanding of how the health system works). For further information, see Gigerenzer et al. (2007) for a detailed definition of "minimal statistical literacy in health" and Bachmann et al. (2007), who have designed a short test for minimum health literacy.

The term "century of the patient" refers to a society where greater investments in health do not mean more profit for the industry, but rather more knowledge for doctors and patients. In fact, shortage of money (e.g., due to the recent financial crises) can be an enabler for the revolution we envision.

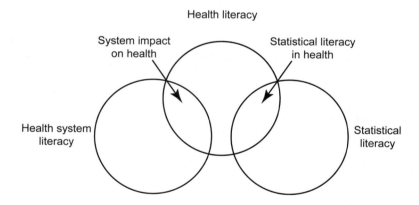

Figure 1.1 Three basic competencies for doctors and patients in the 21st century. Health system literacy entails basic knowledge about the organization of a system and the incentives within it, such as the widespread practice of defensive medicine as a reaction to the threat of litigation. Health literacy entails basic knowledge about diseases, diagnostics, prevention and treatment, and ways to acquire reliable knowledge. Statistical literacy involves the ability to understand uncertain evidence, including concepts such as 5-year survival rates and false positives. The health care system inherited from the 20th century has done little to develop these basic competences in doctors and patients, promoting drugs, patents, and health technology instead.

Biased Funding

The formation of misinformed doctors and patients begins with the funding of research. Given the increasing role of private industry, profitability has become a primary motive for funding and guides the selection of research topics. In 2008, an estimated US$160 billion was spent on health research and development (R&D) in the United States, and more than half originated from industrial sources; that is, pharmaceutical, biotechnology, and medical technology companies (see Nelson, this volume, for other countries). The rapid rise of the industry began with the election of Ronald Reagan in 1980, when Congress enacted a series of laws, including the Bayh–Dole Act, which enabled universities and small businesses to patent discoveries sponsored by the National Institutes of Health (NIH). Before 1980, taxpayer-financed discoveries belonged in the public domain and could be used by any company (Angell 2004). Today, discoveries made by taxpayer-funded research are no longer public; they can be patented and sold to industry, which in turn can charge large sums until the patent expires or competitors are allowed to introduce generic drugs. Before 1980, medical researchers worked largely independently of the companies that sponsored their work, but this is no longer the case. The Reagan years gave a tremendous boost to the "technology transfer" between universities and industry, where medical schools and their faculties entered into lucrative financial arrangements with drug companies. By funding research at universities and outside, industry is able to introduce bias in three ways: by determining the topics that are funded, the design of clinical trials, and the reporting of the results in journals.

The term "biased funding" refers to research funded because it is likely to be profitable, not because it is likely to be relevant for patients. Profitability and relevance can coincide, but often do not. The James Lind Alliance (www.lindalliance.org), for instance, identifies unanswered relevant questions from patients to ensure that those who fund health research are aware of what matters to patients. We illustrate biased funding by pinpointing three blind spots: patient safety, innovative drugs, and physicians' statistical literacy.

Patient Safety

Checklists provide a simple, inexpensive tool for improving safety. Introduced by the U.S. Air Force after the B-17 proved to be too much of an airplane for any one person to fly, checklists have become the safety backbone in commercial aviation. For instance, during the successful emergency landing of US Airways Flight 1549 in the Hudson River, the two pilots relied on the relevant checklists, including those for engine failure and evacuation (Gawande et al. 2009). Whereas customer safety is a priority in aviation, and all pilots are trained to use checklists, neither is the case in medicine. For instance, each year, central venous catheters cause an estimated 80,000 bloodstream infections and, as a result, up to 28,000 deaths in intensive care units (ICU) in U.S. hospitals. Total costs of these infections are estimated at US$2.3 billion annually. To save lives, Peter Pronovost developed a simple checklist of five steps (including hand washing and cleaning the skin with chlorhexidine) for ICU doctors to follow before inserting an IV line to prevent the introduction of bacteria. The checklist reduced the infection rate to almost zero at some one hundred ICUs in hospitals in Michigan (Pronovost et al. 2006). One might think that funding would focus on such strong effects and that hospitals would rush to implement checklists. Yet most ICU physicians do not use them. Infection control has not been a priority of administrators, who focus on hospitals' profits rather than on patient safety. Nor is the hierarchical structure in hospitals fertile ground for checklists, which might require a nurse to remind a surgeon to follow the instructions. But a fundamental reason why so little funding has been made available to develop and implement checklists appears to be that they are cheap, and thus do not promise high-profit patents.

Patient safety is a major problem. The Institute of Medicine estimated that some 44,000 to 98,000 patients are killed every year in U.S. hospitals by documented, preventable medical errors (Kohn et al. 2000). In 2009, the WHO reported that nearly 1 in 10 patients are harmed while receiving care in well-funded and technologically advanced hospitals (WHO 2009a). Little is known about non-hospital settings, where the majority of care is delivered. In 2008, the WHO Patient Safety initiated a grants program to provide seed funds for twenty to thirty small research projects on safety. Patient safety needs to become a major focus of funding.

Me-too Drugs

To gain approval by the U.S. Food and Drug Administration (FDA), a company needs only to show that its drug is better than a placebo, not that it is better than an already existing drug. The same is true in Germany and other European countries. As a result, there is little incentive for a company to fund innovative research for better drugs; all they need to do is to change a few molecules of an old, already approved one and produce a "me-too" drug. Research on me-too drugs has a smaller risk of failure than innovative research. Of the 78 drugs approved by the FDA in 2002, 71 were me-too drugs (Angell 2004:17). Research that results in drugs that are not better than already existing ones—only more expensive as long as the patent lasts—is not in the interest of the patient.

Research that is relevant for patients has a different goal: Is the new drug better or worse than the old one? Sometimes, such comparative effectiveness research is conducted. For instance, consider high blood pressure (hypertension), a condition for which about 25 million Americans are treated. A trial not sponsored by a drug company compared four drugs for treating hypertension: Norvasc® (amlodipine besylate), the fifth best-selling drug in the world in 2002 sold by Pfizer; Cardura® (doxazosin), also from Pfizer; an ACE inhibitor sold by AstraZeneca as Zestril® (lisinopril) and by Merck as Prinivil®; and a generic diuretic ("water pill") of a type that has been on the market for over fifty years. The study found that the old-time diuretic was just as effective in lowering blood pressure and better for preventing heart disease and stroke (ALLHAT Collaborative Research Group 2002). Last but not least, diuretics were priced at about US$37 a year in 2002, while Norvasc® costs $715. Comparative studies are, however, rare. Drug companies do not like head-to-head comparisons with older drugs and use their influence to make certain that the FDA or similar institutions do not request that research answers the comparative question relevant for the patient. The design of research is directly influenced when pharmaceutical companies require researchers to compare a new drug with a placebo rather than with an already existing drug (Angell 2004).

If comparative research is conducted, the drug of the supporting manufacturer is sometimes given at a higher dose than the comparator drugs. (This can make a new drug look good even if it might actually be worse than the older one; yet in the absence of proper studies, no one will know.) Consider Prilosec® (omeprazole), a heartburn drug made by AstraZeneca which was once the top-selling drug in the world with US$6 billion in annual sales. When the blockbuster was set to go off patent in 2001, the company faced competition from generic manufacturers who would sell Prilosec® at a much lower price. To avoid loss in sales, AstraZeneca patented a virtually identical drug, Nexium®, and spent a half billion dollars the same year on advertisements, discounts to managed care plans and hospitals, free samples to doctors, coupons in newspapers, and other ways of persuading consumers to switch from Prilosec® to Nexium®. AstraZeneca conducted four comparative trials; in two of these, Nexium® came out marginally better than Prilosec®. But the company had loaded the die by using different doses: 20 mg of Priolosec® were compared with 40 mg and 20 mg of Nexium®. Biased comparative research is not helpful for patients, who could simply double the dose of Priolosec® or buy a much cheaper generic.

Research on me-too drugs that does not conduct comparative studies with existing drugs is not in the interest of the patient. Ironically, the patient pays twice: as a taxpayer for the research supported by the NIH or other government organizations, and as a patient for the overpriced drugs sold by the pharmaceutical companies that acquired the patents without conducting innovative research.

Physicians' Statistical Literacy in Health

The general public believes that every physician understands medical evidence such as health statistics. Yet the few existing studies indicate that this is not the case, even in the physicians' own specialty. For instance, one of us (GG) trained about 1,000 German gynecologists in risk communication as part of their continuing education in 2006 and 2007. The majority of gynecologists falsely believed that among every 10 women with a positive screening mammogram, 8 or 9 actually have breast cancer, whereas the best estimate is only about 1 (Gigerenzer et al. 2007). These gynecologists' lack of statistical literacy causes unnecessary fear and panic in women with false positive results. More generally, studies indicate that most physicians confuse an increase in 5-year survival rates in screening with a decrease in mortality (Wegwarth et al., submitted) and do not understand how to determine the positive predictive value of a test (Hoffrage and Gigerenzer 1998), and about a third of physicians overestimate benefits if expressed as relative risk reductions (Gigerenzer et al. 2007). Moreover, physicians often confuse concepts such as sensitivity and specificity, and do not know the scientific evidence for benefits and harms of standard tests and treatments (Gigerenzer 2002).

Funding has focused on new technologies and drugs, not on physicians' understanding of these technologies. Although we have developed framing methods to help doctors understand health statistics quickly (Gigerenzer et al. 2007), there is relatively little research on these and even less implementation. In this way, biased funding contributes to ever more technology and less health literacy.

Manifesto for Action to Make Research More Relevant for Patients

During the second half of the 20th century, a system of funding research was created whose primary goal does not appear to support medical research relevant for the patient. Because the causes are multiple and hard to change, a solution might focus on identifying what we call a "triggering factor," that is, a causal factor that takes care of multiple others like a domino effect. Here are three triggering factors for patient safety, me-too drugs, and doctors' statistical literacy.

1. Research funders, such as the NIH in the United States, the National Institute for Health Research (NIHR) in the United Kingdom, and the Deutsche Forschungsgemeinschaft in Germany, should invest in research on why professional practices that harm patients continue to exist, even when there are evidence-based interventions such as checklists to reduce these harms.

2. Regulatory agencies, such as the FDA in the United States, the Medicines and Healthcare Products Regulatory Agency (MHRA) in the United Kingdom, and research funders all over the world, should adopt the principles of comparative effectiveness research and make the approval of a new drug contingent on whether it is substantially more effective, safer, or has fewer side effects than those already in existence—not on whether it is better than a placebo. This single factor could not only stop the stream of me-too drugs, which wastes research money and resources, but also encourage innovative research to

develop better products. The change in the U.S. system as evidenced by the support for comparative effectiveness research in major medical journals, such as *JAMA*, is a welcome sign of change.

3. Research funders should invest in research on the causes and the cure of statistical illiteracy in health care providers. A problem that is so widespread and with such direct detrimental consequences to patients' health can be classified as a pandemic, affecting more people than bird flu and SARS combined.

Biased Reporting in Medical Journals

To foster complete and transparent reporting of research, medical journals have ethical guidelines. These include CONSORT for randomized trials and MOOSE for systematic reviews. Similarly, the Declaration of Helsinki specifies that authors, editors, and publishers have an ethical obligation to report honestly. One would therefore assume that the top medical journals always report results in a transparent and complete manner; however, this is not the case (Nuovo et al. 2002).

Transparent Reporting

Every health statistic can be reported in a transparent or misleading way. For instance, absolute risks, mortality rates, and natural frequencies are transparent, whereas relative risks, 5-year survival rates, and conditional probabilities (e.g., sensitivities) tend to mislead physicians and patients alike. At issue is not one of lying, but rather the art of saying something correctly in a way that most listeners will understand incorrectly.

For instance, consider *mismatched framing* (Gigerenzer et al. 2007): The benefits of a test or treatment are featured in *big* numbers as relative risks while harms are displayed in *small* numbers as absolute risks. Assume that a treatment reduces the probability of getting disease A from 10 to 5 in 1,000, while it increases the risk of disease B from 5 to 10 in 1,000. The journal article reports the benefit as a 50% risk reduction and the harm as an increase of 5 in 1,000; that is, 0.5%. An analysis of the articles published in the *British Medical Journal* (*BMJ*), the *Journal of the American Medical Association* (*JAMA*), and *The Lancet*, 2004–2006, showed that mismatched framing was used in one out of every three articles (Sedrakyan and Shih 2007). We believe it is ethically imperative for editors to enforce transparent reporting: no mismatched framing, no relative risks without baseline risks, and always in absolute numbers. Absolute risks or numbers needed to treat may not look as impressive, but the goal of a medical journal must be to inform—not persuade.

Complete Reporting

If results are not completely reported, it is impossible to judge whether a treatment is appropriate for a patient. Reporting can be biased in several ways. The first is to report just the favorable trials, not all trials. For instance, if two studies showed a positive effect of a treatment, but eight others showed negative results, it is essential that all are reported. However, complete reporting of all studies is neither enforced nor required in most countries. In the United States, the FDA requires a company to submit all trials that it has sponsored; it does not require that all studies be published. For example, the agency typically requires evidence that the drug worked better than a placebo in two clinical trials, even if it did not in the other trials (Angell 2004). As a result, treatments tend to look better than they are.

A second bias is introduced when only the favorable part of the data is reported, but not all data. For instance, consider the clinical trial of the arthritis drug Celebrex®, sponsored by Pharmacia (since acquired by Pfizer). Only after publication in *JAMA* did the outraged editors learn that the results were based on only the first six months of a year-long trial. An analysis of the entire year showed no advantage of Celebrex® (Angell 2004).

A third bias is introduced when researchers "cherry-pick" and report only those variables or subgroups that showed favorable results. Companies' attempts to prevent researchers from publishing their results when they are not favorable are one of the reasons why cherry-picking occurs (e.g., Rennie 1997). Finally, complete reporting is violated and biases are introduced when high-impact medical journals carry advertisements that make promotional statements, but the statements are not supported by the evidence in the bibliographic references given (Villanueva et al. 2003).

Why do editors of major journals not strictly enforce transparent and complete reporting? One answer is conflicting interests, just as in funding of research. It may not be accidental that one-third of the trials published in *BMJ* and between two-thirds and three-quarters published in the major North American journals were funded by the pharmaceutical industry (Egger et al. 2001). Studies funded by the pharmaceutical industry more often report results favorable for the sponsoring company than do studies funded by other sources (e.g., Lexchin et al. 2003). It is in the very interest of companies to frame the results in a way that impresses doctors. Richard Smith (2005), former editor of *BMJ*, explains that a publisher depends not only on the advertisements paid by the industry, but even more on the tens of thousands of reprints that the pharmaceutical industry often purchases to distribute to physicians. "Journals have devolved into information laundering operations for the pharmaceutical industry," wrote Richard Horton (2004:9), editor of *The Lancet*. Biased reporting does not begin in press releases or the media, as it is sometimes assumed. It already exists in the top international medical journals. In the 2003 *BMJ* Christmas issue, David Sackett and Andrew Oxman published a satirical article on distorted reporting of evidence, offering their services on "how to achieve positive results without actually lying to overcome the truth" (Sackett and Oxman 2003:1442).

Manifesto for Action to Stop Biased Reporting in Medical Journals

1. Research funders should (a) structure research application forms so that researchers have to submit their application following the guidelines for their research method, such as CONSORT for randomized controlled trials; (b) ensure that a systematic review of the evidence has been done before new data are collected; and (c) require a research protocol that specifies all research hypotheses and how they are being tested in advance to guarantee completeness of reporting.
2. Journal editors and publishers should sign up to the principles and practices agreed upon by the Sixth International Congress on Peer Review and Biomedical Publication, using the tools made openly available through the EQUATOR Network, *and* strictly enforce these. These principles need to be extended to include transparent reporting of health statistics. Editors should clearly announce that evidence framed in relative risks (without base lines), 5-year survival rates for screening, mismatched framing, and other nontransparent formats will no longer be published (Gigerenzer et al. 2007).
3. Institutions that subscribe to medical journals should give journal publishers two years to implement the previous action and, if publishers do not comply, cancel their subscriptions.

Biased Reporting in Health Pamphlets and Web Sites

In a recent poll of 10,228 people from nine European countries, 21% responded that they sometimes or frequently consult leaflets and pamphlets from health organizations, with the highest number (41%) coming from Germany (Gigerenzer et al. 2009). Yet the amount of biased reporting that stems from this material—typically omissions of harms and overstatement of benefits—is staggering. For instance, analyses of 150 pamphlets (including invitations) on mammography screening showed that benefits are mostly reported in relative risks (108 cases) but rarely in absolute risks (26 cases) or number needed to treat (11 cases), while the harms from overdiagnosis and unnecessary treatment were only mentioned in 37 cases (Gigerenzer et al. 2007). This combination of nontransparency and incomplete reporting hinders informed decision making. Many pamphlets appear to be designed to increase participation rates rather than inform the public. In fact, in Germany, where consulting rates of medical pamphlets were the highest, there is a *negative* correlation between frequency of consulting pamphlets and understanding the benefit of mammography screening (Gigerenzer et al. 2009). Moreover, 98% of German women overestimate the cancer-specific mortality reduction of mammography screening or do not know, consistent with a high reliance of information from pamphlets.

Mismatched framing spreads from medical journals to health pamphlets, web sites, and patient information. For instance, the National Cancer Institute's Risk Disk is intended to help women make informed decisions about whether to use tamoxifen for the primary prevention of breast cancer (Schwartz et al. 1999b). The benefit is framed as a relative risk reduction: "Women [taking tamoxifen] had about 49% fewer diagnoses of invasive breast cancer." The harm of increased uterine cancer, in contrast, is framed as an absolute risk increase: "The annual rate of uterine cancer in the tamoxifen arm was 30 per 10,000 compared to 8 per 10,000 in the placebo arm" (NCI 1998). Transparent reporting would express both as absolute risks. Analyzing the study data reveals that in absolute terms, the 49% refers to a reduction from 33 to 17 in 1,000; that is, 16 in 1,000. Moreover, the Breast Cancer Prevention Study Fact Sheet (NCI 2005) reports only the 49% statistic and no numbers at all for the increased risk of uterine cancer.

Analyses of web sites showed similar degrees of biased reporting, specifically web sites from advocacy groups and governmental organizations. Those from consumer organizations, however, contained more balanced reporting (Jorgensen and Gøtzsche 2004).

For a busy doctor with limited time to keep abreast of medical research, leaflets from the pharmaceutical industry are a major source of information. Pharmaceutical companies dispatch thousands of well-dressed representatives with leaflets and samples in their hands to persuade doctors to prescribe their drugs. A leaflet typically summarizes the results of a published study in a convenient form. A comparison of 175 leaflets with the original studies showed surprisingly that the summaries could be verified in only 8% of the cases. In the remaining 92%, key results were systematically distorted, important details omitted, or the original study could not be found or was not mentioned (Kaiser et al. 2004). In general, leaflets exaggerated baseline risks and benefits, enlarged the length of time in which medication could safely be taken, or did not reveal severe side effects of medication pointed out in the original publications.

Manifesto for Action to Stop Biased Reporting in Health Pamphlets and Web Sites

1. Every hospital and health care provider should nominate a member of their senior management team to take responsibility for ensuring that all patient information is (a) unbiased from an evidence-based standard and (b) transparent for the patient. Transparent reporting includes the use of absolute risks as opposed to relative risks (without base lines), mortality rates for screening (as opposed to 5-year survival rates), natural frequencies (as opposed to conditional probabilities), and techniques

to present these clearly (e.g., diagrams, as in Gigerenzer 2002:45). Health care payers, such as governments and health insurance companies, should ensure that providers implement this action. Doing so will both reduce waste of taxpayers' money and improve patient well-being.

2. National ministries of health that determine strategy and policy should make an explicit commitment to quality of patient information, as announced by the U.K. Prime Minister David Cameron when the new policy for the National Health Service (NHS) was introduced (Dept. of Health 2010:13): "The Government intends to bring about an NHS information revolution, to correct the imbalance in who knows what. Our aim is to give people access to comprehensive, trustworthy, and easy to understand information." Health care regulators, such as the state governments in Germany and the Care Quality Commission in England, should add monitoring the quality of information given to patients to their range of services.

3. Members of institutions that support the democratic ideal of educated patients should make biased information a public issue. The lever is the reputation of organizations that produce health pamphlets, such as patient organizations and charities. For instance, in a number of public lectures, one of us (GG) showed how the widespread misinformation about cancer screening among doctors and patients could be traced back to biased reporting in the pamphlets of the Deutsche Krebshilfe and offered to help rewrite the pamphlets in a complete and transparent way. The institution accepted, and since late 2009, an entirely new set of short brochures was published, in which all misleading relative risk reductions and 5-year survival rates were replaced by transparent absolute numbers and the evidence for harms is no longer omitted.

Biased Reporting in the Media

Europeans consult the general media (television, radio, popular magazines, and daily newspapers) for health information more often than specialized medical sources such as pamphlets and leaflets (Gigerenzer et al. 2009). Yet journalism schools tend to teach everything except understanding evidence, even though health is the leading science topic in U.S. and European media. A survey of health reporters in five Midwestern states found that 80%[1] had no training in covering health news or interpreting health statistics (Voss 2002). Combined with the fierce competition for journal space and the attention of readers, this lack of training results in waves of unnecessary fears and hopes. To illustrate, consider one of the recurring contraceptive pill scares in the United Kingdom.

---

[1] Surveys were sent to 165 reporters from 122 newspapers in 5 Midwestern states to assess the association of training, newspaper size, and experience with reporter's self-perceived reporting ability (Voss 2002).

In 1995, the U.K. Committee on Safety of Medicines issued a warning that third-generation oral contraceptive pills increased the risk of potentially life-threatening blood clots in the legs or lungs twofold; that is, by 100%. The news caused great anxiety, and many women stopped taking the pill, which led to unwanted pregnancies and abortions—some 13,000 additional abortions in the following year in England and Wales, and an extra £4–6 million in costs for the National Health Service. Yet how big was the 100% risk? The studies revealed that out for every 7,000 women who took the earlier, second-generation pills, 1 had a thrombosis, and this number increased to 2 among women who took third-generation pills. The difference between a relative risk increase (100%) and an absolute risk increase (1 in 7,000) was—and still is—not explained to the general public. The losers were the women, particularly adolescent girls, the taxpayers, and the pharmaceutical industry. The only winners were the journalists who got their story on the front pages.

Systematic analyses of media reports reveal three major biases: the omission of numbers, the use of nontransparent numbers (as in the pill scare), and the lack of cautionary notes. These biases do not always originate in the mind of journalists; they may already exist in journal articles. Moreover, press releases suffer from many of the same problems (Woloshin and Schwartz 2002). They often fail to quantify the main effect (35% of 127 press releases), present relative risks without base rates (45%), and make no note on study limitations (77%).

After doctors, pharmacists, and friends, television is the most frequented source of health information in European countries. In a recent survey (10,228 participants), 43% stated that they relied on TV reports sometimes or frequently. Yet when it came to understanding the benefits of breast and prostate cancer screening, those Europeans who relied more often on TV, radio, magazines or daily newspapers were not better informed (Gigerenzer et al. 2009). Although a few informative TV programs do exist, our personal experience with producers and talk show hosts is that most prefer entertaining stories, in particular about celebrities, and poignant pictures to the task of informing the public.

A few newspapers have begun to promote correct and transparent reporting in place of sensationalism and confusion. In the United States, journalists are taught at MIT's Medical Evidence Boot Camp, the Medicine in the Media program sponsored by NIH and the Dartmouth Institute for Health Policy and Clinical Practice's Center for Medicine and the Media.

Manifesto for Action to Stop Biased Reporting in the Media

1. Departments of journalism at universities should teach epidemiological principles and transparent risk communication. No journalist should be left behind.

2. Governments and public health professionals at national, regional, and local levels should accept that the population they serve needs clean and clear knowledge as much as it needs clean and clear water. They

should use their existing channels for health communication not only for transmitting unbiased evidence, but also to counter misleading and sensational media stories quickly and authoritatively. Examples of this approach can be found on the web sites of Behind The Headlines Service, which is part of NHS Choices, and Media Watch.

3. Health professionals and professional bodies should support the work of freelance writers who produce resources such as the blog sites Bad Science and Selling Sickness when they are attacked or sued by industry or other pressure groups.

Conflicts of Interest

Germany spends about 240 billion Euros on health care annually, about 11% of its GDP, whereas the United States spends 17%, about double the expenditure in the United Kingdom. In 2002, for instance, the ten drug companies in the Fortune 500 made more profit (US$35.9 billion) than all the other 490 businesses together (US$33.7 billion; Angell 2004). Conflicts of interest are to be expected when so much money is at stake.

A conflict of interest occurs when a doctor, hospital, or industry cannot simultaneously improve care for patients and its own revenues, but has to choose. Such conflicts arise elsewhere in business and politics, but with a different outcome. When Toyota built better cars for less money, for example, it won new customers. Rivals such as Honda either matched its quality and success, or like General Motors, lost their market share. This basic economic principle—better quality, higher profits—holds in most markets, but health care is a big exception. If a hospital provides better quality by reducing unnecessary and potentially harmful treatments, it reduces costs, but it may also reduce its revenues even more. Patients, in particular in the United States, show little inclination to buy better *and* less expensive care, although they would buy better and less expensive cars. When one of us (GG) attended an internal talk at a leading pharmaceutical company, the speaker, a health economist, said jokingly, "Assume we discovered a drug that is both better and cheaper than what we have. Is there anyone who believes that it would get on the market?" The audience exploded into laughter. Yet the demanding consumers who nearly brought the U.S. automobile industry to its knees could do the same to the medical industry.

Why is Western health care not like the Japanese car industry? One factor is the incentive structure that can conflict with the goal of providing the best service to the patient. If doctors are paid for each extra test and treatment, as in fee-for-service payment systems, they have conflicting interests. Services for which physicians get little pay from health insurances (e.g., taking time to inform patients or paying home visits) are discouraged, whereas those that increase the flow of income (e.g., such as surgery and imagery) are encouraged.

The doctor achieves higher earnings by ordering unnecessary tests and treatments, which may harm rather than help the patient. If physicians were paid a salary rather than for each service, as at the Mayo Clinic in Minnesota, such conflicts of interest would be resolved and patients could get better quality care for less money. Some hospitals have followed the Mayo model and investigated their own overuse of tests. For instance, hospital leaders from Cedar Rapids, Iowa, examined the overuse of CT scans and found that in just one year 52,000 scans were done in a community of 300,000 people. A large proportion was unnecessary and potentially harmful, as the radiation exposure of a CT scan can be about 1,000 times as large as a chest X-ray (Gawande et al. 2009).

A second source of conflict for doctors is (pseudo-)research contracts offered by industry. After a new drug has been approved, a company offers doctors a certain amount of money for each patient they put on the new drug. The research part consists of a summary form that is typically short and simple. Such studies can be sometimes useful for learning more about a new drug, but they create a conflict between monetary incentives and the best health care for the patient. In 2008, German doctors participated in such studies in 85,000 cases (out of about 150,000 doctors in private medical practice), and earned between 10–1,000 Euros per patient, often without informing patients why they were put on the new drug. The conflict is this: Doctors who refuse to be paid for putting their patients on the new drug earn less money.

Financial incentives are not the only source of conflicting interests for doctors. For instance, the formal requirement of completing a certain number of surgeries to qualify as a specialist can cause a conflict between persuading a patient to have a surgery and providing the best care for the patient.

Hospitals are subject to conflicts of interest as well. These appear to be a cause of the striking phenomenon of unwarranted practice variability, as recorded in the Dartmouth Atlas of Health Care. Since the 1970s, Jack Wennberg and his collaborators have systematically documented large and unwarranted variability in practice in North America and Europe. For instance, 8% of the children in one referral region in Vermont had their tonsils removed while in another area 70% underwent tonsillectomies. In Maine, the proportion of women who have had a hysterectomy by the age of 70 varies between communities from less than 20% to more than 70%. In Iowa, the proportion of men who have undergone prostate surgery by age 85 ranges from 15% to more than 60%. Wild variability in surgery is not limited to the United States. In Magdeburg, Germany, similar "small area variations" were reported for elective surgical procedures (back and hip) (Swart et al. 2000). In Hessen, the rate of breast-conserving surgery conducted under similar conditions varied widely (from 0–100%) in 78 clinics, suggesting that treatments are based neither on the best science nor on women's preferences (Geraedts 2006).

More is not better. In the United States, regions with high utilization and expensive care show slightly worse mortality outcomes, lower perceived access, and less patient satisfaction (Fisher et al. 2003a, b). Among the factors that drive this variability are the number of unoccupied hospital beds available, the number of imaging techniques, and other available supply in a hospital, as well as the number of physicians in a region. Once an expensive capacity has been built, a conflict arises between using it for the best profit of the hospital and providing the best health care for the patient.

When Wennberg and his colleagues first published their results, the most surprising reaction was that no public outcry ensued. When, on the occasion of the U.S. health care reform plan in 2009, the physician–writer Atul Gawande made some of these results accessible to a wider audience in the *New Yorker*, they were met once again largely with silence. We need better doctors and better patients: people who react to practice variation rather than allow themselves to be acted upon.

Manifesto for Action to Reduce Interests Conflicting with Best Care

1. Those who determine physician reimbursement should move away from fee-for-service payments to good salaries. There is evidence that fees-for-service encourage unnecessary tests and treatments, including surgery and imaging, leading to more harm done to patients and a waste of taxpayers' money. Salaries encourage better quality, better risk communication, and free time for doctors to take care of their patients' needs, including time to talk without decreasing doctors' income.

2. Those who pay for health care, such as governments and insurance companies, should discontinue payment incentives that increase the rate of interventions unless there is very strong evidence that an increased rate of interventions does more good than harm. For example, it is appropriate to use incentives to increase immunizations to nearly 100%, whereas incentive schemes that would increase the rate of elective surgical operations on the knee may do more harm than good.

3. Medical organizations responsible for continuing medical education should stop using industry funding to sponsor educational programs.

Defensive Medicine

One might assume that doctors who succeed in circumventing biased information and conflicts of interest would be free to treat their patients according to the best evidence. Yet this is not so. Tort law in many countries and jurisdictions not only discourages but actively penalizes physicians who practice evidence-based medicine (Monahan 2007). For instance, Daniel Merenstein (2004), a young family physician in Virginia, was sued in 2003 because he had not automatically ordered a PSA test for a patient, but instead followed the recommendations of leading medical organizations and informed the patient about its pros and cons. The patient later developed an incurable form of prostate cancer. The plaintiff's attorney claimed that the PSA tests are standard in the Commonwealth of Virginia and that physicians routinely order the test without informing their patients. The jury exonerated Merenstein, but his residency was found liable for US$1 million. After this experience, Merenstein felt he had no choice but to practice defensive medicine, even at the risk of causing unnecessary harm: "I order more tests now, am more nervous around patients; I am not the doctor I should be" (Gigerenzer 2007:161).

The term "defensive medicine" refers to the practice of recommending a diagnostic test or treatment that is not the best option for the patient, but one that protects the physician against the patient as a potential plaintiff. Defensive medicine is a reaction to the raising costs of malpractice insurance premiums and patients' bias to sue for missed or delayed diagnosis or treatment. The saying goes: "No one is ever sued for overtreatment." Ninety-three percent of 824 surgeons, obstetricians, and other U.S. specialists at high risk of litigation reported practicing defensive medicine, such as ordering unnecessary CTs, biopsies, and MRIs, and prescribing more antibiotics than medically indicated (Studdert et al. 2005). Being sued costs time and money for the doctor, including the time away from patient care that litigation entails as well as possible damage in reputation. An analysis of a random sample of 1452 closed malpractice claims from five U.S. liability insurers showed that the average time between injury and resolution was five years. Indemnity costs were US$376 million, defense administration costs $73 million, resulting in total costs of $449 million (Studdert et al. 2006). The system's overhead costs were exorbitant: 35% of the indemnity payments went to the plaintiffs' attorneys, and together with defense costs, the total costs of litigation amounted to 54% of the compensation paid to plaintiffs.

U.S. physicians are at highest risk of being sued, and overtreatment is common. In 2006, Americans underwent 60 million surgical procedures, 1 for every 5 Americans (Gawande et al. 2009). No other country operates on their citizens so frequently. Nobody knows whether Americans are better off because of this, but it seems unlikely; we also do not know how many of these surgeries qualify as defensive treatments. We know, however, that every year, hundreds of thousands of Americans die from surgical complications—more than from car crashes and AIDS combined.

In Switzerland, where litigation is less common, 41% of general practitioners and 43% of internists reported that they sometimes or often recommend PSA tests for legal reasons (Steurer et al. 2009). The practice of defensive medicine also expresses itself in discrepancies between what treatments doctors recommend to patients and what they recommend to their own families. In Switzerland, for instance, the rate of hysterectomy in the general population is 16%, whereas among doctors' wives and female doctors it is only 10% (Domenighetti et al. 1993).

One triggering factor that could reduce the practice of defensive medicine is to replace the custom-based legal standard of care by evidence-based liability.

As the case of Merenstein illustrates, even if doctors deliver best practice to a patient, their clinics can be successfully sued, because medical custom ("what most other doctors do"), not scientific evidence, defines the legal standard of care. Malpractice suits are often seen as a mechanism to improve the quality of care, but with custom-based liability, they actually impede the translation of evidence into practice, harming patients and decreasing the quality of care. In the United States, state courts are "gradually, quietly, and relentlessly" abandoning the custom-based standard of care (Peters 2002), yet a clear commitment to scientific evidence is needed. One factor that impedes change is that lawyers and judges, similar to doctors, receive little if any training in understanding evidence. One of us (GG) trained U.S. federal judges in statistical literacy in 2004–2005, but these courses, carried out under the continuing education program organized by George Mason School of Law, appear to have been the only ones ever conducted. Out of some 175 accredited law schools in the United States, only one requires a basic course in statistics or research methods (Faigman 1999). As a consequence, judges, jurors, and attorneys are continuously misled by nontransparent statistics presented in court (Gigerenzer 2002).

Manifesto for Action to Protect Patients from Defensive Medicine

1. Ministries of health should identify features of the legal system that increase the likelihood of being sued for not performing a clinical intervention that has no evidence of benefit. Unlike the European legal systems, the U.S. tort law encourages malpractice suits, which has the unintended consequence of decreasing quality of care by forcing physicians to practice defensive medicine. The resulting exorbitant fees for malpractice insurance and lawyers add to the costs of health care.

2. Those who pay for health care (governments and insurance companies) should make explicit to clinicians and patients the care pathways that give the best balance of benefit and harm with the resources available. They should also state explicitly which interventions (e.g., PSA screening tests, imaging) are more likely to do harm than good, and should therefore not be conducted. Evidence-based shared decision-making tools (e.g., those developed by the Foundation for Informed Medical Decision Making) should be used for patients' decisions when either options have dramatically different outcomes or when patient values about the balance of benefits and risks are particularly important (e.g., elective surgery). To ensure that all options and their consequences have been clearly transmitted, health care providers should start recording patient knowledge before and after the consultation. Dartmouth–Hitchcock Medical Center is already doing this for women's decisions about breast cancer treatment.

3. All agencies and professionals who are in the position to help improve health system literacy should make it clear to the public and the media

that concern about overuse of medical care has primarily to do with the resulting harms and that this would be a matter of equal concern even if finances were unlimited. More is not always better.

Doctors' Statistical Illiteracy

The last element in the chain that leads to misinformed patients is probably the least known. It is commonly assumed that only patients have problems with health statistics, not their physicians. Most legal and psychological articles on patient–doctor communication assume that the problem lies in the patient's mind. Doctors may be said to not listen carefully to their patients' complaints, consult with them only five minutes on average, or withhold information. However, rarely is it considered that doctors themselves might not understand medical evidence (e.g., Berwick et al. 1981; Rao 2008). Yet most doctors that have been studied do not understand health statistics and thus cannot evaluate the evidence for or against a treatment, or critically judge a report in a medical journal (Gigerenzer et al. 2007). Lack of statistical literacy in health makes doctors dependent on the biased information contained in leaflets distributed by pharmaceutical companies (see above) or the continuing education organized by the industry. In the United States, there is 1 drug representative or detailer, as they are known, for every 5 or 6 doctors. Every week the average doctor is visited by several, who provide information, free samples, gifts such as golf balls or tickets to sporting events, and sometimes a free lunch for doctors and their staff (Angell 2004).

Consider Rudi Giuliani's statement mentioned at onset: that the 5-year survival rate for prostate cancer is 82% in the United States compared to only 44% in the United Kingdom under socialized medicine. Any physician should know that these figures tell us nothing about whether screening saves lives, because differences in 5-year survival rates do not correlate with differences in mortality rates (Welch et al. 2000). Yet would physicians see through Giuliani's misleading claim? To test this, Wegwarth et al. (submitted) gave 65 physicians practicing internal medicine the actual changes in 5-year survival rates from the Surveillance, Epidemiology and End Result (SEER) program for prostate cancer, which showed differences similar to those reported by Giuliani. Seeing the 5-year survival rates, 78% judged the screening as effective. When the same SEER data was given to the same physicians in terms of mortality rates (as mentioned before, the mortality rates are about the same), only 5% judged the screening to be effective. Only 2 out of 65 physicians understood the lead-time bias, and not a single one understood the overdiagnosis bias.

Five-year survival rates are not the only kind of health statistics that confuse doctors. Conditional probabilities such as sensitivities and specificities provide another challenge. For instance, Gigerenzer et al. (2007) provided 160 German gynecologists with the relevant health statistics needed for calculating the chances that a woman with a positive screening mammogram actually has breast cancer: a prevalence of 1%, a sensitivity of 90%, and a false positive rate of 9%. The physicians were asked: What would you tell a woman who tested positive that her chances were of having breast cancer? The best answer is that about 1 out of 10 women who test positive actually have cancer; the others are false positives. Yet 60% of the gynecologists believed that 8 or 9 out of these 10 women actually have cancer, and 18% that the chances are 1 in 100. Similar lack of understanding among physicians has been reported in the evaluation of positive HIV tests (Gigerenzer et al. 1998), in diabetes prevention studies (Mühlhauser et al. 2006), and other medical tests and treatments (Eddy 1982; Casscells et al. 1978; Ghosh and Ghosh 2005; Hoffrage et al. 2000; Young et al. 2002).

The inability of so many physicians to understand evidence in their own specialty is a disturbing fact. But medical schools and continuing education programs do not seem to acknowledge this collective statistical illiteracy as a fundamental problem of health care. Framing techniques have been developed to enable physicians to understand health statistics by representing the numbers in a transparent form (Gigerenzer 2002; Wegwarth and Gigerenzer, this volume). For instance, consider mammography screening again. It is easy to teach physicians to translate conditional probability information into *natural frequencies*: Think of 1,000 women. Ten are expected to have breast cancer, and of these, 9 test positive. Of the 990 women without cancer, about 89 nevertheless test positive. Now, almost all (87%) gynecologists understood that 9 + 89 will test positive, and only 9 of these actually have breast cancer, which amounts to roughly 1 out of 10 (Gigerenzer et al. 2007). This and other mental techniques can be efficiently taught in a few hours and—most important—unlike standard statistical training, the training effects do not fade away after a few weeks (Sedlmeier and Gigerenzer 2001). Some medical schools are presently adopting these techniques, but most still produce physicians who lack the ability to understand evidence. Without statistical literacy in health, informed medical decision making will remain an illusion.

Manifesto for Action to Protect Patients from Statistically Illiterate Doctors

1. Medical schools should ensure that students are taught transparent risk communication in addition to evidence-based skills. Evidence is necessary but not sufficient, given that doctors and patients alike are misled by nontransparent health statistics. For instance, the Charité in Berlin is currently introducing not only evidence-based medicine but also transparent risk communication for all medical students. The transparency program is outlined in Gigerenzer (2002) and Gigerenzer et al. (2007).

2. Organizations responsible for continuing medical education and recertification programs should ensure that practicing doctors receive the same education in transparent risk communication as medical students.
3. Patients should have the courage to ask questions about the range of options, their quantitative benefits and harms, and insist on transparent answers from their doctors, just as if they were speaking to a school teacher about their child's progress. Patients can be resourceful, provided they are given the resources in the first place (Gray 2002). This will not only benefit patients but will also lead to a change in clinician behavior and reduce the risk of litigation for the institution. In this century of the patient, patients have responsibilities as well as rights.

Creating the Century of the Patient

The professionalization of modern medicine began in the 19th century. In most developed countries, people's health improved from a combination of clean water, better hygiene, and healthier and sufficient amounts of food. It also involved abandoning harmful procedures that had been popular for centuries, such as the extensive bleeding of patients to get rid of "bad" blood. This can be considered the first health care revolution.

The second half of the 20th century witnessed enormous scientific advances that gave us miracles such as the artificial hip and a cure for childhood leukemia, combined with the immense investment of resources in service expansion, professional education, and management. This second health care revolution created powerful systems of health care management. The 20th century became the century of the doctor, the clinics, and the medical industry. Knowledgeable patients were not the primary goal of the second revolution, as illustrated by the pill scares in the United Kingdom and the striking misinformation of the general public in Europe and the United States about the pros and cons of cancer screening (Gigerenzer et al. 2009). Despite great advancements, the 20th century left us with uninformed doctors and patients, unwarranted practice variation that turns geography into destiny, waste of resources, and safety problems. Most countries can no longer afford such a wasteful system, and the recent financial crises provide a unique opportunity for change.

A third health care revolution is now needed. Whereas the first revolution brought clean water, the third should bring clean information. It should turn the 21st century into the *century of the patient*—a genuinely democratic ideal. Citizens have the right to know the basic facts and a responsibility to base their health care decisions on the best available evidence. Our vision of a healthy health care system is that of a democracy where knowledge is distributed across all levels of society. It is not a new idea and has been expressed at various times in the past. Making good use of dispersed knowledge was essential for the first known successful democracy in Athens (Ober 2008). The costs of participatory political practices in Athens were more than matched by superior returns in social cooperation. This democratic ideal was also expressed by the second president of the United States, John Adams (2000/1765): "The preservation of the means of knowledge among the lowest ranks is of more importance to the public than all the property of all the rich men in the country." As the economist Friedrich Hayek (1945) has argued, liberty and democracy demand that a general knowledge be dispersed among the people. When it comes to health, the 20th century failed to promote educated citizens in modern democracies. Even worse, the current system itself causes, supports, and profits from the uninformed patient.

To achieve this third revolution, major efforts on many levels will be needed to reach its goals (Table 1.2). A critical mass of informed patients will not resolve all problems of health care, but they will constitute the major triggering factor for better care. Informed patients will ask questions that require doctors to become better informed and provide better care. They will be able to see through deception and attempts to create undue expectations and fears. The century of the patient requires the funding of research that is relevant for patients rather than for patents. It entails the enforcement of ethical guidelines about complete and transparent reporting in journals, brochures, and the media, and demands a legal system to protect patients and doctors alike against defensive medicine. Finally, it obliges medical schools to teach statistical literacy in health and transparent risk communication.

The century of the patient will involve more ways to transform the patient from a problem to a solution. For example, to improve the care of epilepsy, an excellent way would be to bring together patients, their parents, caretakers, and teachers with neurologists and other clinicians to develop solutions that reflect the practical and theoretical knowledge of all involved. This can lead to hypotheses about treatments that can be investigated in systematic research. The century of the patient will also involve a change in the doctor–patient relation, from frightened and ignorant patients who blindly trust their doctors toward shared decision making. Shared decision making has been promoted as an alternative to paternalism for some time, but given defensive decision

Table 1.2   Goals of the century of the patient.

	Funding of research relevant for patients
+	Transparent and complete reporting in medical journals
+	Transparent and complete reporting in health pamphlets
+	Transparent and complete reporting in the media
+	Incentive structures that minimize conflicts of interest
+	Best practice instead of defensive medicine
+	Doctors who understand health statistics
=	Informed patients

making and statistical illiteracy in health, *informed* shared decision making has rarely been possible.

Calls for better health care have been typically countered by claims that this demand implies one of two alternatives, which nobody really wants: raising taxes or rationing care. The problem, however, is not lack of money, and the cure is not more money. At issue is a better health system. The century of the patient is the third alternative: better doctors, better patients, and better care for less money.

2

When Misinformed Patients Try to Make Informed Health Decisions

Wolfgang Gaissmaier and Gerd Gigerenzer

Abstract

Statistical illiteracy in health—the inability to understand health statistics—is widespread among the general public. Many people find it hard to accept uncertainty in the first place and, even if they do, basic numerical information is difficult to understand. The problem is aggravated when the benefits and harms of treatment options must be evaluated or test outcomes understood.

Statistical illiteracy results not only from a lack of education but from the nontransparent framing of information that is sometimes unintentional, but which can also be used deliberately to manipulate people. In health care, nontransparent framing of information seems to be the rule rather than the exception. Patients have difficulties finding reliable information—on the Internet, in invitations to screening, medical pamphlets, or media reports—yet this situation can be corrected. Statistical thinking must be taught to the public, and health care workers and journalists must be trained in transparent framing. Knowing what questions to ask, what information is missing, and how to translate nontransparent statistics into transparent ones would empower an educated citizenry to reject attempts to persuade rather than inform.

Introduction

A recent press release advertised the results of an international randomized controlled trial on the benefits of using PSA tests for prostate cancer screening. It stated that PSA screening would reduce the risk of dying from prostate cancer by 20% (Wilde 2009). But what does that really mean? Just how big is 20%, and how many people does it equate to? It meant that out of every 1,410 men who regularly participated in prostate cancer screening, 1 less person died of prostate cancer than in an equally large group of men who did not participate (Schröder et al. 2009). What the press release did not report, however, is that out of these 1,410 men, 48 were unnecessarily treated and hence subjected to potential incontinence and impotence. In addition, it omitted the fact that there is no evidence that PSA screening reduces overall mortality at all. That is, the 1 man (out of 1,410) who was saved from dying from prostate cancer likely died from something else in the same time frame. The press release also failed to mention that there was a second large clinical trial, published in the same issue of that medical journal, where no reduction in prostate cancer mortality was found to be attributable to screening (Andriole et al. 2009).

This example illustrates two key problems in the communication of clinical evidence: communication is often made nontransparent through the use of, what is called, relative risks ("20%") instead of more transparent absolute risks ("1 in 1,410"), and it is often incomplete as only those facts which suit the interests of the communicator are reported. Together with lack of statistical education, nontransparency and incomplete reporting contribute to what we call statistical illiteracy in health; that is, the inability to understand health statistics. One major cause of statistical illiteracy is conflict of interest on the part of those communicating health statistics, who push an agenda instead of informing citizens.

The problem of statistical illiteracy is a collective one (Gigerenzer 2002; Gigerenzer et al. 2007; Reyna and Brainerd 2007). It exists not only in patients but also in physicians, politicians, and journalists. In this chapter, we focus on the extent of statistical illiteracy in the general public, explain the major causes, and offer some remedies on how it could be overcome. We do not intend to provide a comprehensive survey, but use evidence to exemplify the general situation in health care.

Extent of Statistical Literacy among Patients

To be health literate, patients need to have at least four basic abilities. They need to (a) accept living with uncertainty, (b) have a basic understanding of numerical information, (c) grasp the benefits and harms of treatment options, and (d) understand test results.

The Illusion of Certainty

To appreciate the importance of health statistics, patients need to understand that in the first place, there is no such thing as certainty. As Benjamin Franklin once said: "In this world, there is nothing certain but death and taxes." Yet living with uncertainty can be extremely difficult when health statistics, as opposed to baseball statistics, are at issue. The term "illusion of certainty" refers to an emotional need for certainty when none exists. This feeling can be attached to test results that are taken to be absolutely certain and to treatments that appear to guarantee a cure. One might think that physicians routinely inform patients that even the best tests are not perfect and that every test result needs therefore to be interpreted with care, or may need to be repeated. Studies indicate, however, that clinicians rarely communicate the uncertainties about risks and benefits of treatments to patients (Braddock et al. 1999).

In a nationwide survey conducted in 2006, 1,000 German citizens over the age of 18 were asked: "Which of the following tests are absolutely certain?" While only 4% believed that an expert horoscope could give absolutely accurate results, a majority of Germans believed that HIV tests, fingerprints, and DNA tests were absolutely certain, even though none of these are (Gigerenzer et al. 2007). In contrast to these tests, which tend to make relatively few errors, a mammography (positive or negative mammogram) has a miss rate of about 10%, and its false positive rate is nearly as high. Nonetheless, it was rated as "absolutely certain" by 46% of the women and 42% of the men. Higher education is only a slight safeguard against the illusion of certainty: One-third of women with a university degree also believed that mammograms are absolutely certain.

Once one accepts that uncertainty is unavoidable in the world, the next challenge is to understand numbers that express uncertainties. This most elementary skill is called *basic numeracy*.

Basic Numeracy

Schwartz, Woloshin, Black, and Welch (1997) developed a simple three-question scale to measure basic numeracy:

1. A person taking Drug A has a 1% chance of having an allergic reaction. If 1,000 people take Drug A, how many would you expect to have an allergic reaction? ___ person(s) out of 1,000
2. A person taking Drug B has a 1 in 1,000 chance of an allergic reaction. What percent of people taking Drug B will have an allergic reaction? ___ %
3. Imagine that I flip a coin 1,000 times. What is your best guess about how many times the coin would come up heads in 1,000 flips? ___ times out of 1,000

The test was applied to a random sample of female veterans in New England, 96% of whom were high school graduates and whose average age was 68. Only 54% were able to convert 1% to 10 in 1,000; 20% were able to convert 1 in 1,000 to 0.1%; and 54% were able to answer that one would expect the coin to come up heads 500 times out of 1,000, with the most common incorrect answers to the last being 25, 50, and 250. The number of correct answers was strongly related to women's ability to accurately interpret the benefit of mammography after being presented with standard risk reduction information: Only 6% of women answering just one basic numeracy question correctly could accurately interpret the data, compared to 40% of those answering all three questions correctly. Thus, basic numeracy seems to be a necessary precondition for making informed decisions (cf. Reyna et al. 2009), and although physicians do better on this test, even they are far from perfect (see Wegwarth and Gigerenzer, this volume).

Table 2.1 shows the prevalence of low numeracy skills in representative samples of the general population of U.S. and German adults. Note again the great difficulty that large parts of the public, just as the female veterans, had in translating small frequencies into percentages. The left column in Table 2.1 shows that only 25% of U.S. citizens correctly converted 1 in 1,000 to 0.1%. Even among the highest education groups, this percentage was merely 27%. In another study, Lipkus, Samsa, and Rimer (2001) found that only 21% of well-educated adults were able to calculate this problem correctly. Comparable results have been found recently in a survey of probabilistic, representative national samples in the United States and in Germany (Table 2.1, columns 3 and 4), and this question was again found to be the most difficult one. It was answered correctly by only 24% of U.S. and 46% of German adults. In addition, overall numeracy on an extended version of the original questionnaire was higher in Germany than in the United States. Education predicted numeracy in both countries, but the gap between those with low education (less than high school) and those with high education (college or more) was much larger in the United States (40% overall accuracy vs. 83%) than in Germany (62% vs. 81%).

Statistical literacy becomes even more important when interpreting the benefits and harms of treatments, which are often communicated using more complicated health statistics, such as relative risks. Recall that in the introductory example above, a 20% relative risk reduction (RRR) in prostate cancer

Table 2.1 Basic numeracy in the United States and Germany based on nationally representative samples. The table shows data from two studies and separately includes U.S. citizens with highest educational attainment for one study.

	U.S. adults ages 35–70[a] n = 450	Postgraduate degree[a] n = 62	U.S. adults ages 25–69[b] n = 1009	German adults ages 25–69[b] n = 1001
	% Correct answer			
Convert 1% → 10 in 1,000	70	82	58	68
Convert 1 in 1,000 → 0.1%	25	27	24	46
Heads in 1,000 coin flips	76	86	73	73

[a] Schwartz and Woloshin (2000, unpublished data)
[b] Galesic and Garcia-Retamero (2010)

mortality was the same as an absolute risk reduction (ARR) of 1 in 1,410. Are patients aware of the difference between these two formats?

Understanding Benefits and Harms of Treatments

Patients need realistic estimates of the benefits and harms of treatment options to be able to evaluate whether the benefits outweigh the harms. Often they do not have realistic estimates, however, as highlighted by a recent representative survey of more than 10,000 citizens from nine European countries (Gigerenzer et al. 2009). In this survey, using face-to-face interviews, men and women were asked to estimate the benefits of prostate and breast cancer screening, respectively. As shown in Figure 2.1, about 90% of both men and women overestimated the benefits of screening, by tenfold, hundredfold, or more, or did not know.

One reason for such misunderstandings is that benefits and harms of treatments are often communicated as relative risks, which, as we will illustrate, are difficult for people to understand. But there is a simple solution: Use absolute risks instead.

Is perceived treatment efficacy influenced by framing information in terms of RRR and ARR? In a telephone survey in New Zealand, respondents were given information on three different screening tests for unspecified cancers (Sarfati et al. 1998). The benefits were identical, except that they were expressed either as RRR, ARR, or the number of people needed to be treated (NNT) or screened to prevent 1 death from cancer (which is 1/absolute risk reduction):

- RRR: If you have this test every two years, it will reduce your chance of dying from this cancer by around one-third over the next ten years.
- ARR: If you have this test every two years, it will reduce your chance of dying from this cancer from around 3 in 1,000 to around 2 in 1,000 over the next 10 years.
- NNT: If around 1,000 people have this test every two years, 1 person will be saved from dying from this cancer every 10 years.

When the benefit of the test was presented as an RRR, 80% of 306 New Zealanders said they would likely accept the test. When the same information was presented as an ARR and NNT, only 53% and 43% wanted the test, respectively. Medical students also fall prey to the influence of framing (Naylor et al. 1992), as do patients (Malenka et al. 1993) and health professionals (Mühlhauser et al. 2006). In a meta-analysis on the effect of presenting information in terms of absolute risks versus relative risks, Covey (2007) analyzed 31 experiments that either investigated physicians, other health professionals, students, or patients which showed that all of them can be consistently manipulated by framing the treatment effect differently.

(a) Perceived benefit of breast cancer screening

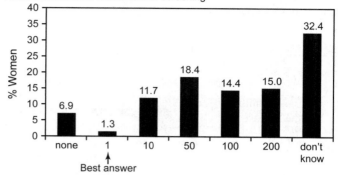

(b) Perceived benefit of prostate cancer screening

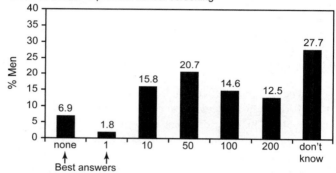

Figure 2.1 Results of a survey (Gigerenzer et al. 2009) on the perceived benefits of cancer screening in nine European countries (Austria, France, Germany, Italy, Netherlands, Poland, Russia, Spain, and the United Kingdom). Over 90% of men and women overestimated the benefits of mammography or PSA screening, or did not know. The data shows the results for the age group for which the screening is usually offered. (a) Perceived benefit of mammography screening by women age 50–69, summed across nine countries (n = 1467). Bars show the percentage of women who believed that out of 1,000 women participating in screening, X fewer will die from breast cancer compared to women who do not participate. The available evidence indicates that the best answer is 1 in 1,000 (Woloshin and Schwartz 2009). (b) Perceived benefit of PSA screening by men age 50–69, summed across the eight EU countries (n = 1291). Russia is excluded here, because Russian men estimated the benefits much more accurately than anyone else and thus would distort the EU picture here (for Russia, see Gigerenzer et al. 2009). Bars show the percentage of these men who believed that out of 1,000 men participating in screening, X fewer will die from prostate cancer compared to men who do not participate. Because estimates vary between 0 in 1,000 (Andriole et al. 2009) and 0.7 in 1,000 (= 1 in 1,410) (Schröder et al. 2009), we marked both 0 and 1 in 1,000 as correct.

The problem with relative risks is that, unlike absolute risks, they remain silent about the baseline risk. A 50% risk reduction, for instance, can mean a reduction from 2 to 1 out of 100,000 people. However, it can also mean a reduction from 20,000 to 10,000 out of 100,000 people, which would be a much more relevant effect. Particularly for low probability risks, communicating changes in relative terms makes effects loom larger than they actually are.

Understanding Test Results

Patients in a clinic in Colorado and Oklahoma were asked about standard tests for diseases such as strep throat infection, HIV, and acute myocardial infarction (Hamm and Smith 1998). Each patient judged (a) the probability that a person has the disease before being tested (prevalence or base rate), (b) the probability that a person tests positive if the disease is present (sensitivity), (c) the probability that a person tests negative if the disease is absent (specificity), and (d) the probability that a person has the disease if test results are positive (positive predictive value). Most patients estimated the four probabilities to be essentially the same—independent of whether the base rate was high or low, or the test accurate or not. Even experienced patients did not understand health statistics, which suggests that their doctors either never explained risks or failed to communicate them properly. Studies with university students show that they too have difficulties drawing conclusions from sensitivities and specificities (Gigerenzer and Hoffrage 1995).

The problem is that the relevant pieces of information, such as the chance of detecting a disease, are usually communicated as conditional probabilities (e.g., sensitivities and specificities). For instance, a 30-year-old pregnant woman took a nuchal scan for testing whether her unborn child has Down syndrome. She is told that the chance of a positive test result if the child actually has Down syndrome is 80% (sensitivity). That is, 80% is the conditional probability of testing positive given Down syndrome. However, this probability is often confused with the positive predictive value of the test; that is, the probability of the child having Down syndrome given a positive test result, which is, of course, not the same. This can be illustrated with a more intuitive example. Until now, every American president has been male; that is, the probability of being male given that one is president of the United States has been 100%. The reverse, obviously, does not hold: Given that one is male, chances of being the president of the United States are rather low.

The question is how to get from the sensitivity of the test to the positive predictive value, which is the information one really wants. Two further pieces of information are necessary. First, one needs to know the base rate of the disease; for a pregnant woman at the age of 30, this rate is about 0.15%. Second, one needs to know the false positive rate of the test; that is, the probability of getting a positive test result given that the child actually does not have Down syndrome, which is about 8%. Formally, the sensitivity, the base rate, and the false positive rate can be combined to calculate the positive predictive value by applying Bayes's rule. However, both physicians and laypeople often have trouble with these probabilities, and it is much simpler to think about such problems in terms of what we call natural frequencies.

Instead of combining conditional probabilities such as sensitivities and false positive rates, natural frequencies are about concrete cases; for instance, 10,000 pregnant women. Out of these 10,000 women, we expect 15 to carry a child with Down syndrome (= 0.15% base rate); the remaining 9,985 women are not affected. Of the 15 women whose child has Down syndrome, we expect that 12 will receive a positive test result (= 80% sensitivity). From the remaining 9,985 women, about 799 women will also test (falsely) positive (= 8% false positive rate). Thus, there are 811 women who receive a positive test result, out of which 12 actually carry a child with Down syndrome. Therefore, the probability of a child having Down syndrome given a positive test—the positive predictive value—is about 12 out of 811, which is about 1.5% (Figure 2.2).

Estimating the probability of disease given a positive test (or any other posterior probability) has been repeatedly shown to be much easier with natural frequencies than with conditional probabilities in students (e.g., Gigerenzer and Hoffrage 1995, 1999), physicians (Gigerenzer et al. 2007), and the elderly (Galesic, Gigerenzer et al. 2009). Even fifth graders can consistently solve Bayesian problems with natural frequencies (Zhu and Gigerenzer 2006).

Note that natural frequencies refer to situations where two variables are considered: Natural frequencies are joint frequencies, as shown in Figure 2.2. In contrast, relative frequencies (which are numerically identical to the conditional probabilities in Figure 2.2) do not facilitate judgments (Gigerenzer and Hoffrage 1995), a fact sometimes misunderstood in the literature (Hoffrage et al. 2002).

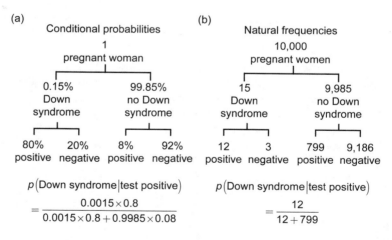

Figure 2.2 A 30-year-old pregnant woman gets a positive nuchal scan for Down syndrome. What are the chances that her child actually has Down syndrome (Kurzenhäuser and Hoffrage 2002)? The information in (a) is expressed in terms of conditional probabilities, and the formula is known as Bayes's rule. The information in (b) is expressed in terms of natural frequencies, which simplify the computations and foster insight.

In summary, relative risks and conditional probabilities tend to confuse patients, whereas absolute risks (and NNTs) help them understand the benefits and harms, just as natural frequencies help communicate what a test result means.

Causes

There are various players in public health whose goals can conflict with transparent risk communication: pushing a political agenda, attracting media attention, selling a new drug, increasing compliance with screening, or trying to impress physicians. We will argue that a major reason for statistical illiteracy can thus be found not only in patients' minds and lack of training, but in their environment. Statistical illiteracy is fostered by nontransparent framing of information that is sometimes an unintentional result of lack of understanding, but can also be an intentional effort to manipulate or persuade people.

As the above examples have shown, two number formats are particularly hard to understand for the general public: relative risks and conditional probabilities. These two formats can easily be replaced by transparent formats (absolute risks and natural frequencies), but unfortunately seldom are. Despite the general belief that one can find everything on the Internet or in other media, it is in fact difficult to find information about health care that is both transparent and complete. As Gigerenzer and Gray (this volume) emphasize, the problem already starts with nontransparent information in medical journals and is amplified by leaflets containing confusing, incomplete, or even wrong information. We will demonstrate that patients have a hard time finding good information, be it in searching through invitations to screening, medical pamphlets, the Internet, or media reports about medical research. All of these sources suffer from nontransparent information and are more likely to confuse people than to enlighten them.

Are Patients Likely to Find Transparent Information in Medical Pamphlets or on the Internet?

Patients only rarely consult first-hand sources such as medical journals. Instead, besides asking their physician, they rely on other sources of information. To illustrate the quality of information available to patients, consider the case of breast cancer screening. First of all, women who contemplate participating need some basic information about breast cancer. The mortality rate, not the incidence rate, is most relevant for screening, given that the goal of screening is to reduce mortality, whereas it cannot reduce the risk of getting breast cancer (incidence). Naturally, the incidence rates loom larger than the mortality rates and thus contribute to raising anxiety; campaigns that selectively report incidence rates have been criticized for this reason (Baines 1992). Most importantly, information on breast cancer screening should provide information about the potential benefits and harms, so that a woman can make an informed decision as to whether she wants to participate or not. Table 2.2 provides the essential information about the benefits and harms. Benefits can be expressed in terms of both total cancer mortality and breast cancer mortality. For women who participate in screening, there is no difference in total cancer mortality, but a reduction of breast cancer mortality of 1 in 1,000. At the same time, screening may lead to two major harms: false positives resulting in unnecessary biopsies and unnecessary treatments, such as lumpectomies. A third harm is getting radiation-induced cancer from the mammography, but since no reliable estimates of the actual danger exist, we have decided not to include this in the facts box (Table 2.2).

The facts box is a transparent way to communicate the major benefits and harms of screening and treatments in general (see Schwartz and Woloshin, this volume). What information do women actually get on breast cancer screening, and in what format do they get it? There are three sources of information we focus on here: invitations to screening, pamphlets, and web sites. In countries with publicly funded screening, eligible women are often made aware of these programs by letters of invitation. Thus, by sheer numbers of people reached, such letters are—alongside physicians—potentially the most important source of information about screening. Invitation letters would be the ideal opportunity to provide patients with balanced, transparent information about screening, so that they can make informed decisions. Jorgensen and Gøtzsche (2006) investigated such invitations to attend breast cancer screening in seven countries with publicly funded screening: Australia, Canada, Denmark, New Zealand, Norway, Sweden, and the United Kingdom (Table 2.3). Other studies have investigated the information that medical pamphlets and web sites provide about breast cancer screening in many countries (Table 2.3).

Table 2.2   Facts box for mammography screening; potential benefits and harms are 10-year risks. Based on Woloshin and Schwartz (2009) and Gøtzsche and Nielsen (2006).

Breast Cancer Screening with Mammography		
	Women aged 50 years	
	1000 women not screened	1000 women screened annually for 10 years
Benefits?		
• Total cancer mortality	No difference	
• Breast cancer mortality	5	4
Harms?		
• False positives with biopsies	—	50 to 200
• Overtreatment[a]	—	2 to 10
Positive predictive value?[b]		1 out of 10

[a]   For example, unnecessary lumpectomy.
[b]   That is, proportion of women with breast cancer among those who test positive.

Table 2.3 Information about breast cancer screening available for patients in invitations to screening, pamphlets, and web sites. Adapted from Gigerenzer et al. (2007). Numbers are percentages.

	Invitations n = 31; 7 countries[a]	Pamphlets n = 58; Australia[b]	Pamphlets n = 27; Germany[c]	Pamphlets n = 7; Austria[d]	Web sites n = 27; 8 countries[e]
Baseline risk					
• Lifetime risk of developing breast cancer	32	60	37	43	44
• Lifetime risk of dying from breast cancer	n/a	2	4	0	15
Benefits?					
• Relative risk reduction of death from breast cancer	23	22	7	0	56
• Absolute risk reduction of death from breast cancer	0	0	7	0	19
• Number needed to screen to avoid 1 death from breast cancer	0	0	4	0	7
Harms?					
• Overdiagnosis and overtreatment	0	n/a	11	n/a	26
• Harms from X-rays	n/a	n/a	44	100	15
Positive predictive value?	0	0	15	0	15

[a] Jorgensen and Gøtzsche (2006)
[b] Slaytor and Ward (1998)
[c] Kurzenhäuser (2003)
[d] Rásky and Groth (2004)
[e] Jorgensen and Gøtzsche (2004)

Most of the invitations (97%) stated the major benefit of screening is the reduction in breast cancer mortality. However, the very few (23%) that also mentioned the size of the benefit always did so by using RRRs rather than ARRs. None of the invitations included information about potential harms or the positive predictive value. Instead, most invitations used persuasive wording and prespecified appointments. Thus, the invitation letters clearly aim at compliance rather than at informing the public, which is probably a result of a built-in conflict: those who are responsible for the screening program are also responsible for designing the invitations, which puts their goal of increasing compliance at odds with increasing transparency.

In medical pamphlets, numbers are very often not given at all. In the few cases where quantitative estimates of the benefits are provided, they are almost exclusively presented as RRRs. Many of these sources of information also remain mute on the harms. However, some pamphlets (German and Austrian) do include information about harms from X-rays, even if mostly to reassure patients that these are negligible (Rásky and Groth 2004). Almost no pamphlet explains what a positive test result means.

Given this imbalance in reporting, it is probably not surprising that the survey conducted in nine European countries about the perceived benefits of cancer screening (Gigerenzer et al. 2009) found that those who said they sometimes or frequently consulted health information in pamphlets had no better understanding than those who did not. In Germany, where pamphlets were consulted by a record 41% of the public, those who consulted pamphlets sometimes or frequently showed even a higher overestimation of benefits than those who did not.

Web sites—in particular, those of advocacy groups and governmental institutions (24 web sites in total)—recommended screening and favored information that shed positive light on it. Only few mentioned the major potential harms of screening: overdiagnosis and overtreatment. Three web sites of consumer organizations had a more balanced perspective on breast cancer screening and included information on both the potential benefits and harms. In total, very few sites met the standards of informed consent, as specified by the General Medical Council's (1998) guidelines for patient information. This problem is not limited to information about cancer and has been shown for other conditions as well (Impiccatore et al. 1997; Rigby et al. 2001). These results are alarming, given that many people use the Internet to acquire information about health issues—in the European Union, this number is 23% (see Jorgensen and Gøtzsche 2004).

Do the Media Provide Balanced Information about Health Topics?

The press has a powerful influence on public perceptions of health and health care; much of what people—including many physicians—know and believe about medicine comes from the print and broadcast media. However, journalism schools tend to teach everything except understanding numbers. Journalists generally receive no training in how to interpret or present medical research (Kees 2002). A survey of health reporters at daily newspapers in five U.S. Midwestern states (Voss 2002) reported that very few found it easy to interpret statistical data and less than a third found it easy to put health news in context. This finding is similar to that of the Freedom Forum survey, where nearly half of the science writers agreed that "reporters have no idea how to interpret scientific results" (Hartz and Chappell 1997:30).

Lack of education inevitably affects the quality of press coverage, particularly in the reporting of health statistics about medical research, as has been repeatedly documented (e.g., Moynihan et al. 2000; Ransohoff and Harris 1997; Schwartz et al. 1999a). One disturbing problem associated with how the media report on new medications is the failure to provide quantitative data on how well the medication works. Instead, many of these news stories present anecdotes, often in the form of patients describing miraculous responses to the new medication. If the benefits of a medication are quantified at all, they are commonly reported as an RRR. The situation is similar when it comes to the harms of medications: Typically, less than half of stories name a specific side effect and even fewer actually quantify it. This is most dramatic in direct-to-consumer advertisements, which often display the RRR from the medication in prominent, large letters, but present harms in long lists in very fine print. Television ads typically give consumers more time to absorb information about benefits than about risks, resulting in better recall of benefits (Kaphingst et al. 2004, 2005).

In general, journalists do not seem to help the public understand health statistics, at least with regard to cancer screening. In none of the nine European countries surveyed by Gigerenzer et al. (2009), about the perceived benefits of cancer screening, were estimates of the benefits any better by those participants who reported sometimes or frequently using television or newspapers as a source for health information.

Remedies

The facts reviewed so far might be discouraging. It seems that many players in the field of health avoid transparency and complete reporting—ranging from the major medical journals (Nuovo et al. 2002; Schwartz et al. 2006) to governments and health organizations to the media. Yet this does not mean that there is nothing to be done. The most important means of improvement is teaching the public statistical thinking combined with training health care providers and journalists in transparent framing. But that necessitates rethinking how statistical thinking is taught.

Teaching Statistical Literacy

Statistical thinking is the most useful part of mathematics for life after school. In most countries, however, almost all of the available classroom time is spent on the mathematics of certainty—from algebra to geometry to trigonometry. If children learned to deal with an uncertain world in a playful way, much of collective statistical illiteracy would be history. The U.S. National Council of Teachers of Mathematics (NCTM) has announced its commitment to teaching data analysis and probability in grades prekindergarten to 12, as described in its Principles and Standards for School Mathematics (NCTM 2000), and declared data analysis and probability its "professional development focus of the year," providing additional resources and continuing education. The NCTM prefaced its Principles with a simple truth: "Young children will not develop statistical reasoning if it is not included in the curriculum."

Today, the mathematics curriculum in many countries includes probability and statistics. Yet research on the effect of teaching showed that although students learn how to compute formal measures of averages and variability, even those with good grades rarely understand what these statistics represent or their importance and connection to other concepts (Garfield and Ben-Zvi 2007). Few learn to see a connection between statistics in school and what is going on in their world, which is exactly how one could grab their attention: by teaching real-world problems instead of throwing dice and flipping coins. Adolescents love baseball statistics, want to know about HIV, have heard about probabilities of rain, worry about the chance of a major earthquake, and when they get older, become interested in graphs about stock indices and develop concerns about cholesterol and blood pressure. How safe is the contraceptive pill? What is the error margin for polls and surveys? Personal relevance is what makes statistics so interesting. This would, of course, also require educating teachers first.

Teaching statistical literacy in school would lay the ground for also improving training doctors in medical statistics. Even back in 1937, an editorial in *The Lancet* noted that the use (or abuse) of statistics "tends to induce a strong emotional reaction in non-mathematical minds." It complained that for "most of us figures impinge on an educational blind spot," which "is a misfortune, because simple statistical methods concern us far more closely than many of the things that we are forced to learn in the six long years of the medical curriculum." Improvements have been made since then, although there are still medical organizations, physicians, and students who tend to see statistics as inherently mathematical and clinically irrelevant for the individual patient (Gigerenzer 2002; Altman and Bland 1991; Wegwarth and Gigerenzer, this volume).

Provide Complete and Transparent Information

An important response to statistical illiteracy is to give the public numbers. Patients have a right to learn how large the benefits and harms of a treatment are. Verbal descriptions of risks, however, are notoriously unclear and lead to misunderstandings (Steckelberg et al. 2005; Trevena et al. 2006). Contrary to popular belief, studies report that a majority of patients prefer, in fact, numerical information to care alone (Hallowell et al. 1997; Wallsten et al. 1993). As indicated above, there are simple ways to make numbers easier to grasp (see also Fagerlin et al. 2007). In this chapter we have addressed two of them: using absolute risks instead of relative risks, and using natural frequencies rather than conditional probabilities. There is more to transparency than can be covered in this chapter. Pictorial, icon, and graphic representations are other formats that can foster insight (Galesic, Garcia-Retamero et al. 2009; Hawley et al. 2008; Kurz-Milcke et al. 2008; Lipkus 2007; Paling 2003; Zikmund-Fisher, Fagerlin et al. 2008; Zikmund-Fisher, Ubel et al. 2008). Bunge et al. (2010) provide a review about evidence-based patient information.

Conclusion

Despite the growth of information technology, the problem of statistical illiteracy in health is widespread. Patients and doctors alike often lack skills in basic numeracy, and the problem is further aggravated when the benefits and harms of treatment options need to be evaluated or test results assessed. In the literature, statistical illiteracy is often presented as if it were largely a consequence of cognitive limitations (Kahneman et al. 1982). However, if such "probability blindness" were simply caused by faulty mental software, then we would just have to live with a miswired brain. The only remedy taken thus far has come in some form of paternalism; that is, people have been inhibited from making important health decisions and instead nudged toward outcomes determined by others (Thaler and Sunstein 2008).

Most causes of statistical illiteracy that we discussed, however, are found in the external environment. The majority of information directed at patients is either incomplete, nontransparent, or both. Consequently, the easiest and most effective remedy is to use transparent representations, such as absolute risks or natural frequencies, when presenting health information. This should happen in association with a change in school curricula, so that the next generation is equipped to deal with risk and uncertainty. An educated society must know what questions to ask, what information is missing, and how to translate nontransparent statistics into transparent ones. An educated citizenry will drive change in the media and other institutions by exerting pressure to supply complete and transparent information.

We believe that statistical literacy is a necessary precondition for educated citizens in a functioning democracy. Understanding risks and asking critical questions also has the potential to shape the emotional climate in a society and protect its members from external manipulation. In such a society, citizens can develop a better informed and more relaxed attitude toward health.

3

Reducing Unwarranted Variation in Clinical Practice by Supporting Clinicians and Patients in Decision Making

Albert G. Mulley, Jr., and John E. Wennberg

Abstract

Variation in clinical practice in seemingly similar populations of patients has been described for more than seventy years. International collaboration to increase understanding of the sources of practice variation and respond constructively have spawned efforts to expand and better manage professional knowledge, and to elicit and accommodate the personal knowledge of patients about what matters most to them when they face medical decisions under conditions of uncertainty. The approach, which has come to be known as shared decision making, can move us toward assurance that patients receive the care they need and no less and the care they want and no more. The use of decision aids to support shared decision making can effectively address the limitations in statistical thinking among clinicians as well as patients and thereby help establish informed patient choice as a standard of practice and improve the quality of medical decision making and the efficiency of health care.

When Geography Is Destiny

In 1938, J. Allison Glover reported on the incidence of tonsillectomy among school children in England and Wales (Glover 1938). He meticulously documented peculiar increases and decreases in rates over the preceding 15 years as well as unexplained differences by age, gender, and social status. Most striking was a tenfold variation in tonsillectomy from one region to another. To explain these "strange bare facts of incidence," Glover hypothesized that the conspicuous success of the operation in the occasional case had led to its adoption in many more doubtful cases, and he endorsed the earlier conclusion of a report from the Medical Research Council that there was a "tendency for the operation to be performed…for no particular reason and for no particular result."

Glover noted that between 1931 and 1935, for every death caused by complications of enlarged tonsils treated medically, there were more than 8 deaths attributable to tonsillectomy.

Rediscovering Practice Variation

More than thirty years later, Wennberg and Gittlesohn independently observed the same phenomenon in the United States (Wennberg and Gittelsohn 1973). Tonsillectomies varied almost 12-fold between the Vermont counties with the lowest and highest rates of the procedure. Subsequent work comparing the United States, the United Kingdom, and Norway, which focused on ten surgical procedures, including hysterectomies and tonsillectomies, noted that rates of these surgical procedures could vary as much as 10- to 15-fold between regions (McPherson et al. 1982). Although the use of surgery was generally highest in the United States, the amount of variability observed within the three countries was very similar, irrespective of the differences in how health care was financed. For each country, the observed variations could not be explained by variations in demographics and disease prevalence. Variation in surgical rates between and within countries was associated with the level of uncertainty about the probabilities of outcomes after surgery (Wennberg et al. 1980).

Since those early surgical studies, Wennberg and colleagues have used data from Medicare, the system that provides universal coverage to Americans 65 and older, to document variations in the use of surgical procedures and other clinical services across the entire United States (Dartmouth Atlas of Health Care 2010). The observed variations remain as striking as those documented by the initial studies.

Untangling the Clinical Sources of Practice Variation

Many of the highly variable surgical procedures were undertaken to improve quality of life by reducing symptoms associated with common conditions such as benign prostatic hyperplasia (BPH), benign uterine conditions, and disorders of the lumbar spine. In each case, evidence for comparative effectiveness was inadequate, and the resulting uncertainty allowed clinicians' ample discretion in making their recommendations. In the case of surgery for BPH in the early 1980s, most surgeons held that the goal of surgery was to improve life expectancy by reducing the risk of chronic obstruction of the bladder and kidneys, although others believed the treatment was primarily to improve the quality of life. For these latter clinicians, the goal of surgery was to reduce bothersome symptoms, which were presumed to increase inexorably over time. There was little evidence to support either the preventive or the quality of life theory, and clinicians in both camps of opinion preferred objective measures, such as urinary flow rates, rather than measures of the impact of surgery on symptoms. No matter what their clinical theories, the more aggressive surgeons believed that it was best to operate sooner rather than later when peri-operative risk would be higher because of advancing age and concomitant comorbidity.

In a series of research initiatives extending over more than five years, an international multidisciplinary team comprised of experts in biostatistics, decision analysis, survey research, epidemiology, and ethics as well as urology undertook an evaluation of these untested clinical hypotheses using many of the tools of the evaluative sciences: meta-analysis of existing clinical research, claims data analysis to capture additional clinical experience, decision analysis to model uncertainty and assess the sensitivity of decisions to probabilities, and eventually randomized trials and preference trials for the most plausible and relevant clinical hypotheses.

It became apparent that the preventive theory—operate early to avoid urinary tract obstruction and higher mortality—was wrong. For most men, the goal of surgery should be to improve the quality of life by reducing urinary tract symptoms. In addition, it became clear that uncertainty about the outcomes was not the only source of complexity for decisions about treatment of BPH. Some patients were greatly bothered by their symptoms—much more so than other men, even with the same or lower level of symptoms. Individual men thus felt differently about the probability and the degree of symptom relief afforded by treatment and the probability and impact of side effects. Patients also differed in their concern about the mortality risks associated with surgery: what was an acceptable risk to some was not for others (Wennberg et al. 1988; Fowler et al. 1988; Barry et al. 1988).

Untested medical theories and poor management of professional knowledge were thus identified as major sources of unwarranted variation. By contrast, differences among patients in subjective assessments of health states, risks, and time trade-offs (utilities, risk attitudes, and discount rates in the vocabulary of economists) were identified as sources of "warranted" variation. For example, men with BPH felt differently about the bother of urinary dysfunction: some men with mild symptoms were very bothered; others with severe symptoms were not bothered much at all. Men also felt very differently about the prospect of retrograde ejaculation, a form of sexual dysfunction that occurs in the majority of men who elect surgery for BPH. In fact, this side effect was so common that it was often not described to men because the surgeons did not consider it a "complication."

Given this explication of the sources of practice variation, the challenge was to make clinical decisions as knowledge-based or informed as possible by minimizing the sources of unwarranted variation while making them as patient-centered or personal as possible by recognizing and accommodating the warranted sources of variation. That challenge was met with the development of computer-based interactive laser videodisc technology interventions to support decisions. These shared decision-making programs (SDPs) managed the best available clinical evidence for the clinician and made information most relevant to the clinical decision comprehensible for patients. SDPs also provided a balanced appreciation for the variable impacts on quality of life that different treatment choices might have for different patients. This formulation of the problem and its solution was described in 1988 (Wennberg et al. 1988; Fowler et al. 1988; Barry et al. 1988). These three papers won the national health services research award and were the first three references in the first request for proposals from the Agency for Health Care Policy and Research, which sought to extend and replicate the approach through the funding of patient outcomes research teams (PORT). As a result, the outcomes research collaboration expanded to include many more colleagues and was extended to other conditions, including back pain and coronary artery disease in the first round of PORT funding. SDPs were developed for these conditions as well as for prostate cancer, breast cancer, and benign uterine conditions, among others.

Supporting Clinicians and Patients in Decision Making

The SDP development agenda raised new questions for the collaborators which spanned even further disciplines. Should patients' subjective assessments of health states, or utilities, be measured? Could they be with any reliability and accuracy? How could the gist of decisions made in the face of unavoidable uncertainty be communicated to people with variable levels of health literacy and numeracy? How could risks be best communicated? What about time trade-offs and discount rates? As early as 1989, a national group of experts in cognitive psychology and risk communication were convened at Dartmouth to bring together the best available understanding of these challenges. The accumulating interdisciplinary knowledge shaped each successive SDP (Kasper et al. 1992; Mulley 1989, 1990).

The coronary artery disease SDP, "Treatment Choices for Ischemic Heart Disease," was one of the most sophisticated of the early programs. It was developed by collaborators at Duke, University of California at San Francisco, University of Minnesota, New England Medical Center, and University of Toronto as well as Massachusetts General Hospital and Dartmouth. Cox hazard models and logistic regression models were developed to estimate patient-specific probabilities of good and bad outcomes, including 5-year survival curves with each of the available treatment options. Graphs, figures, and animation were used to present information with comprehension demonstrated by sequential formative assessments with multiple groups of patients (Mulley 1995a). A published summative evaluation showed high levels of patient comprehension and satisfaction in a population with low levels of educational attainment (Liao et al. 1996).

Two breast cancer SDPs demonstrated further the need for decision support among clinicians as well as patients (Mulley 1993a, b). Development of the SDP to support surgical decisions for patients with early-stage invasive cancer uncovered a misunderstanding of the clinical evidence that was widely prevalent among clinical oncologists and surgeons. In the early publications of results of the NSABP-06 trials, which demonstrated equivalent survival with either mastectomy or lumpectomy followed by radiation, it appeared that local as well as distant recurrence of cancer was also equivalent with the two treatment options. However, the earliest reports of those trials excluded consideration of local recurrence within the breast previously treated with lumpectomy. When these outcomes were considered, survival and nonlocal recurrence were indeed equivalent. But the women who received lumpectomy and radiation had an absolute increase in risk of all forms of recurrence of greater than ten percentage points over a ten-year period (Mulley 1993b).

Development of the SDP for adjuvant therapy of breast cancer raised similar challenges in correcting clinicians' current conventional wisdom. The prodigious meta-analyses produced by the Early Breast Cancer Trialists Group could not be readily brought to bear by clinicians without being reduced to simplified standard clinical policies that all too often relied on the relative reduction in recurrence risk achieved rather than the absolute reduction, which could be quite small for women with negative axillary nodes and small tumors (Mulley 1993a).

The Impact of Shared Decision-making Programs

The original SDP for men with BPH had profound effects. Men who worked with the program achieved a high understanding of the relevant knowledge. They were able to describe clearly their levels of discomfort with existing urinary symptoms and concern about future sexual dysfunction. When so informed and given help to reflect on how they felt about the outcomes, they made choices that were concordant with those feelings: men who were very bothered by their symptoms were seven times more likely to choose surgery; men who were bothered by the prospect of sexual dysfunction were one-fifth as likely to choose surgery. With decisions informed by both the evidence and personal knowledge, the rate of surgery fell 40% from baseline levels in the United States (Barry et al. 1995). It appeared that surgeons had systematically overestimated patients' preference for symptom relief and underestimated their preference to avoid sexual dysfunction. It is likely that such faulty assumptions about patients' preferences varied from one region to another, contributing to regional variation in rates.

Randomized trials of other SDPs and similar decision aids showed similar declines in demand for surgery for benign uterine conditions in the United Kingdom, and for herniated lumbar disk in the United States. (Deyo et al. 2000; Kennedy et al. 2002; O'Connor et al. 2003). Rates of surgical intervention for spinal stenosis increased (Deyo et al. 2000). An international Cochrane Review of more than fifty randomized trials of decision aids included seven trials involving major elective surgery; demand decreased by 21–44% as knowledge increased (O'Connor et al. 2003). A small trial among men with prostate disease in England showed an increase (O'Connor et al. 2003). When expert opinion was used to define ideal candidates on clinical grounds for joint replacement in Canada, 85% in high-rate regions and 92% in low-rate regions did not want surgery (Hawker et al. 2001).

The effect of the coronary artery disease SDP is particularly notable. In a randomized trial conducted in Ontario, where the rate of surgery was roughly one-half that in New York and one-third that in areas of California and Texas, exposure to the SDP reduced the rate of revascularization by roughly 25% (Morgan et al. 2000). The per capita rate of revascularization surgery in the SDP group in Ontario was lower than the rate in any of the 306 hospital referral regions in the Dartmouth Atlas of Health Care.

The need for informed decision making is particularly acute in the case of diagnostic tests and screening exams, which are often recommended with inattention to the events that inevitably follow, each with the potential for error and harm as well as benefit. As with the early SDPs, clinicians may need as much help as patients. For decades, studies have shown that clinicians are often inept at dealing with the conditional probabilities that determine the predictive value of test results or communicating uncertainty among themselves or to patients (Hoffrage and Gigerenzer 1998; Gigerenzer et al. 2007). Because there is little room for uncertainty in the "if–then" standard clinical policies that facilitate the work of practice, they often respond reflexively to the positive result with more tests or treatment (Eddy 1984).

This diagnostic-therapeutic cascade is especially evident when radiographic images reveal visible pathology that is incidental to presenting symptoms. Such findings often lead to overdiagnosis of conditions that would be of no consequence to future health and well-being had they not been discovered (Lurie et al. 2003; Wennberg et al. 1996).

The appeal of early detection of disease, combined with limitations in statistical thinking, creates a special case of the clinical cascade. There is a strong tendency for clinicians and patients to want to believe in the value of screening, often with little or no attention to the potential for harm in the overtreatment that follows. An early, simple SDP for prostate cancer screening was shown in a randomized trial to improve dramatically men's knowledge and reduce the rate at which they chose screening from more than 95% to roughly 50%. Concern about prostate cancer decreased (Frosch et al. 2001).

Practice Variation and the Effect of Regional Supply

The early SDPs focused on decisions that are highly sensitive to patients' utilities for health states, risk attitudes, and willingness to make time trade-offs. What about the decisions that clinicians make countless times each day in the flow of clinical practice? How do they decide on the interval between a patient's return visit for follow-up of an acute problem or monitoring of a long-term condition? What about diagnostic imaging and laboratory tests for early detection, diagnosis, or monitoring? And when should a patient see a specialist consultant, be sent to the hospital, or to the intensive care unit (ICU)? There are few or no randomized trials that define the comparative effectiveness of different levels of these services. Here, too, clinicians cope by adopting standard clinical policies (Eddy 1984). Over time, these clinical policies mask the underlying uncertainty for clinicians and their patients even as they vary markedly at the level of individual clinicians and practices as well as regions.

Across a range of national health care economies, with different degrees of reliance on government and private insurance, strong associations exist at the regional level between per capita supply and per capita use of physician visits, diagnostic images, hospital bed-days, and intensive care (Dartmouth Atlas of Health Care 2010; Fisher et al. 2003a, b; Richardson and Peacock 2006). After major investments have been made in building capacity to deliver particular services, the marginal cost perceived at the point of care can be sufficiently low to encourage routine use of increasingly service-intensive standard clinical policies, even when the potential for benefit is small. Clinicians are accustomed to practicing within the context of local capacity and are usually surprised to learn that the frequency of use of physician visits, hospitals, and ICUs in their region is so radically different from other regions. Though invisible, capacity profoundly affects behavior. When clinicians from different regions are presented with standardized patient vignettes, they make decisions consistent with their local service intensity (Sirovich et al. 2008).

In the United States, it is the difference in capacity and resulting rates of these services that explain most of the nearly threefold regional variation in per capita expenditures for care (Dartmouth Atlas of Health Care 2010). The relationships between capacity, volume of services, per capita spending, and mortality, however, are counterintuitive. More does not equate to better. Rather than being associated with mortality reductions, high utilization and spending regions show, in fact, slightly worse mortality outcomes. High-cost regions also experience lower perceived access and less satisfaction among patients and clinicians (Fisher et al. 2003a, b). The effects of capacity on the quality of the patient's experience are most dramatically displayed in the example of end of life care. In some U.S. regions, more than 30% of deaths involve a stay in an ICU, whereas in other regions only 6% do (Dartmouth Atlas of Health Care 2010). Assuring that patient preferences are respected at this stage in life may be the greatest challenge facing advocates for informed patient choice.

Finding a Way Forward: Democratizing the Clinician–Patient Relationship

At the heart of the shared decision-making approach is the recognition that professional knowledge is necessary but not sufficient for good decision making. The patient's personal knowledge about what matters most is often as or more important. Greater investments should be made in systems that support clinicians and patients in their respective decision-making roles, including measures of decision quality and outcomes (Sepucha et al. 2004). Decision quality measures designed to assure that decisions are not made in the face of avoidable ignorance and which are personalized in a manner consistent with the preferences of patients could stimulate greater recognition among clinicians and patients of the complexity of decision making and the need for decision support. By focusing on the degree to which patients are informed and treatment is concordant with their informed preferences rather than on utilization, these measures protect against biasing decision support to control costs.

Over the longer term, more radical transformation will be necessary to create learning health care systems capable of capturing the collective experience of patients and continuously generating and using evidence about what works for whom and what is valued by whom. Learning health care systems that include multiple providers will shine light on practice variation generating hypotheses for improvement. Some such systems will use the point of care to assemble cohorts of patients who choose or are assigned (with randomization for major decisions when at personal equipoise) to different treatments or care patterns (Mulley 1995b; Olsen et al. 2008). The feasibility of this approach has been demonstrated in research settings for improving evidence for surgical interventions (Weinstein et al. 2006).

Learning health care systems which take full advantage of electronic medical and health records that support clinicians and patients could amass collective experience sufficient to determine the effectiveness of the clinical practice policies that are not likely to be subjected to randomized trials. They could also measure outcomes of the seemingly inconsequential decisions that trigger clinical cascades of great consequence. Support for informed patient choice could reveal patient preferences and thereby provide invaluable information for policy makers' decisions about expanding or contracting capacity to deliver different services.

These ideas are not new. The importance of "truth-telling" to avoid overuse by informing patients about options and outcomes, and the need to capture collective experience by measuring "end results" was articulated a century ago at the dawn of science-based diagnosis and treatment (Cabot 1903; Mulley 2009). Together, these principles of professionalism form the basis for the learning health care system. Barriers to implementation, then and now, were and are neither conceptual nor technical. Success will depend on clinicians, patients, and policy makers finding the competences, curiosity, and courage to confront the implications of practice variation and change the context and culture of clinical decision making.

4

Do Patients Want Shared Decision Making and How Is This Measured?

Martin Härter and Daniela Simon

Abstract

Shared decision making is an approach where clinicians and patients communicate together using the best available evidence when faced with the task of making decisions. The chapter presents an overview of current research that focuses on patient participation, the level to which patients want to be involved in medical decisions, and strategies that assess the measurement of these preferences. While most patients (> 80%) want detailed information and physicians often underestimate this need, some patients clearly indicate a strong preference to participate in decision making. Patients' preferences for participation can vary depending on factors such as age, gender, experience of illness, and relationship with the physician. At present, only a few psychometrically sound instruments are available to measure patients' preferences for participation.

Introduction

Shared decision making has been advocated as an appropriate approach to involve patients in decision making. Since the late 1990s, when several publications on conceptual definitions of shared decision making emerged (Charles et al. 1997; Coulter 1997; Towle 1997), interest in this approach has steadily grown, especially for diseases for which more than one treatment option exists and the best choice depends on how a person values the benefits and harms of each option (O'Connor et al. 2009). Shared decision making is an approach where clinicians and patients communicate together using the best available evidence when faced with the task of making decisions. Patients are supported to deliberate about the possible attributes and consequences of options, to enable them to reach informed preferences about the best action to take—one which respects patient autonomy, where this is desired, as well as ethical and legal standards. Shared decision making is closely associated with the use of decision support interventions, also known as decision aids (Edwards and Elwyn 2009).

Charles described a set of principles for shared decision making, stating "that at least two participants, the clinician and patient be involved; that both parties share information; that both parties take steps to build a consensus about the preferred treatment; and that an agreement is reached on the treatment to implement" (Charles et al. 1997). These principles rely on an eventual arrival at an agreement but this final principle is not fully accepted by others in the field (Makoul and Clayman 2006). Elwyn and colleagues described a set of competences for shared decision making composed of defining the problem that requires a decision, the portrayal of equipoise and the uncertainty about the best course of action, thereby leading to the requirement to provide information about the attributes of available options and support a deliberation process (Elwyn et al. 2000).

Many publications that cover aspects of shared decision making prefer to use the terms "patient involvement" or "patient participation." This conceptual variety implies problems of inconsistent measurement, of defining relationships of shared decision making and outcome measures, and of comparisons across different studies (Makoul and Clayman 2006).

Intervention studies on better involvement of patients in medical decisions use basically three different approaches (Haywood et al. 2006). First, the training of health professionals can enhance patient involvement, patient and physician satisfaction, and treatment adherence (Loh et al. 2007; Maguire and Pitceathly 2002). Second, the use of patient decision aids leads to improved knowledge, more realistic expectations, less decisional conflict, greater patient satisfaction, and improved treatment adherence (O'Connor et al. 2009). Third, patient education can be accomplished through the use of leaflets, video tapes, or direct communication training; it can result in patients asking more questions during the consultation, perceiving more control over their health, showing a higher preference to play an active role in their treatment; and it can lead to a better understanding and recall of information and treatment recommendations (Brown et al. 1999; Cegala et al. 2001).

Patients' Need for Information and Participation

While most patients want detailed information and physicians often underestimate this need, some patients indicate a strong preference to participate in decision making (Degner and Sloan 1992; Guadagnoli and Ward 1998; Auerbach 2001; Kaplan and Frosch 2005). Early studies with cancer patients reported that more than 60% expressed a desire to participate in clinical decisions (Cassileth et al. 1980; Blanchard et al. 1988). However, other studies indicate that the majority of cancer patients preferred their physician to make the actual decision (Beaver et al. 1996; Degner and Sloan 1992). Vogel et al. (2009), in one of the rare longitudinal studies, showed that breast cancer patients who rated their level of information at baseline as high were less depressed and experienced higher quality of life after three and six months. Patients who participated as much as they had wanted were more satisfied with the decision-making process and had lower stress/depression scores three months later. In early studies of primary care, only 19% of patients with hypertension wanted to be involved in decision making (Strull et al. 1984). A representative survey among citizens in eight European countries found that approximately 59% of respondents wanted shared decision making (Coulter and Magee 2003; Dierks and Seidel 2005). When compared to actual results of involvement in the decision-making process over the past 12 months, only 44% of patients claim that they were adequately involved (Dierks and Seidel 2005).

Patients' preferences for participation are not fixed and can vary depending on factors such as age, sex, education, experience of illness and medical care, health status, type of decision, attitude toward decision making, relationship with the physician, and preference for information (Elwyn et al. 2003; Say et al. 2006). Nonetheless, socio-demographic and disease-related variables have been shown to account for only 6.9% of the variance in participation preferences (Gillespie et al. 2002), and no differences in preferences could be found between acute and chronic conditions (Hamann et al. 2007).

In addition, qualitative studies have found that engagement in decision making is a developmental process enhanced by access to information, the development of personal expertise, and the relationship with the health care professional. Barriers that inhibit preference for participation are patients' lack of understanding of their potential role in decision making as well as a lack of knowledge and understanding that there is not always a right decision (Say et al. 2006). Thus, patients fear that they lack the expertise, knowledge, and clinical experience needed for decision making as well as the support to identify their preferences.

It is often debated that patients' expressed preferences for participation are only valid if patients have a clear understanding of the concept of preference-sensitive decisions and the impact that their own preferences and participation in decision making might have (Llewellyn-Thomas 2006; Fraenkel and McGraw 2007). Studies suggest, however, that there are different conceptualizations of participation. Levinson et al. (2005) found that many patients want to be offered choices even though they prefer to leave the final decision up to their physician. This corresponds with earlier work by Deber and Baumann (1992), who distinguish between two aspects of choice behavior: problem solving focuses on finding solutions; decision making refers to trade-offs from a number of possible alternatives and relies on preferences. In their study on patients who undergo an angiogram, Deber et al. (1996) found that most patients want their physician to do the problem solving but wish to be involved in the decision making. However, patients' involvement in decision making does not necessarily mean that they are also the final decision maker. Thus, participation in the decision-making process needs to be differentiated from participation in the final decision.

Others emphasize the importance of balancing patients' desired amount of participation with the way they are actually involved by the physician. For example, Cvengros et al. (2007) showed that patients who were engaged in decisions that ran contrary to their preference displayed more resistance to and refusal of the physician's recommendations. As patients' preferences for involvement cannot be clearly predicted, physicians need to explore thoroughly the extent to which a patient desires to be involved.

Measuring and Assessing Shared Decision Making

A review of psychometric instruments for the measurement of shared decision making found four instruments for the assessment of patients' preferences for participation (Simon et al. 2007).

The *Autonomy Preference Index* measures patients' preferences regarding information and participation in treatment decision making (Ende et al. 1989). The entire scale consists of 23 items with five response categories. Eight items evaluate the need for information, while the preference for participation is measured by six statements on participation, in general, and nine questions on the preference for participation in the case of upper respiratory tract illness (representing mild disease), hypertension (moderate disease), and myocardial infarction (severe/most threatening disease). The reliability of the English-language scale shows a Cronbach's α of 0.82 (Ende et al. 1989). Validity has only been tested for the participation scale and shows correlations with a single item on patient control ($r = 0.54$) and higher scores for a highly motivated sample of patients. A German translation has been employed under different medical conditions. To retain the factor structure, three items had to be deleted. High ceiling effects were found, especially on the subscale "preference for information" (Simon et al. 2010).

The *Krantz Health Opinion Survey* on patient preferences consists of two subscales and refers to routine aspects of care. "Behavioral involvement" includes nine items relating to attitudes toward self-treatment and active behavioral involvement of patients, and "information" comprises six items on the desire to ask questions and wanting to be informed about medical decisions (Krantz et al. 1980). The total scale of 15 items, with a binary response format, has a Kuder-Richardson 20 reliability of 0.77, and the subscales have reliability scores of 0.74 and 0.76, respectively. Test–retest reliability scores are 0.74 for the total scale, 0.71 for "behavioral involvement," and 0.59 for "information" for a seven-week period of time. Moderate correlations were found with health locus of control ($r = 0.31$), which was even lower for the subscales, thus indicating relatively independent constructs. Correlations close to zero were found with social desirability. The scale discriminates in terms of the use of clinic facilities ($r = -0.28$), enrolment in a medical self-help course ($t = 2, 69$; $p < 0.5$), and patients' verbal behaviors in a clinic setting ($r = 0.30$). Krantz et al. recommend further testing of the scale before the full validity and predictive potential can be assessed (Krantz et al. 1980).

The *Control Preference Scale* contains five statements on the extent of patients' preferred participation in decision making, ranging from an autonomous treatment decision to complete physician responsibility for the decision (Degner and Sloan 1992). There are two different formats of the scale. In the questionnaire version, a rank order of five statements on the preferred level of participation needs to be indicated. In the card-sorting version, five cards relating to the desired extent of participation need to be placed in a rank order. The English-language scale has been validated on a sample of cancer patients. The Coombs criterion, a measure of reliability for ordinal data, has been sufficiently met. Validity tests have not yet led to satisfactory results (Degner and Sloan 1992).

The *Patient Attitudes and Beliefs Scale* comprises twelve items on patients' attitudes and beliefs regarding participation in decision making (Arora et al. 2005). Seven items relate to the factor "pros" for participation, with the remaining five items forming the basis for the factor "cons." The score "decisional balance" can be calculated by subtracting cons from pros. The validation of this English-language scale was carried out on a convenience sample of primary care patients in a large hospital. Both factors have acceptable internal consistency (Cronbach's $\alpha = 0.71; 0.72$) (Arora et al. 2005). All three subscales discriminate between patients at different levels of readiness to participate.

Comment on Instruments

The instruments that are available to assess patients' preferences have been developed in English and validated only on one or a small number of samples by the original authors. They have been used in intervention studies without further psychometric testing for different settings. In terms of psychometric quality, many of the presented instruments show satisfactory, good, or even excellent internal consistency (= reliable responses); however, construct validity has not, in several cases, been sufficiently investigated (Ende et al. 1989; Krantz et al. 1980; Degner and Sloan 1992). Furthermore, several authors point out limited implications of their validation samples. This is also confirmed in validation studies for the same scales in different languages and health care settings, suggesting different factor structures and high ceiling effects of items (Giersdorf et al. 2004; Simon et al. 2007, 2010).

Variations in patients' preferences for involvement may be due to a number of methodological factors, as there is no entirely satisfactory way of measuring decision-making preferences (Kaplan and Frosch 2005; Say et al. 2006).

Different constructs and psychometric instruments with differing scores of reliability and validity have been used to assess preferences. A study conducted by Fraenkel and McGraw (2007) indicates that patients' perception of the concept of involvement in decisions might be different from what is measured with existing instruments. In addition, the common measurement categories of "passive," "active," and "shared" are difficult to compare with mean scores on an ordinal scale. Furthermore, instruments usually contain only a small number of statements which might not reflect the complexity of decision-making preference, and several instruments use vignettes that refer to theoretical preferences which may not reflect patients' preferences in real situations (Say et al. 2006; Ende et al. 1989).

Conclusions

Most patients want detailed information about their disease, the probable course, and effective therapeutic options to be taken. While physicians often underestimate this need, some patients indicate a clear preference to participate in decision making. Engagement in decision making is a developmental process enhanced by access to information, the development of personal expertise, and a positive relationship with the health care professional. Barriers that inhibit preference for participation are patients' lack of understanding of their potential role in decision making as well as a lack of knowledge and understanding that there is not always a right decision. Additional research is needed on patients' preferred roles in decision making, with a particular emphasis on international comparisons. Patients' concepts of participation need to be thoroughly explored in qualitative studies to inform the further development of existing quantitative measures of preferences or to stimulate new ways to assess these constructs.

Health Illiteracy:
Roots in Research

5

Health Research Agendas and Funding

David E. Nelson

Abstract

There is a large range of national public funding support for health research across countries. By contrast, allocations for overall funding for health literacy and related research areas are limited. Health research agendas and resource allocation are policy decisions that involve the use of power. There are strong incentives to maintain the status quo, especially in the face of level or declining funding. Many macro- and micro-level factors influence research agendas and funding support. These range from broader societal values and health care delivery systems, to the individuals themselves who make decisions. There is a great need for more research in areas such as implementation of simple interventions in "real-world" settings and the effects of communication technologies on receipt, processing, and seeking of health information by the public. There is some reason for optimism: awareness and support for more transdisciplinary and applied research relevant to health literacy is increasing, and some countries have adopted effective approaches to assess new health technology and treatment prior to introduction into clinical and public health practice.

Introduction

There is increasing concern that the results from health research do not lend themselves to information that is practical and understandable by patients and other members of the public, clinicians, policy makers, and journalists. In other words, there is a gap between what health researchers study and communicate among themselves, and what lay audiences and clinicians want and need to know. Regardless of whether one looks at levels of funding for health literacy itself, or of funding for related topics such as health services research, health technology assessment, or dissemination and implementation, there are currently few resources being devoted to conduct research on these critical topics.

Before examining some of the more specific issues regarding research and practices to improve health literacy, we need to examine critically what type of health research gets conducted and funded. In other words, how, what, and why do some health issues and items become included on research agendas and receive funding, and what are the implications for increasing research needed to improve health literacy?

In this chapter, I provide a broad review of the extent to which financial resources are currently allocated for health research across different countries. I then examine how health research funds are distributed, and the content of national health research agendas. Thereafter I consider the major factors that influence the development and funding of research agendas, and their implications for health literacy and related research. To conclude, I consider potentially fruitful issues or topics directly relevant to improving health literacy for which more research is needed.

First, however, I offer a few caveats: There is not much empiric research on health research agenda development or on how such funding decisions are made (CIHR 2004; Shaw and Greenhalgh 2008; Tetroe et al. 2008). Definitions and categorizations of research agendas and funding areas across countries or in the scientific literature are inconsistent (e.g., what is considered to be applied, clinical, translational, prevention, or public health research). This review was conducted using resources available in the English language. Finally, more information was identified and used from the United States (particularly the National Institutes of Health [NIH]), Australia, Canada, and the United Kingdom than from other countries or sources.

Overall Health Research Funding Levels

A useful starting point is to consider international funding estimates of health research, sometimes referred to as research and development (R&D), from a 2008 report published by the Global Forum for Health Research based on 2005 data (Burke and Matlin 2008). Health R&D investments accounted for 21.6% of R&D funding across all economic sectors, compared with 11.5% in 1986. In 2005, an estimated $160 billion (U.S. dollars) was spent on health R&D worldwide, and this amount has grown considerably since 1986 (Figure 5.1). A total of 51% of health R&D funding in 2005 came from the private sector, 41% from public funds, and 8% from not-for-profit organizations.

Of the total funding, $155.3 billion (97%) came from high income countries. The United States accounted for 50% of health R&D funding; the combined amount from Japan, the United Kingdom, Germany, and France accounted for another 27% (Table 5.1). For the 6% of funding from the category "all other countries" in Table 5.1, most of it was from the so-called innovative developing countries of Argentina, Brazil, India, and Mexico. However, a different picture of funding emerges when examined as a percentage of national health expenditures. Health R&D accounted for more than 6% of national health expenditures in Sweden, Switzerland, Denmark, and the United Kingdom.

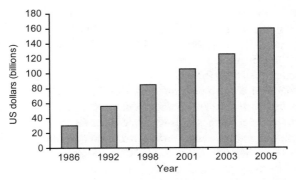

Figure 5.1 Global funding for health R&D from 1986–2005 (after Burke and Matlin 2008).

It should be noted that there are some limitations to global health R&D estimates. In countries such as Finland and Canada, for example, a substantial portion of funds is provided by state or provincial governments, not by the national government. Furthermore, in addition to funding attributable to individual countries, the European Union (EU) also funds health research (EC 2009). The Seventh Research Framework Program (FP7) announced by the EU in July 2009 provided a total budget of €620.5 million to support health research (EC 2009).

Table 5.1 Health R&D expenditures in 2005 for selected countries. NA: not available. After Burke and Matlin (2008).

Country	Global distribution of health R&D expenditures (%)	Health R&D as a percentage of national health expenditures (%)
United States	50	3.8
Japan	10	4.4
United Kingdom	7	6.1
Germany	6	3.0
France	5	3.2
Canada	3	4.4
Switzerland	2	9.0
Italy	2	2.3
Sweden	2	9.3
Spain	2	2.7
Australia	1	NA
Belgium	1	5.0
Denmark	1	7.3
Netherlands	1	0.4
China (with Taiwan)	1	0.7
All other countries	6	NA

Estimates of the extent of private funding for health research are available for a limited number of countries. In Australia, of the estimated $2.8 billion funded for health R&D in 2004–2005, 26% ($730 million) came from the business sector; this was an increase from 1992–1993, when it was only 20% (Access Economics 2008; Research Australia 2009). In Canada, as of 2007 an estimated $6.3 billion was spent on health R&D, with expenditures on health R&D increasing by more than 2.5-fold from 1996 through 2007 (SIEID 2008). A total of 30% of R&D ($1.9 billion) came from business enterprises (SIEID 2008). Industry as a source of all health R&D funding has increased substantially since 1988, when this sector funded only 16% of such research, although overall industry financial support has changed little since 2004 (Madore and Norris 2006; SIEID 2008).

Health research funding in the United States accounted for an estimated $122.4 billion in expenditures in 2008 (see Table 5.2; Research!America 2008). Health research expenditure tripled in the United States from 1994 through 2004 (Moses et al. 2005). Private sources accounted for nearly 60% of total funding, an amount that has remained relatively constant since the mid-1990s (Research!America 2008; Moses et al. 2005).

The pharmaceutical, biotechnology, and medical technology industries are especially generous research funders. Although Table 5.2 contains U.S. data, the impact of private industry research funding is evident globally. The proportion of the global drug development pipeline from organizations based in the United States is estimated at 70% (Moses et al. 2005), and increasingly, clinical research trials funded by pharmaceutical companies are being conducted in countries outside of North America and Western Europe (Glickman et al. 2009).

Although the total amount of funding by nonprofit organizations is much less than funding from for-profit industries and public sources, it can play a pivotal role in some situations and for some research topics. For example, the Gates Foundation has played a critical role in providing substantial resources for health research funding of important issues in less developed countries (e.g., malaria, enteric diseases, and tobacco control). Nonprofit organizations

Table 5.2 Funding of health research in the United States, 2008 (adapted from Research!America 2008).

Funding source	Amount (billions of US$)
Industry[a]	68.2
Other private sources	3.3
Federal government	38.1
All other	12.8
Total	122.4

[a] Pharmaceutical companies ($35.8 billion), biotechnology companies ($23.0 billion), and medical technology companies ($9.5 billion). Sums are rounded.

have the advantage of being nimble and more focused in what types of research they choose to fund.

Distribution of Health Research Funding

The previous section provided an overview of health research funding but did not address what type of research is actually funded. To put it more succinctly: Is the balance correct? Comprehensive reviews of how health research funding is distributed are available from Australia, Canada, the United Kingdom, and the United States and are discussed below. Note that most of these data are based on funding from federal government sources.

Australia

A review of health research funding in Australia was published in 2009 (Research Australia 2009). The two major funding organizations are (a) the National Health and Medical Research Council (NHMRC), which exclusively focuses on health and medical research ($542 million) and (b) the Australian Research Council, which primarily funds research in the sciences and humanities ($510 million). The majority of NHMRC funds are allocated through competitive grants to individual scientists or research institutions (NHMRC 2009; Research Australia 2009).

The allocation of NHMRC research funding by broad research areas and by national health priority topics are listed in Table 5.3. Basic science received

Table 5.3   Health research funding allocations for Australia's national health and medical research council (after Research Australia 2009).

	Funding (%)[a]
Broad research area	
Basic science	49
Clinical medicine and science	30
Public health	16
Health services research	3
Preventive medicine	1
National health priority disease areas	
Cancer	30
Cardiovascular disease	22
Diabetes	14
Mental health	13
Injury	6
Arthritis and osteoporosis	6
Obesity	5
Asthma	4

[a]   Percents may not total 100 due to rounding.

slightly more than half of the funds, with clinical medicine/science and public health the next largest areas. When examined by national health priority area, the combined expenditures for cancer and cardiovascular disease totaled more than 50% of the budget, with the combined funds for diabetes and mental health being slightly more than 25%.

In 2008, the Australia Research Council provided 34% of its budget for research on psychology, 20% for public health/health services, 12% to biomedical engineering, and 12% to neurosciences. The remaining funding was allocated among six different areas (all of which received 5% or less), including behavioral and cognitive sciences, which received 3% (Research Australia 2009).

Of the $762 million allocated in Australia for health-related R&D in 2006–2007 by the business sector, an estimated 30% was for pharmacology/pharmaceutical sciences; 28% for clinical sciences; and 42% for other medical and health sciences.

Canada

Reviews of the allocation of all Canadian federal funding for health research are available from several sources (CIHR 2004, 2009a; Madore and Norris 2006). The Canadian Institutes of Health Research (CIHR), a federal agency similar to the NIH in the United States, is the major national health research agency in Canada, accounting for about 56% of all such funding (CIHR 2004). A total of 70% of the CIHR research budget is reserved for investigator- or organizational-initiated peer-reviewed research, with 30% for strategic initiatives (CIHR 2009a, b).

The CIHR funds research in one of four broad areas: biomedical or basic (70% of funds), clinical (14%), social/cultural/environmental/population health (11%), and health systems/services (5%) (Kondro 2009). The three strategic initiatives and the percentage of CIHR dollars allocated for each were (a) advances in health knowledge (65%); (b) people and research capacity (28%); and (c) knowledge translation and commercialization (7%). In 2004–2005, it was estimated that knowledge translation research accounted for 0.2% of all federal health research funding (Madore and Norris 2006).

United Kingdom

A comprehensive analysis of health research funding allocation of £950 million in the United Kingdom (primarily by the Medical Research Council and the Department of Health) and major private research foundations (British Heart Foundation, Cancer Research UK, and Wellcome Trust) was published in 2006 (UKCRC 2006). Approximately two-thirds of funding was for basic sciences and etiologic research, with the remaining allocated to other areas (Table 5.4). Twenty-five percent was considered applicable for research on

Table 5.4 Health research funding allocation in the United Kingdom (adapted from UKCRC 2006).

	Funding (%)[a]
Broad research area	
Etiology	35
Basic science (underpinning)	34
Treatment development and evaluation	17
Detection and diagnosis	5
Health services	5
Prevention	3
Disease management	2
Disease category	
Cancer	28
Neurological or mental health	22
Infectious diseases	13
Blood, cardiovascular disease, or stroke	12
All other	25

[a] Percents may not total 100 due to rounding.

general health and well-being (e.g., all diseases), with 75% related to specific diseases or areas of health.

Further analyses by type of disease found that cancer and neurological diseases/mental health accounted for about half of funding (Table 5.4). When compared with disability-adjusted life year (DALY) estimates in the United Kingdom, cancer and infectious diseases received disproportionately greater funding. By comparison, neurological or mental health; blood, cardiovascular disease, or stroke; oral and gastrointestinal disorders; and respiratory disorders received less funding. An estimated 3% of all health research funding was categorized as being for psychological, behavioral, or socioeconomic processes.

United States

Some data are available on the allocation of research funding by private industry. Pharmaceutical, biotechnology, and medical device companies invest 14–21% of their revenue in R&D (Moses 2009; Pisano 2006), which is a larger share than other industries. For pharmaceutical companies in 2007, prehuman and preclinical research (basic science) accounted for 27% of funding; Phase 1 through Phase 4 clinical research trials for 62%; and 11% for other types of research (PhRMA 2009). By comparison, basic science research accounted for 57% and clinical trial research for 33% of funding in 1994 (Moses et al. 2005).

Federal funding of biomedical research in the United States in 2008 was distributed broadly across ten different agencies (Research!America 2008). The dominant U.S. government funder is NIH, with its $29 billion accounting for more than three-fourths of all health research dollars. A total of $10.4 billion of extra funding for two years was appropriated by Congress to NIH for fiscal years 2009–2010 as part of U.S. federal stimulus bill, with an additional $1.1 billion allocated across three federal agencies for comparative effectiveness research.

NIH research funding has been categorized in several different ways. More than 80% of NIH funding is allocated through competitive grants to individual scientists or research institutions (about 50,000 grants annually). About 55% of NIH research funding is for basic science and 45% for applied science; these percentages varied little from 1994 through 2008 (Moses et al. 2005; Zerhouni 2007). An estimated 10.5% of the 2009 NIH research budget was for behavioral and social science research (Silver and Sharpe 2008). Health services research funding across all U.S. federal agencies totaled $1.68 billion in 2008 (CHSR 2009), with $1 billion of this for the NIH, accounting for 3% of its research budget.

A study from 1999 examined NIH research funding levels for 29 specific diseases by measures of disease burden (Gross et al. 1999). There was strong correlation between research funding and DALY, moderate correlation for mortality and years of life lost, but no correlation with disease incidence, prevalence, or hospitalization days. Disproportionately more funding was allocated to HIV/AIDS, breast cancer, and diabetes; disproportionately less funding was allocated for chronic obstructive pulmonary disease, perinatal conditions, and peptic ulcer disease.

The NIH Roadmap for Medical Research, a plan to address roadblocks to research and fill knowledge gaps, was initiated in 2004 (NIH 2009b). Funding has been provided to support networks of researchers to develop and conduct collaborative research projects. Roadmap-related research now receives about 1% of all NIH funding. This effort was designed to address roadblocks to research by supporting funding for areas such as higher risk research, interdisciplinary efforts (including public/private partnerships), and attempting to change the clinical research enterprise (e.g., through translational research and clinical research networks). It has created numerous research centers and networks to conduct translational and interdisciplinary research, including public–private partnerships primarily designed to move knowledge from laboratory findings to the discovery of new methods for diagnosis, therapy, and prevention in clinical settings. For example, the NIH began the Clinical and Transitional Science Award (CTSA) program in 2006. There are currently 24 CTSA-funded academic centers established, and the NIH expects to fund 60 by 2012.

An important component of the NIH Roadmap is an initiative for clinical outcomes assessment called the "Patient-Reported Outcome Measurements Information System," or PROMIS. PROMIS involves researchers in multiple institutions who are systematically reviewing and conducting research on survey item outcome measures used in clinical practice and research. Patient outcome measures include pain, fatigue, physical functioning, emotional distress, and social role participation. The PROMIS collaboration was developed to encourage researchers to use similar and validated outcome measures in research studies, and to select measures relevant to patients. This initiative provides strong motivation and incentives for researchers to work together and use measures that are relevant to patients and comparable across studies. An encouraging aspect is that the PROMIS model could be adapted for researchers, patients, and members of the general public for other research and practice areas, including prevention.

Formal or official estimates of NIH funding levels for health literacy and related areas (e.g., patient–provider communication) do not exist. However, I have conducted a research portfolio analysis to examine currently funded grants with a major emphasis on health literacy. Several search terms were employed, including "health literacy," "numeracy," and "doctor–patient communication." A total of 57 grants were identified that received a total funding amount of \$13.5 million; 26% of these grants were awarded by the National Cancer Institute (NCI).

The NCI has made some commitment to conduct research on health literacy and related topics. The NCI has administrative units (branches) responsible for grants on outcomes; basic and biobehavioral science; applied cancer screening; and health communication and informatics research. The NCI has also supported specific research funding initiatives and research syntheses related to health literacy. For example, the Outcomes Research Branch supports a Patient-Centered Communication Initiative and published a monograph on this topic (Epstein and Street 2007). The Basic and Biobehavioral Research Branch has supported conferences, monographs, and special issues of scientific journals that summarize or synthesize relevant research on decision making and related areas. Since 2003, the NCI has funded academic centers of excellence in cancer communication research to extend the reach, improve the effectiveness, and increase the efficiency of cancer communication (NCI 2006).

National Health Research Agenda Plans

Agendas for health research have been developed by the World Health Organization (WHO strategy on research for health) and by the European Union (FP7) (EC 2009; WHO 2009b). Many countries have engaged in comprehensive reviews or planning activities to guide health research agendas and funding, including the four countries previously discussed in more detail. Instead of individually reviewing the WHO, EU, and each of the four countries' research agendas, this section provides an overview of similar themes that emerged.

In Australia, international commissions have been convened in recent years to review and make recommendations about federally funded health research.

The NHMRC has a draft National Strategy for health research that was published in 2009 (NHMRC 2009). In Canada, a draft of the Health Research Roadmap, which is the strategic plan for the CIHR from 2009–2014, was also published in 2009 (CIHR 2009b). In 2006, a review of U.K. health research funding was conducted under the auspices of venture capitalist David Cooksey (2006). The Cooksey Report contains a series of recommendations about improving research organizations and performance. As mentioned previously, the NIH in the United States began the Roadmap for Medical Research in 2004.

Five common themes were evident from the review of these various reports and other materials. First, there is great optimism and much enthusiasm about the state of scientific and technologic advancements, particularly in areas such as biomedical engineering, genomics, and informatics. These advances are viewed as having promising health benefits for society, along with economic benefits, such as increased private investment and employment.

Second, there is interest and desire among many health research leaders to support applied research, as there is concern whether the increases in research funding in recent years has resulted in health improvements (Glasgow et al. 2007). For example, one of the four WHO research strategies specifically focuses on *translation* (described as "evidence into practice") (WHO 2009b), and two of the three pillars of EU-funded health research are *translating research for human health* and *optimizing the delivery of healthcare to European citizens* (EC 2009).

Individuals and organizations in many scientific, health practitioner, and advocacy communities, as well as some political leaders and members of the public, are increasingly clamoring for results with practical implications to reduce suffering. Terms such as knowledge translation, translational research, and evidence-based syntheses are mentioned as important research agenda and funding priorities. However, it must be noted that these terms have widely different meanings among different groups. For example, knowledge transfer can have the connotation of commercialization, and translational research often implies getting new technologic or pharmaceutical products and services into medical practice more rapidly, as opposed to insuring that evidence-based and cost-effective practices are adopted (Glasgow et al. 2007).

Third, there is awareness and support for the large and growing role that private industry plays in influencing public research agendas and funding. This includes a strong interest to work closely with private industry leaders to increase public research funding, and public–private collaborations, to assist industry. Examples include support for partnerships to facilitate bringing products and services (e.g., new treatments or screening techniques) into broad use in a more rapid manner.

Fourth, there is support for interdisciplinary research and better coordination of public funded research efforts among government agencies. There is awareness that major breakthroughs are more likely to occur through "big science," which is heavily dependent on collaborative and interdisciplinary work rather than through individual researcher enterprise. In practical terms, this includes such things as financially supporting research centers of excellence within universities that cross multiple scientific disciplines, networks that link researchers across institutions, and cooperative international efforts.

Fifth, there is little or no mention that the proposed changes would likely require reallocating existing funding or a substantial restructuring of existing governmental research funding agencies. Increasing support for applied research would likely result in reduced funding for basic research. The U.K. Cooksey Report, for example, proposed more funding for translational research but no reduction in basic research funding, and more funds for higher risk investigator-initiated research but also that funding for national priority research areas would be instigated (Black 2006). Furthermore, a funding emphasis on transdisciplinary and other types of collaborative research could radically change professional advancement systems for individual scientists (e.g., tenure) that have existed for decades.

Research Agenda Development and Funding Decisions

What does or does not receive health research funding, and why, are straightforward questions. Unfortunately, there is a noticeable lack of empirical research in this area from which to draw, although insights are available from research in other fields (Shaw and Greenhalgh 2008; Tetroe et al. 2008).

Creating health research agendas and allocating resources are policy decisions. This means they are based on the values and social contexts of decision makers and involve the use of political power (Nelson et al. 2009). Decisions are not solely the result of a "rational" process based on objective data, but are strongly influenced by underlying ideologies and assumptions, most of which are not openly discussed or challenged among scientific researchers or practitioners (Shaw and Greenhalgh 2008). Taking into account prior studies in this area and the current and planned national research agendas and funding, six highly influential factors were identified that strongly influence what is more or less likely to be included on research agendas and their subsequent funding levels.

Broad Societal Values and Health Care Delivery Systems

Scientists operate within distinctive scientific cultures and share many similarities; areas of research interest among statisticians, for example, are likely to be comparable across countries (Kuhn 1996). Nevertheless, scientists are part of, and influenced by, their national cultures and subcultures in the same way as other citizens. Broad societal and cultural standards and beliefs in all countries affect how health care is delivered, what research topics are studied, how they are studied, and funding levels. There is substantial intercountry variation in

72   D. E. Nelson

the level of trust for governmental leaders, institutions, and authority figures, including scientists and doctors, as well as how much health research is valued. Similarly, there are substantial country-to-country differences in how health care services are delivered, and how health research is funded, including the research infrastructure (e.g., indirect costs).

The current economic recession affecting many countries has influenced how much public funding for health research is valued compared to other public funding priorities. Factors such as public versus private funding of research and health care services, the mix of physician specialties (generalists versus specialists), restrictions on public availability or funding of health care products and services, and support for specific prevention or treatment approaches are all influential.

Some countries are more individualistic, whereas others are more cooperative; some countries have a culture more supportive of public funding to address societal problems, whereas others tend to prefer private funding. This can help explain, for example, why individual-oriented research projects, individual-level interventions (as opposed to governmental or organizational mandates), and private industry funding are more common in the United States than elsewhere. Research priorities can vary across countries based on preferences for using approaches or interventions viewed as "new" or "different," and beliefs about scientific or technologic progress (e.g., "magic bullets" such as surgery or medications for complex problems such as obesity). In Finland, for example, the process of health technology assessment is based on a careful and deliberative review of the scientific evidence of effectiveness conducted by a national board of experts. Decisions about adopting and funding newly developed health care products, procedures, and services are closely tied to that country's health care delivery system. There is variability in research funding based on societal preferences for addressing a health issue or current concern that is perceived as an acute concern, as opposed to prioritizing research and funding for long-established challenges, such as improving health decision making by patients.

Level of Support or Opposition for a Health Topic by Lay Audiences and Health Care Providers

The level of interest among individuals and organizations from beyond the scientific research community influences research agendas and funding. Support is higher for research on certain health issues (e.g., cancer, heart disease, HIV/AIDS) because of their burden, visibility, and pressure from the general public (e.g., as measured by mortality rates, disability) or efforts of powerful interest groups or individuals. Acute infectious disease outbreaks, because they can generate a lot of media interest and fear in the general public, can also result in funding increases for research. In some instances, research agendas or funding may be specific or circumscribed, especially for private funding of research.

Powerful political leaders, media representatives, philanthropists, organizations (especially advocacy organizations), and celebrities (e.g., Bono, Lance Armstrong) influence research priorities and funding. Such individuals and organizational representatives help to raise awareness about specific health problems or issues and can help to allocate public funding or raise private funds for health research. Since the 1980s, advocacy organizations have been extremely instrumental in supporting research funding for HIV/AIDS in the United States and elsewhere. In contrast, in Germany there is substantial opposition among many members of the public and political leaders to stem cell research, resulting in no public funding for research in that country.

Advocacy groups and organizations often consist of individuals with a high level of personal involvement. Some of the most powerful advocates have been persons affected by a disease or condition in some way. Canadian Terry Fox in the 1980s, who had metastatic bone cancer, became an effective fundraiser for cancer research after he began a cross-country run that received prominent media attention. Katie Couric, a prominent television journalist in the United States, became a forceful public advocate for colon cancer screening after her husband died of this disease (Cram et al. 2003).

Health care providers and their organizations can also influence research agendas and funding. Perceived threats to professional autonomy can generate fear and opposition. In the United States, for example, research and evidence-based scientific reviews on medical care practices and comparative effectiveness research have generated substantial opposition from organized medical provider groups such as orthopedists. This has resulted in Congress placing restrictions on the type and funding of certain areas of health services research supported by the federal government (Wennberg 1996).

Profitability

Given the large and generally increasing role of private industry in health research, profitability is the dominant concern. Corporate leaders and stockholders are most interested in the financial bottom line; thus decisions about what ends up on research agendas and how much funding is allocated is based on the potential return on investment. This means that most of the research in private industry is designed for applied or practical applications, such as the development of new pharmaceuticals or other products. However, a patent discovered through research in one company may also serve as sources of revenue if other companies need to pay to use the patent in their own research.

When profit is the dominant motivation, there are certain approaches and types of research that are more or less likely to be conducted. The major emphasis of research is likely to be on treatment (i.e., persons who already have a problem) rather than on prevention, as this is where the greatest profits exist. Furthermore, health problems that affect a large number of people (e.g., hypertension, high cholesterol levels, acne, or menstrual abnormalities) have potentially large markets for private industry products or services. Major research breakthroughs from private industry have occurred in each of these areas. By contrast, other health conditions or topics have had limited profitability and are less likely to be funded. Rare diseases are not commonly selected for further research by private companies because of small markets. Similarly, research funding for vaccine research by private companies lagged for many years because of concerns about low profitability or financial loss, particularly as a result of prominent lawsuits based on safety concerns.

The issue of profitability also affects research agenda and funding decisions for public (government) resources. There is great interest in many countries to foster public and industry partnerships at the individual, institutional, and governmental level. This is partly driven by wanting to pool resources for projects, and partly by the desire to increase the speed at which research discoveries are applied in clinical or public health practice.

Another reason for the growing public–private research efforts is because of a belief that such research will have economic benefits. One aspect is a desire to increase employment, which is a particular concern during the current economic downturn: increasingly health research is viewed as a growth industry. Another aspect of the perceived economic benefits stems from a concern that private corporations will physically move and conduct their research "elsewhere," whether within another geographic area of a country or in another country considered to be more business friendly. This concern is understandable, given the globalization of pharmaceutical and medical technology companies that has occurred with other industries.

Personal and Professional Interests of Scientists and Scientific Organizations

For public funds, research agenda items and the allocation of funds are most commonly delegated to scientists or scientist-dominated committees. This makes much sense, given the technical nature of scientific research. Certain prominent researchers, disciplines, and their respective organizations often have a dominant role in developing health research agendas and making funding allocation decisions within governmental agencies and private foundations or charities.

This is especially true for research funding awarded through granting mechanisms. While these nearly always have competitive processes reviewed by scientific peers, once financial resources are granted, scientists and research institutions have much freedom as to what research is conducted and how it is done. Currently, in most countries there are few or no incentives to ensure that health research has practical applications; the "production" of research is decentralized (Green et al. 2009).

Although many scientists believe they hold completely neutral viewpoints ("objective") and that research is solely driven by altruism (Kuhn 1996), neither of these are accurate descriptions of how research agendas are developed and funding decisions made (Shaw and Greenhalgh 2008; Tetroe et al. 2008). Scientists and health care providers, and their respective organizations, have their own professional and personal areas of interest. A further challenge is the specialization of scientists, making intra-scientific communication across (and sometimes within) disciplines difficult (Braun 1994). Personal and discipline-specific interests of scientists have a strong influence on what is considered worthy of research. Furthermore, like other people most scientists are interested in professional advancement, job security, or prestige for themselves and their institutions. Similarly, research, scientific-specific disciplines, and other organizations desire to attain or retain their own power and prestige.

What this means is that the status quo is preferred by many scientists and their organizations; that is, there is a desire to retain current research processes, infrastructure, and other arrangements. The academic tenure system in many countries is usually based on individual measures of scientists, such as receiving funding as a primary investigator and publication of research findings in scientific journals.

Thus without positive or negative incentives to change, there is inherent conservatism when it comes to changing existing research arrangements, agendas, and funding allocations. Scientists who have historically been successful competing for unrestricted research grants are not likely to want to be mandated to work on certain research topics in certain ways (e.g., strategic national initiatives). Absent a change in reward systems, such as some type of formal recognition for transdisciplinary or team scientific research or practical use of research findings by patients, substantial changes in existing research agendas or financial allocations are unlikely.

Allocating New versus Existing Resources

Not unique to government funding, decisions about health research agendas and funding are strongly influenced by whether available resources are declining, unchanged, or increasing. From a political perspective, in an environment of increasing fiscal resources it is far easier for decision makers to allocate resources to newer areas or priorities. Such times tend to foster more collaborative climates, with an increased willingness by more well-funded programs and individuals to share resources with newer and less well-funded researchers and research areas. Decisions about funding are quite different in the face of level or declining resources. Persons and organizations working in research areas that receive lower funding levels to begin with, or that are subject to larger budget cuts become especially interested, not surprisingly, in collaborating with programs with more funding. However, a well-known organizational- and individual-level characteristic of those in leadership positions slated to receive level or reduced funding is to ensure that they meet the needs of their current constituents ("everyone for themselves") (McDonough 2000).

This tendency to try and retain resources during more challenging economic times means that it is much more difficult to convince decision makers to support new research agenda items or reallocate existing resources. This was demonstrated in Canada in 2009: although the CIHR health research plan called for increasing interdisciplinary research (CIHR 2009b), the federal budget eliminated funding for open competition for team science research grants that year. Furthermore, the call for increased funding for applied research in the CIHR plan resulted in concerns and opposition from some basic scientists (Annan 2009).

Who Participates Directly in Decision Making?

The final major factor influencing research agendas and funding are the individuals who participate in decision making. This is also related to the scientific disciplines, institutions, organizations, or agencies of decision makers. As with all resource allocation situations, available funding is finite, which means that the power of the constituencies represented by individual decision makers has substantial influence over what issues are researched, the types of research conducted, and the level of funding received.

A major reason why more health literacy-related research is not conducted is that such individuals rarely participate in direct decisions about research agendas and funding. In some countries and organizations there is more effort to attempt to gather this information, and there may be representation in grant review sessions or similar meetings. In the United Kingdom, for example, there is a major effort to involve patients and members of the public in all stages of health research (from developing research agendas through the publication of results) that is funded by the National Health Service (NHS 2009). However, it is usually scientists themselves who make most decisions about what research is needed, and many of them are not well-versed in what physicians or the public see as high-priority research needs. Thus, large gaps have developed as to what scientists, physicians and other health care practitioners, and members of the public deem most worthy for researching and funding. Furthermore, scientists may insist on research purity (e.g., internal validity) of studies that is not plausible in practice settings (external validity) (Green et al. 2009).

As mentioned previously, individuals have their own individual scientific or professional interests. They also have loyalty to their professional colleagues and scientific disciplines. Persons who represent a specific institution or organization (e.g., a government agency) have biases that tend to support the work, and the individuals, within their organizations, as well as their own self-interests. Hence it would be extremely unlikely that an organizational representative would support an option to eliminate or substantially reduce resource allocation for his or her own organization.

Health Literacy–relevant Topics Needing More Research

Transdisciplinary Syntheses with Context-based Recommendations

Over the past thirty years there have been substantial advances in analyzing and synthesizing research studies (e.g., meta-analyses and rules for study inclusion in literature reviews). There is also an abundance of guidelines about what doctors and other health care practitioners should or should not do, many of which have had a minimal impact. Nevertheless, there remains a need for research syntheses that not only provide summaries of what research shows but also deliver specific, simple, and realistic recommendations for practitioners and the public.

Evidence-based recommendations should not be solely directed to health care practitioners, but need to extend to health care system administrators and to the general public to provide them with tools to help them better understand health issues and make decisions. Evaluation research is needed about the effectiveness of practical tools designed to help various individuals, improving the tools, and how they can be more widely disseminated and adopted in real-world settings.

Dissemination and Implementation Research

Research syntheses with recommendations are essential but do little to ensure that evidence-based recommendations are used in practice. Rather than acknowledging the difficulties and challenges of implementation and incorporating these into research agendas, many researchers place the burden of using research evidence on health care practitioners (Proctor and Rosen 2008).

Despite increased attention to the importance of dissemination and implementation, this is an area of research where much more work is needed. This has been referred to as Phase 5 or Translation 2 research (Green et al. 2009), which involves implementing interventions and evaluating their effectiveness in real-world (nonexperimental) settings. In the United States, trans-NIH program announcements and special emphasis panels to fund dissemination and implementation research have been made available, along with specific research initiatives within certain institutes (e.g., National Institute of Mental Health, the NCI). However, the former Deputy Director for Research Dissemination and Diffusion at the NCI referred to such funding as "decimal dust" in percentage terms when compared to the entire NIH budget (Kerner et al. 2005).

There are many reasons why research findings that are based on scientific consensus are not adopted by the practice community or the public at large (Green et al. 2009). These reasons often transcend individuals, being strongly influenced by organizations and systems in which information and health care is delivered. More research is needed that moves beyond describing barriers to implementation and identifies solutions. Such work is context-specific and often slow and laborious. It involves small and simple changes, and thus requires long-term funding commitments and multi-level research (e.g., systems approaches) which reach beyond the attempt to simply educate individuals. In many fields of engineering, failure analysis is commonly conducted. This type of research is used to identify problems and explain why adverse events occurred. In health research, there is no equivalent of conducting research on intervention implementation failures in practice environments. If such research was funded, common themes might be identified and shared more broadly.

Conversely (and likely to be met with greater enthusiasm), there is a need for more research to identify implementation successes and why they were successful. Much knowledge can be gleaned from research in fields besides health (e.g., education and agriculture) (Fixsen et al. 2005). Taken together, both failure and success analyses of intervention implementation in the areas of decision making and communication could lead to the development and adoption of more useful approaches. A starting point might be the four principal characteristics of successful implementation identified in a research synthesis by the National Implementation Research Network in the United States (Fixsen et al. 2005):

1.   selection, training, and coaching of those implementing the intervention,
2.   presence of an organizational infrastructure,
3.   full participation by communities and individuals in selection and evaluation of programs and practices, and
4.   supportive political and regulatory environments.

Research on Reducing Cognitive Burden
Related to Understanding Statistics

An area in great need for additional research is whether, and how, the problem of reducing cognitive burden can be addressed among health care providers and the public. Ample research has shown the difficulties that many patients and doctors have in understanding and applying numbers commonly used in health, particularly probability (Nelson et al. 2009). These problems are likely to be magnified for persons with low levels of involvement or limited time to weigh findings, as well as biased reporting of health statistics.

One of the major challenges is that this type of research is conducted across multiple disciplines without sufficient interaction among scientists. Those who study narratives differ markedly from those who study computer science, yet both contribute to research on the selection and presentation of data. More research is needed to classify or categorize people on their preferences for receiving information in the form of data and the "dose" of data that is sufficient, as well as on simple educational techniques or approaches to improve statistical knowledge. Given the technological advances in visualization, there is a great need for more research on how to improve data visualization to enhance understanding (Kurz-Milcke et al. 2008).

On the other hand, because transparent framing of probability helps doctors and patients alike to understand health statistics, research is needed to investigate and implement the necessary tools in medical schools, continuing education programs, and the patient–doctor interaction. Moreover, research is needed to understand how people select information intermediaries (e.g., individuals, web sites) and to evaluate approaches to assist them in making better intermediary choices.

Research on the Effects of Communication Technologies on Receiving, Processing, and Seeking Health Information

A worldwide natural experiment has been underway over the past twenty years or so with the explosion of new communication technologies. With the development and wide adoption of the Internet, mobile technologies such as cell phones, and advances in photography and visualization, people are exposed to, and can readily seek and find, information about health and other topics in ways previously unimaginable.

There is a need for more research on how the communication revolution influences health care providers, the public, and media representatives. Specifically, given the plethora of sources available, limited research is being conducted on information seeking and information source preferences (including triangulation of sources). Furthermore, more research is needed to determine if there are changes in how people process information and make decisions. For example, heuristics may play a more important role now, and in the future, as people seek, select, process, understand, and act on health information (Wegwarth et al. 2009).

Conclusions

Many factors influence decisions about health research agendas and funding. They influence not only the overall support for research, but the distribution or mix of what is funded and not funded. It is essential to recognize the impact of differences in social priorities, health care delivery systems, and overall effects of economic climate, as this is truly a multilevel and complex process. There is a long-recognized gulf between the research community and health practitioners and the public with regard to research priorities; furthermore, as with persons and systems in other areas besides health, there is an underlying resistance to change by many researchers.

Concerning the current situation and making projections for the near-term future regarding agendas and funding for health research, particularly as it pertains to health literacy and prevention, there are reasons for pessimism and optimism. Unlike the relative economic prosperity of the 1990s and earlier this decade, when health research funding increased in some countries, the present economic climate is much less favorable. This may result in level or even reduced public funding for health research, as there is competition for these resources from other sectors. Support for new initiatives, or changing existing research agendas and redistributing research funding that is currently heavily oriented toward discovery, will be extremely difficult.

Private industry funding of health research, while increasing, is a mixed blessing. On one hand, research is oriented toward application with the goal of developing products or services. Some educational efforts, as well as products and services to improve health literacy, have been conducted by private industry (WHCA 2010). However, the need for a financial return on investment is paramount, and it can result in pressures for marketing and use of products and services that may not be indicated or as beneficial as alternatives (e.g., when research indicates that persons in certain age groups should be counseled not to receive a screening test or immunization).

There are, however, some reasons for optimism. There are growing demands and funding for more team science and collaborative transdisciplinary projects. There is interest and pressure to translate research into practice; for some projects this may increase the involvement of behavioral scientists and health care practitioners in research decision making. There is growing awareness among many researchers and practitioners of the importance of health literacy, as evidenced by reports and recommendations from the WHO and the U.S. Surgeon General (WHCA 2010). While levels of funding for research on health literacy, health services research, health technology assessment, and dissemination and implementation are low, there is some research occurring in these areas. Coupled with the increasing costs associated with health care products and services and the aging population in the developed world, there is likely to be support for research to discover and implement simple approaches to improve health literacy not only as a "public good," but also as a potential means to help control health care expenditures.

Finally, there are approaches used by some countries that provide useful models or frameworks for helping ensure that research findings are being utilized in health care decision making and practice. In 2004, Italy created a national organization called the Italian Medicines Agency (AIFA) with funding from a levy on the pharmaceutical industry (Addis and Rocchi 2006; Folino-Gallo et al. 2008). AIFA has authority to fund and assess research pharmaceutical products (i.e., for efficacy, safety, and post-marketing surveillance of adverse effects), and to approve medications for use in clinical practice for which the Italian government-funded health care system will pay. This has resulted in a close connection between level of research evidence, regulatory action, and clinical practice (Addis and Rocchi 2006).

In Sweden, the Scientific Council on Health Technology Assessment (SBU) has existed for more than 15 years (SBU 2009). SBU is an independent national public authority that assesses health technology for treatment effectiveness, diagnostic accuracy, prevention, and optimal utilization of health care resources. Reports by the SBU review the available scientific evidence to support decision making in health care with an eye toward identifying approaches that offer the most benefits and the least risk; they also focus on the most efficient ways to allocate resources. Information and conclusions in reports are intended for persons who make decisions about what health care options will be used, such as health professionals, administrators, planners, purchasers, policy makers, as well as patients and family members. Findings are widely disseminated through multiple communication channels, including the news media.

Acknowledgments

I thank Gerd Gigerenzer, Deborah Greenberg, Kara Hall, Brad Hesse, Marjukka Mäkelä, Stephen Marcus, Gloria Rasband, Scott Ratzan, Linda Peterson, Holger Schünemann, and Jonathan Wiest for their assistance.

6

Reporting of Research

Are We in for Better Health Care by 2020?

Holger Schünemann, Davina Ghersi, Julia Kreis,
Gerd Antes, and Jean Bousquet

Abstract

Background: Logical arguments support the view that complete, transparent, and objective reporting of research results avoids systematic error, misinformation, and unrealistic expectations. Evidence about publication bias (selective publication of research results on the basis of the obtained results), selective outcome reporting bias (reporting on outcomes research depending on the obtained results), increased demand for information by consumers, and ethical considerations supports these logical arguments. Based on requests from the organizing committee of this Strüngmann Forum, we addressed the following questions: Should there be a requirement to publish or report all results? If so, who or what should require the results to be published? What protocols and standards exist for publication and reporting, and how can they help to address the problem? Is the problem solvable? We conclude by summarizing whether the current suggestions are real solutions.

Methods: Using logical arguments informed by electronic searches of PubMed and web sites of the U.S. Food and Drug Administration (FDA), the European Medicines Agency, and the EQUATOR Network as well as reviews of references lists, we informed the discussion at this Strüngmann Forum. After the Forum, based on resulting dialog, we refined the answers to these key questions.

Results: In addition to appealing to researchers to report all research results, there are three key strategies to improve reporting of research results: (a) mandatory complete reporting to oversight agencies (regulatory agencies and ethics boards), (b) prospective study registration, and (c) requirements by journal editors for complete and standardized reporting of research. Enforcement of complete reporting by regulatory agencies is a simple solution for those interventions for which approval is requested. This data should be made public. Prospective registration of clinical trials should reduce the risk for reporting bias and a number of initiatives exist. Biomedical journal publishers can enhance reporting by enforcing, for example, the *Uniform Requirements for Manuscripts Submitted to Biomedical Journals* developed by the International Committee of Medical Journal Editors (ICMJE). The EQUATOR Network is a resourceful collaboration that focuses on complete and accurate reporting of research results. Protocols and guidelines (supplemented by checklists) for the reporting of various research study types exist, and include the CONSORT statement for randomized controlled trials, the STARD for diagnostic research studies, STROBE for observational studies, and PRISMA and MOOSE for systematic reviews. Developers of clinical practice guidelines can use the GRADE approach to ensure transparent and standardized development of guidance documents, which can be evaluated using the AGREE or the COGS instrument. However, while these and many other checklist and reporting criteria exist, there is limited evidence to show that reporting has improved as a result. In fact, journals often fail to adhere to their own reporting guidelines.

Conclusions: Complete reporting and publishing of research results has become increasingly recognized as a way to reduce bias when interpreting research. However, there is much room for improvement. Prospective study registration offers one way to improve the situation and should go beyond the field of clinical trials to include observational studies and all systematic reviews. New processes and mechanisms that implement reporting requirements for all research are needed. The usual candidate is an appropriate platform on the Internet that limits the influence of conflict of interest, and those who make profit with the Internet should fund it.

Introduction

Authors, editors and publishers all have ethical obligations with regard to the publication of the results of research. Authors have a duty to make publicly available the results of their research on human subjects and are accountable for the completeness and accuracy of their reports. They should adhere to accepted guidelines for ethical reporting. Negative and inconclusive as well as positive results should be published or otherwise made publicly available. Sources of funding, institutional affiliations and conflicts of interest should be declared in the publication. Reports of research not in accordance with the principles of this Declaration should not be accepted for publication.
—Declaration of Helsinki (WMA 2009)

Clinical research, like any research, is driven by highly trained people who are motivated, for the most part, by intellectual curiosity and academic advancement. Research is also driven by financial gains and the aspiration for power. The currency of research for academic promotion and advancement as well as profit and power is publicizing research results in scientific journals. Reporting the results of clinical research, thus, would appear to be a key to success. In addition, logical and ethical arguments emphasize that complete, transparent, and objective reporting of research results avoids systematic error, misinformation, and unrealistic expectations of consumers of health care information. Evidence about publication bias and selective outcome reporting bias supports these arguments. Despite the various motivations, not all research is reported or, if it is, it is reported differently than planned. In other words, the Helsinki Declaration on complete and transparent reporting is not adhered to by many researchers, who thereby fail to meet their ethical obligations.

Table 6.1 Reasons for lack of reporting of research results.

1. Negative financial implications due to less positive-than-expected effects of the evaluated intervention or strategy.
2. Lack of time or skills (time invested provides less benefit than the anticipated positive outcomes).
3. Belief that the results are not correct because they do not confirm stated hypothesis.
4. Disagreement about conclusions between investigators/authors.
5. No interest by journal editors. Peer review filters out:
   • results that are not along the lines of widely held beliefs,
   • theories, or
   • results from competing investigators.
6. Multiple testing of hypothesis, in particular in observational studies, with aim of reporting statistical significant results.
7. Change in professional environment.

Regardless of what the underlying reasons are (see Table 6.1 for examples), the lack of reporting of clinical research results can have extremely deleterious consequences when results indicate lack of net benefit, and potentially harmful application of widely applied interventions and behavior are not stopped (Table 6.2). In fact, paradoxically, since much research (i.e., more than 50%) remains unpublished or goes unreported, our very interpretation of a given research area may be systematically misled or biased as a result of incomplete, nontransparent, selective, or inaccurate reporting (Chan et al. 2004; Mathieu et al. 2009). Lack of reporting constitutes a serious ethical problem if members of the public agree to participate in trials on the understanding that they are contributing to the global body of health-related knowledge and the results of this research are not made publicly available (Krleza-Jeric et al. 2005). Matters of reporting bias get worse with unregulated interventions and diagnostic procedures, such as devices or "over-the-counter" medicinal products that have less stringent requirements of approval or coverage.

Despite increasing attention to the reporting of clinical research results, reporting bias—in the broader sense—is a phenomenon that continues to exist more than fifty years after Sterling's description (Sterling 1959). While a conceptual differentiation of the types of reporting bias on the basis of reasons and consequences is helpful for understanding and evaluating the field (e.g., publication bias, pre-publication bias, and "true" reporting bias; Chalmers 1990), in this chapter we will use "reporting bias" as an overarching term to include all forms

Table 6.2 Consequences of lack of reporting research results.

1. Harm of an intervention may remain unknown.
2. Financial investments are made for interventions that offer no benefit.
3. Research and resources are invested in areas of limited value.

of the problem. We address the following questions and make simple suggestions for how reporting bias could become a "problem of the past" by 2020:

1. Should there be a requirement to publish or report all results? If so, who
   or what should require results to be published?
2. What protocols and standards exist for publication/reporting, and how
   can they help to address the problem?
3. Is the problem solvable?

Although publication by the research community assumes publication in a
peer-reviewed, traditional journal, "publication" in its truest sense means making information available to the public. Reporting can therefore occur in many
shapes and forms, and includes licensing applications, conference abstracts,
web site publication, marketing materials, as well as many other formats. We
examine several of these aspects.

Methods

As a source for compiling the evidence in this article, the first author (HJS)
searched PubMed and the databases of the U. S. Food and Drug Administration
(FDA), the European Medicines Agency (EMEA), and the EQUATOR
Network, and consulted the reference list of identified and relevant literature as
well as textbooks (Guyatt, Rennie et al. 2008) and his own files in consultation
with the second author (DG). In October 2009, some of the authors attended
the focal meeting to this Ernst Strüngmann Forum. Using logical arguments
informed by discussion during this Forum, the three key questions listed above
were determined. Conceptually we separated the aim "complete and unbiased
reporting" from the methods that are used to achieve it.

Should There Be a Requirement to Publish or Report All Results?

There are three key potential mechanisms for achieving public availability of
research results: legal, ethical, and funding. From a legal perspective, there is
no legally binding international requirement for researchers to publish their
research. An increasing number of countries are, however, introducing national
legislation to require public reporting, particularly of clinical trials of regulated drugs and devices. By requiring researchers to conform with the Helsinki
Declaration, ethics review committees (or institutional review boards) are in
the position to demand complete reporting, and funding agencies are in a similar authoritative position. Scientific publishers of biomedical journals are well
positioned to require (and encourage!) the reporting of research results, but
they must adhere to the same ethical principles that allow complete, unbiased,
and non-conflicting reporting.

Regulatory, Oversight, and Funding Agencies

Food and Drug Administration of the United States

The development and approval process for drugs by the FDA is guided by the Center for Drug Evaluation and Research (CDER) as well by U.S. legislation. The CDER's task is to evaluate new drugs before they can be sold. Drug companies seeking to sell a drug in the United States are required to first test it and send CDER the evidence from the clinical research to prove that the drug is safe and effective for its intended use. A team of CDER physicians, statisticians, chemists, pharmacologists, and other scientists reviews the company's data and proposed labeling. The FDA provides detailed guidance on reporting for a number of research and approval areas. The FDA has stringent requirements for post-marketing reporting, in particular for adverse events (FDA 2009). For many drugs, manufacturers, applicants, packer, distributor, shared manufacturer, joint manufacturer, or any other participant involved in divided manufacturing have post-marketing safety reporting responsibilities. If an applicant becomes aware of a reportable adverse experience, the applicant is responsible to prepare a post-marketing safety report and submit it to the FDA.

Following the FDA Amendments Act of 2007, all ongoing clinical trials that involve a drug, biological product, or device regulated by the FDA must be registered. In addition, since September 2008, the results of all trials have been required to be posted in the same registry within one year of the study's termination. This is an important advancement and includes comprehensive information such as tables of baseline and demographic characteristics as well as results for primary and secondary outcomes. As of 2009, tables listing the harms reported during the trial must also be published in the registry (Groves 2008). This applies to all clinical trials of drugs and devices, but excludes phase I drug trials (preliminary safety studies for new products) and small feasibility studies of a device. Furthermore, it covers all trials—regardless of whether they are conducted and sponsored by industry or elsewhere—if the products concerned need approval by the FDA.

The European Medicines Agency

As a regulatory agency in Europe, the primary role of the EMEA is to conduct assessments for the authorization of medicines that are based on an objective, scientific assessment of their quality, safety, and efficacy. "Through its scientific committees, the EMEA assesses every medicine for which a marketing-authorization application has been submitted (in accordance with the centralized procedure), and prepares a recommendation (called an "opinion") that is then relayed to the European Commission, which has the ultimate responsibility for taking decisions on granting, refusing, revoking, or suspending marketing authorizations" (EMA 2010b).

In its roadmap for 2010, EMEA emphasizes improvement of adverse event reporting. In contrast to the FDA, specific mentioning of *complete* reporting (of *all* results) is not included (EMA 2010a). EMEA (2006) also stipulates the following:

1. The Agency shall refuse access to a document where disclosure would undermine the protection of: (a) the public interest as regards public security, defense and military matters, international relations, the financial, monetary or economic policy of the Community or a Member State; (b) privacy and the integrity of the individual, in particular in accordance with Community legislation regarding the protection of personal data.

2. The Agency shall refuse access to a document where disclosure would undermine the protection of: (a) commercial interests of a natural or legal person, including intellectual property; (b) court proceedings and legal advice; (c) the purpose of inspections, investigations and audits, unless there is an overriding public interest in disclosure.

3. Access to a document, produced or received and in possession of the Agency, which relates to a matter where the decision has not been taken, shall be refused if disclosure of the document would seriously undermine the decision-making process, unless there is an overriding public interest in disclosure.

Thus, while EMEA may require complete reporting of results from some applicants with special emphasis on adverse event reporting, these results may not be in the public domain and thus may not be accessible to all decision makers.

Manufacturers in Europe make data available, for example, to national Health Technology Assessment (HTA) agencies such as the Institute for Quality and Efficiency in Health Care (IQWiG) in Germany, only on a voluntary basis. Such voluntary agreements are not always sufficient, as became apparent recently when a drug company withheld information on relevant studies for a benefit assessment carried out by IQWiG (Stafford 2009). As a result, IQWiG called for EU-wide legislation to publish the results of clinical trials, pointing out that this should also apply retrospectively to drugs already approved and be done in timely fashion (IQWiG 2009).

Oversight Agencies

Other oversight agencies, such as ethics boards, committees, and data safety and monitoring boards, may have another major oversight function. Examples show that ethics board approval depends on or leads to monitoring of trial registration (Tharyan 2007). At the Christian Medical College in Vellore, Tamil Nadu, the application form for institutional funding and/or research ethics committee approval was modified to include a declaration that the trial would be prospectively registered in a clinical trial registry. Ethics clearance is provisional until a valid trial registration number is provided to the ethics committee, along with a copy of the details of that registration. The requirement to register prospective trials is an ethical imperative for ethics committees, since safeguarding the rights of trial participants and weighing risks and benefits are cardinal obligations of any research ethics committee (Levin and Palmer 2007). In fact, the demand for the registration of clinical trials has been added to the Helsinki Declaration in 2008: "Every clinical trial must be registered in a publicly accessible database before recruitment of the first subject" (WMA 2009).

Funding Agencies

Funding agencies such as NIH and CIHR require funded trials to be registered. However, as explained below, registration alone, in particular of funded studies, presents only a partial solution to biased reporting.

Publications in the Scientific Literature

In addition to the requirements for reporting data to regulatory agencies, which began with the CONSORT statement approximately a decade ago, a number of reporting guidelines and protocols in the scientific literature have become available, and concerted efforts have led to stricter reporting requirements. For example, many biomedical journals now require authors to adhere to the *Uniform Requirements for Manuscripts Submitted to Biomedical Journals* developed by the ICMJE (2010). The requirements include descriptions of the ethical principles in the conduct and reporting of research and provide recommendations related to editing and writing. One of the key requirements (for later publication) is prospective and public registration of clinical trials of all interventions, including devices. However, although the ICMJE policy requires prospective registration of all interventional clinical studies and their methodology, it does not require the registration of the results for these trials. While the lack of reporting requirements does not eliminate the concern about publication bias, it enables researchers to explore reasons for not publishing research results. Over 700 journals are registered as following the ICMJE guidelines.

The Grey Literature International Steering Committee adapted the ICMJE requirements and created the *Guidelines for the Production of Scientific and Technical Reports* (GLISC 2007). The guidelines cover ethical considerations, publishing and editorial issues, and report preparation. Many other journals have published and endorsed reporting guidelines for various study designs.

However, requirements for registration or *complete* reporting of observational studies do not exist beyond journal reporting guidelines. This constitutes one reason for increasing scrutiny of the evidence from observational studies (in addition to the problem posed by the many tested, and yet unreported, hypotheses in observational studies). Fortunately, there is increasing recognition of the requirement for prospective registration of observational studies, as evidenced by the European Centre for Ecotoxicology and Toxicology of Chemicals position (ECETOC 2010):

> As any scientific endeavor, an epidemiology study should follow a rigorous scientific process to yield reliable results. A protocol should be available describing the specific hypothesis to be tested, the design, study subject selection, measurement of the risk factor, effect parameter and the statistical analysis that will be carried out. Next, the data collection phase can take place and the statistical analysis can be conducted. All results of the study should be included in the report to be submitted for publication....At this moment it is possible that published articles do not report all study results and the study results cannot be weighed against the initial study hypothesis.

Progress is being made with the reporting and publishing of basic research data. The Minimum Information for Biological and Biomedical Investigation portal provides the latest information on data-reporting standards ("minimum information" checklist) for investigations such as the MIAME for microarray experiments (MIBBI 2010). However, there does not appear to be a uniform or mandatory requirement to *publish* results. We believe that such a requirement should exist.

What Protocols and Standards Exist for Publication or Reporting?

Regulatory agencies have their institutional reporting requirements which should be guided by the Helsinki Declaration. Ethics boards are regulated by national laws and institutional bylaws. Credibility in health care research is related to scientific publishing, and thus scientific editors play a central role in ensuring complete and standardized reporting. The following accepted registries are listed by the ICMJE:

- www.actr.org.au
- www.clinicaltrials.gov
- www.ISRCTN.org
- www.umin.ac.jp/ctr/index/htm
- www.trialregister.nl, and
- www.who.int/ictrp/about/details/en/index.html (the primary registry of the World Health Organization).

Review of the registries is conducted by WHO, which has established special advisory committees to monitor both registration and develop accepted processes.

While much progress regarding *registration* has been made for clinical trials (Krleza-Jeric et al. 2005), protocols and standards for the *reporting* of various types of research study exist (for a summary of reporting requirements for journal publications and academic investigators, see EQUATOR Network 2010). The EQUATOR Network is an international initiative that seeks to improve reliability and value of medical research literature through the promotion of transparent and accurate reporting of research studies. It is also developing a library for information about health research reporting. Below we briefly describe the current existing major instruments, which share in common the primary aim of protecting against bias by reminding researchers of key reporting and quality criteria (and biased interpretation). Details are summarized in Tables 6.3–6.6.

For complete reporting of clinical trials, the CONSORT Statement for randomized controlled trials focuses on methodological quality criteria and the follow-up of patients through a trial (Table 6.3; Moher et al. 2001). Diagnostic accuracy studies can be evaluated for both complete reporting and risk of bias (internal validity) using the STARD checklist (Bossuyt et al. 2003; see also Table 6.4). A more recent project, the STROBE initiative, focuses on reporting for observational studies (von Elm et al. 2007), and includes the subcategory of genetic association studies described in the STREGA statement (Little et al. 2009). A revision of the QUOROM statement produced the PRISMA statement. PRISMA aims to help authors report a wide array of systematic reviews to assess the benefits and harms of a health care intervention (Moher et al. 2009). It focuses on ways in which authors can ensure transparent and complete reporting of systematic reviews and meta-analyses. The MOOSE statement provides guidance for systematic reviews of observational studies (Stroup et al. 2000). Developers of clinical practice guidelines can use the GRADE approach (Table 6.5) to ensure transparent and standardized development of guidance documents (Guyatt, Oxman et al. 2008), which can be evaluated using the AGREE (Table 6.6) or the COGS instrument (Burgers et al. 2004; Shiffman et al. 2003).

Other reporting standards include:

- GNOSIS: Guidelines for neuro-oncology: standards for investigational studies which report on surgically based therapeutic clinical trials,
- ORION: Guidelines for transparent reporting of outbreak reports and intervention studies of nosocomial infection (Burgers et al. 2004; Shiffman et al. 2003),
- REMARK: Reporting recommendations for tumor marker prognostic studies (McShane et al. 2005),
- COREQ: Consolidated criteria for reporting qualitative research (Tong et al. 2007),
- TREND: Transparent reporting of evaluations with non-randomized designs (Des Jarlais et al. 2004),
- SQUIRE: Standards for quality improvement reporting excellence guidelines for quality improvement reporting (Davidoff et al. 2008).

Table 6.3 Checklist of items from CONSORT Statement 2001 to include when reporting a randomized trial (after Moher et al. 2001). This checklist is intended to accompany the explanatory document that facilitates its use. For more information, see CONSORT (2010).

Section and topic	Item	Descriptor
Title and abstract	1	How participants were allocated to interventions (e.g., "random allocation," "randomized," or "randomly assigned").
Introduction Background	2	Scientific background and explanation of rationale.
Methods Participants	3	Eligibility criteria for participants and the settings and locations where the data were collected.
Interventions	4	Precise details of the interventions intended for each group and how and when they were actually administered.
Objectives	5	Specific objectives and hypotheses.
Outcomes	6	Clearly defined primary and secondary outcome measures and, when applicable, any methods used to enhance the quality of measurements (e.g., multiple observations, training of assessors).
Sample size	7	How sample size was determined and, when applicable, explanation of any interim analyses and stopping rules.
Randomization: sequence generation	8	Method used to generate the random allocation sequence, including details of any restrictions (e.g., blocking, stratification)
Randomization: allocation concealment	9	Method used to implement the random allocation sequence (e.g., numbered containers or central telephone), clarifying whether the sequence was concealed until interventions were assigned.
Randomization: implementation	10	Who generated the allocation sequence, who enrolled participants, and who assigned participants to their groups.
Blinding (masking)	11	Whether or not participants, those administering the interventions, and those assessing the outcomes were blinded to group assignment. If done, how the success of blinding was evaluated.
Statistical methods	12	Statistical methods used to compare groups for primary outcome(s); Methods for additional analyses, such as subgroup analyses and adjusted analyses.
Results Participant flow	13	Flow of participants through each stage (a diagram is strongly recommended). Specifically, for each group report the numbers of participants randomly assigned, receiving intended treatment, completing the study protocol, and analyzed for the primary outcome. Describe protocol deviations from study as planned, together with reasons.

Table 6.3 (continued)

Section and topic	Item	Descriptor
Recruitment	14	Dates defining periods of recruitment and follow-up.
Baseline data	15	Baseline demographic and clinical characteristics of each group.
Numbers analyzed	16	Number of participants (denominator) in each group included in each analysis and whether the analysis was by "intention-to-treat." State the results in absolute numbers when feasible (e.g., 10/20, not 50%).
Outcomes and estimation	17	For each primary and secondary outcome, a summary of results for each group, and the estimated effect size and its precision (e.g., 95% confidence interval).
Ancillary analyses	18	Address multiplicity by reporting any other analyses performed, including subgroup analyses and adjusted analyses, indicating those pre-specified and those exploratory.
Adverse events	19	All important adverse events or side effects in each intervention group.
Discussion Interpretation	20	Interpretation of the results, taking into account study hypotheses, sources of potential bias or imprecision and the dangers associated with multiplicity of analyses and outcomes.
Generalizability	21	Generalizability (external validity) of the trial findings.
Overall evidence	22	General interpretation of the results in the context of current evidence.

Still, while checklist and reporting criteria for a number of different study designs or research reports exist, there is only limited evidence that reporting has in fact improved. Often, journals fail to adhere to their own reporting guidelines. In fact, the authors of the SQUIRE statement remarked (Davidoff et al. 2008:674–675):

> Unfortunately, little is known about the most effective ways to apply publication guidelines in practice. Therefore, editors have been forced to learn from experience how to use other publication guidelines, and the specifics of their use vary widely from journal to journal. We also lack systematic knowledge of how authors can use publication guidelines most productively. Our experience suggests, however, that SQUIRE is most helpful if authors simply keep the general content of the guideline items in mind as they write their initial drafts, then refer to the details of individual items as they critically appraise what they have written during the revision process. The question of how publication guidelines can be used most effectively appears to us to be an empirical one, and therefore we strongly encourage editors and authors to collect, analyze, and report their experiences in using SQUIRE and other publication guidelines.

Table 6.4 STARD checklist for reporting of studies of diagnostic accuracy (version January 2003).

Section and topic	Item	Descriptor
Title/abstract/ keywords		
	1	Identify the article as a study of diagnostic accuracy (recommend MeSH heading "sensitivity and specificity").
Introduction	2	State the research questions or study aims, such as estimating diagnostic accuracy or comparing accuracy between tests or across participant groups.
Methods		
Participants	3	The study population: The inclusion and exclusion criteria, setting and locations where data were collected.
	4	Participant recruitment: Was recruitment based on presenting symptoms, results from previous tests, or the fact that the participants had received the index tests or the reference standard?
	5	Participant sampling: Was the study population a consecutive series of participants defined by the selection criteria in item 3 and 4? If not, specify how participants were further selected.
	6	Data collection: Was data collection planned before the index test and reference standard were performed (prospective study) or after (retrospective study)?
Test methods	7	The reference standard and its rationale.
	8	Technical specifications of material and methods involved including how and when measurements were taken, and/or cite references for index tests and reference standard.
	9	Definition of and rationale for the units, cut-offs and/or categories of the results of the index tests and the reference standard.
	10	The number, training and expertise of the persons executing and reading the index tests and the reference standard.
	11	Whether or not the readers of the index tests and reference standard were blind (masked) to the results of the other test and describe any other clinical information available to the readers.

Table 6.4 (continued)

Section and topic	Item	Descriptor
Statistical methods	12	Methods for calculating or comparing measures of diagnostic accuracy, and the statistical methods used to quantify uncertainty (e.g., 95% confidence intervals).
	13	Methods for calculating test reproducibility, if done.
Results		
Participants	14	When study was performed, including beginning and end dates of recruitment.
	15	Clinical and demographic characteristics of the study population (at least information on age, gender, spectrum of presenting symptoms).
	16	The number of participants satisfying the criteria for inclusion who did or did not undergo the index tests and/or the reference standard; describe why participants failed to undergo either test (a flow diagram is strongly recommended).
Test results	17	Time-interval between the index tests and the reference standard, and any treatment administered in between.
	18	Distribution of severity of disease (define criteria) in those with the target condition; other diagnoses in participants without the target condition.
	19	A cross tabulation of the results of the index tests (including indeterminate and missing results) by the results of the reference standard; for continuous results, the distribution of the test results by the results of the reference standard.
	20	Any adverse events from performing the index tests or the reference standard.
Estimates	21	Estimates of diagnostic accuracy and measures of statistical uncertainty (e.g., 95% confidence intervals).
	22	How indeterminate results, missing data and outliers of the index tests were handled.
	23	Estimates of variability of diagnostic accuracy between subgroups of participants, readers or centers, if done.
	24	Estimates of test reproducibility, if done.
Discussion	25	Discuss the clinical applicability of the study findings.

Table 6.5   GRADE criteria for assessing the quality of evidence.

Study design	Initial quality	Lower if	Higher if	Overall quality
Randomized trials	High	Risk of bias:	Large effect:	High: ⊕⊕⊕⊕
		−1 Serious −2 Very serious	+1 Large +2 Very large	
		Inconsistency: −1 Serious −2 Very serious	Dose response: +1 Evidence of a gradient	Moderate: ⊕⊕⊕◯

Observational studies	Low	Indirectness:
		−1 Serious
		−2 Very serious
			All plausible residual:
			−1 Confounding
			+1 Would reduce
			      a demonstrated
			      effect
				Low: ⊕⊕◯◯

		Imprecision:
		−1 Serious
		−2 Very serious
			+1 Would suggest a
			      spurious effect
			      if no effect was
			      observed
				Very low: ⊕◯◯◯

		Publication bias: −1 Likely −2 Very likely		

Table 6.6   AGREE instrument for evaluating guideline quality and reporting. Rater is instructed to use a scale from 1–4, where 1 indicates strong disagreement and 4 indicates strong agreement.

Quality criterion	Rating (n/4)
Scope and purpose	
Comment: The overall objective(s) of the guideline is (are) specifically described.	
Comment: The clinical question(s) covered by the guideline is (are) specifically described.	
The patients to whom the guideline is meant to apply to are specifically described.	
Stakeholder involvement	
Comment: The guideline development group includes individuals from all the relevant professional groups.	
Comment: The patients' views and preferences have been sought.	
Comment: The target users of the guideline are clearly defined.	

Table 6.6 (continued)

Quality criterion	Rating (n/4)
Comment: The guideline has been piloted among target users.	

Rigor of development

Comment: Systematic methods were used to search for evidence.	
Comment: The criteria for selecting the evidence are clearly described.	
Comment: The methods used for formulating the recommendations are clearly described.	
Comment: The health benefits, side effects and risks have been considered in formulating the recommendations.	
Comment: There is an explicit link between the recommendations and the supporting evidence.	
Comment: The guideline has been externally reviewed by experts prior to its publication.	
Comment: A procedure for updating the guideline is provided.	

Clarity and presentation

Comment: The recommendations are unambiguous.	
Comment: The different options for management of the condition are clearly presented.	
Comment: Key recommendations are easily identifiable.	
Comment: The guideline is supported with tools for application.	

Applicability

Comment: The potential organizational barriers in applying the recommendations have been discussed.	
Comment: The potential cost implication of applying the recommendations have been considered.	
Comment: The guideline presents key review criteria for monitoring and/or audit purposes.	

Editorial independence

Comment: Guideline is editorially independent from the funding body.	
Comment: Conflicts of interest of guideline development members have been recorded	

Is the Problem Solvable?

In addition to appealing to researchers to report all research results, three key strategies will improve the reporting of research results: (a) mandatory complete reporting to oversight agencies (regulatory agencies and ethics boards), (b) prospective study registration, and (c) requirements by journal editors for complete and standardized reporting of research, regardless of the type of research and interventions that are investigated. Our review has shown that most study designs in health care research are accompanied by authoritative reporting guidelines. In fact, duplicate efforts are beginning to emerge.

CONSORT has been associated with some improvements in the quality of reporting of primary research. A systematic review conducted in 2006 found that journals using CONSORT proved to be significantly better in reporting the method of sequence generation (risk ratio [RR], 1.67; 95% confidence interval [CI], 1.19–2.33), allocation concealment (RR, 1.66; 95% CI, 1.37–2.00), and overall number of CONSORT items than those who did not use CONSORT (standardized mean difference, 0.83; 95% CI, 0.46–1.19) (Plint et al. 2006). Publication of the CONSORT statement appeared to have less effect on items such as the reporting of participant flow and blinding of participants or data analysts in that analysis (Plint et al. 2006). Pre- and postadoption of CONSORT showed an improvement in the description of the method of sequence generation (RR, 2.78; 95% CI, 1.78–4.33), participant flow (RR, 8.06; 95% CI, 4.10–15.83), and total CONSORT items (standardized mean difference, 3.67 items; 95% CI, 2.09–5.25) in journals that adopted CONSORT (Plint et al. 2006).

Innovative models are required because clinical trial results are often manipulated, and this manipulation is resistant to reporting so long as results are not interpreted in a biased fashion. Furthermore, what matters is the totality of the relevant research evidence, less so individual studies. For example, by publishing individual clinical trials ad hoc, medical journals provide a mechanism that can be subverted by funding bodies and researchers with an interest in getting particular trial results (Montori et al. 2004; Smith and Roberts 2006).

As described by Smith and Roberts (2006), the process could start with posting a systematic review of the existing trial evidence on the Internet to show what is already known about a particular intervention and what further research is needed. If there is uncertainty about the effectiveness of the treatment, such that a further trial is needed, a new trial would be registered and the trial protocol would also be posted on the Internet. Everybody with any involvement in the trial would be listed with their contribution explained, abolishing the current need for "paternity testing" of published trials. At any point, observers (i.e., patients, researchers, clinicians, editors, or anyone else) would be able to comment online about the interpretation of the systematic review's data, the importance of the trial question, or the reliability of its methods.

This model currently ignores the requirement for full reporting and the reporting of evidence other than that from trials. It, therefore, requires expansion.

Policy makers around the world must work to ensure that this takes place. We are dealing with health care, and any reasons held against this expansion are feeble compared to the potential benefit and ethical obligations.

Regarding the publication of "negative" research results, journal editors are giving greater attention to this, and there is evidence that some strategies work (Sridharan and Greenland 2009). Yet despite greater awareness of reporting requirements, there is still much room for improvement. For example, Mathieu et al. (2009) searched MEDLINE for reports of randomized controlled trials in three medical areas (cardiology, rheumatology, and gastroenterology) that were published in 2008—three years after mandatory trial registration—in the ten general medical journals and specialty journals with the highest impact factors. Of the 323 articles with trials examined, only 147 (45.5%) had been adequately registered (i.e., registered before the end of the trial, with the primary outcome clearly specified); 89 (27.6%) published trials had not been registered and 45 (13.9%) were registered after the completion of the study; 39 (12%) trials were registered with no or an unclear description of the primary outcome and three (0.9%) were registered after the completion of the study and had an unclear description of the primary outcome. Interestingly, nearly one-third of the articles with trials adequately registered (31% or 46 out of 147) showed some evidence of discrepancies between the outcomes registered and the outcomes published. This work demonstrates that journal editors need to enforce the policies they set (Mathieu et al. 2009).

Smidt et al. (2007) assessed whether the quality of reporting of diagnostic accuracy studies has improved since the publication of the STARD statement. They evaluated reporting in 12 medical journals in 2000 (pre-STARD) and 2004 (post-STARD). The mean number of reported STARD items was 11.9 (range 3.5 to 19.5) in 2000 and 13.6 (range 4.0 to 21.0) in 2004, an increase of 1.81 items (95% CI: 0.61 to 3.01) across 141 articles. This improvement, however, was not associated with whether journals had adopted STARD, and time trends could not be excluded.

What matters is not merely *whether* a trial gets reported, but *how* results are reported. One of the pitfalls of reporting biomedical research relates to spinning research results despite adequate reporting of the results. For many reasons, authors may put special emphasis and interpretation on certain results that obscure or limit objective evaluation of research findings (Montori et al. 2004). Furthermore, conclusions in trials are often influenced by those who fund the study (Als-Nielsen et al. 2003). When using the biomedical literature, people must be equipped to evaluate the validity of results and how they apply to patient care (Guyatt, Rennie et al. 2008). Furthermore, Moher et al. (2009) warn against blind endorsement of reporting guidelines because the development process of reporting guidelines is often poorly reported.

The most important question—whether improved reporting leads to better outcomes for patients as well as more transparency and reduction in reporting bias—remains unanswered. In their recent analysis, Vedula et al. (2008)

showed that there may be rather subtle differences between the primary and other outcomes specified in the protocol and those described in the published report, which may lead to different interpretation of an intervention's effectiveness.

This Strüngmann Forum revealed the need for further attention to the following areas:

- Internet posting of all research and analysis being conducted.
- The demand from patient organizations for complete reporting.
- Mechanisms to ensure that journal editors enforce existing policies for reporting.
- The need for educating those involved in research training programs about the registration of research hypothesis as well as the reporting of analysis and results.
- The requirement to disclose the sale of reprints by journal editors (see also Sepkowitz 2007).
- There is a remaining risk that outcomes associated with interventions may be unknown at the time of study design and implementation. These outcomes are usually adverse in nature and should therefore be recorded with great care. The inclusion of patient-reported outcomes (e.g., generic quality of life measures) will help overcome this problem.
- Funding for enforcement on various levels.
- How can collaboration between relevant parties be fostered? Who should be involved? Who should lead these efforts?
- What, if any, additional evidence is required to convince policy makers?

Conclusions

Ethical principles demand that the research community must adhere to standards of complete and adequate reporting. While the ideal scenario is one that includes scientists adhering to reporting guidelines and ethical principles, history teaches us, and the limitations and challenges outlined in this chapter suggest, that voluntary reporting is insufficient and that enforcement of policies for complete, transparent, and unbiased reporting is required. Better reporting and publication of research results can be achieved. However, the currently preferred method of reporting to regulatory agencies and study registration is insufficient.

Collaboration between the FDA and systematic reviewers and guideline developers will enhance the quality of guidance that can be given to health care consumers if a consequent follow-up is undertaken on registered trials. Guidelines, ideally based on systematic reviews and HTA reports, constitute the foundation upon which health care decision makers are informed and the end stage of health care guidance development (which itself requires evaluation).

Guidelines should be based on complete and best evidence. To avoid misleading conclusions, guideline developers and those evaluating the body of evidence for a given health care question should follow rigorous and transparent standards to ensure the development of transparent guidelines (e.g., GRADE Working Group 2010), which include evaluations of selective reporting bias and publication bias.

7

Medical Journals Can Be Less Biased

J. A. Muir Gray

Abstract

The quality of medical research depends on the use of structured protocols. Problems associated with poor-quality research reports range from poor design to improper management or irrelevant research. Structured protocols have been shown to improve reporting, yet implementation and adherence remain major issues for those who fund research as well as for those who publish the results. In addition, the peer-review process used in research selection and publication contains flaws that must be addressed. Priority needs to be given to systematic reviews of randomized controlled trials, as these yield higher-quality, stronger evidence than the report of any single controlled trial.

Introduction

Over the last ten years, a revolution has occurred in how medical literature is perceived. Instrumental to this change, the Cochrane Collaboration has shifted the emphasis on quality, not just quantity, of medical literature. In the initial stages of the Cochrane Collaboration, people began to learn that when considering evidence about the effects of an intervention, the randomized controlled trial was the method of choice: it was the least likely to include errors due to bias and, if trials were well designed, least likely to include errors due to chance. In addition, Cochrane promoted the idea that a systematic review of randomized controlled trials yielded higher-quality, stronger evidence than the report of any single controlled trial.

For many people, the term "systematic review" has become associated with randomized controlled trials. It is, of course, possible to conduct systematic reviews on any type of research, including qualitative research, and although systematic reviews provide the strongest evidence, they, like all other types of research reports, vary in quality. Even when a review can be clearly classified as a systematic review, and not simply an editorial written by one person without benefit of a systematic literature search and all the other accompanying steps, the quality and strength of the evidence varies.

The Scandal of Poor Medical Research

In 1994, Altman wrote an editorial for the *British Medical Journal* entitled "The Scandal of Poor Medical Research," which highlighted the major problems in clinical research of the day: poor design, badly conducted, or irrelevant research. Unfortunately, some 16 years later, this situation has hardly improved. In fact, the problems associated with poor-quality research reports—whether a systematic review or a "primary" research report—form only part of the continuing scandal.

Recently, Chalmers and Glasziou (2009) identified a number of ways in which resources are wasted:

1. Research is done without having conducted a systematic review prior to commencement.
2. Research is poorly designed.
3. Research is poorly conducted.
4. Research is not completely and accurately reported.

To detect these issues, the patient or clinician must rely on research funders or those responsible for research governance. Patient and clinicians cannot themselves, however, identify the deficiencies in research design and conduct, and must rely on editors and peer reviewers. Due to the inherent weaknesses in the peer-review and editorial process, this trust is not always justified.

Structured Protocols

To improve the reporting of randomized controlled trials, the CONSORT statement established a structured protocol that required authors to provide enough information so that readers would know how the trial was performed (Altman 1996). This was followed by a number of different protocols developed for the various types of research reports.

The EQUATOR Network, funded principally by the British National Health Service, grew out of the work of CONSORT and other guideline development groups. Initiated in 2006, EQUATOR is an international initiative that "seeks to enhance reliability and value of medical research literature by promoting transparent and accurate reporting of research studies" (EQUATOR Network 2010). Currently it is taking steps to develop and disseminate protocols, but voluntary adoption of these protocols is not enough.

Journal editors and publishers are responsible for the adoption and adherence of protocols, yet progress has been slow. Given the significance of reporting, the multiple discussions that have taken place, and the time that has transpired, one would have hoped for more.

There is, however, another way to ensure adoption. Those who pay for journals are in an ideal position to insist that journals conform to standards. Take, for example, a medical institution which purchases electronic access for its clinicians, researchers, and students. Access to high-quality reporting is of paramount importance to these readers, and thus it is in the interest of subscription holders to demand not only adoption but adherence to standards.

It may be necessary to build in a grace period of, say, two years to bring about compliance, because of the need to train peer reviewers and put new processes in place. However, the delivery of concise information for use by clinicians and patients remains an urgent priority. Inadequate reporting has significant implications for those who have been taught to turn to journals for answers and to put their faith in peer-reviewed articles as quality assured and reliable knowledge.

Peer Review

A significant amount of research has gone into analyzing the deficiencies in the peer-review process, and a number of principles have emerged:

1. Peer review remains better than the alternative; namely, the opinion of a single editor.
2. It is not possible for even the most diligent peer reviewer to identify problems unless research reporting is improved, and this requires action on the part of research funders.
3. Peer review can be improved through the training of peer reviewers; however, the use of structured report protocols is critical.

Peer review and editing can improve the quality of medical research reporting (Goodman et al. 1994) but there are severe limitations associated with both. The term "peer reviewed" is often understood to be synonymous with the term "quality assured." Although an improvement over a single editor's scrutiny, the peer-review process has been shown to have many flaws (Mulrow 1987).

Medical journals consist of a number of different types of documents. The two main types consulted by readers in search of evidence are review articles (including editorials) and peer-reviewed articles. For review articles, some senior member of a specialty or profession is approached to review a topic; the result is a published review backed by the reputation and authority of the author. Review articles are often written for the clinician, whereas peer-reviewed reports of research are written primarily by researchers for researchers.

As useful as such reviews and editorials may be, two landmark studies revealed significant deficiencies in the process and highlighted the need for systematic reviews of research, which were explicit in their methods of literature searching, appraisal, and data synthesis (Jefferson and Godlee 1999; Oxman and Guyatt 1988). This culminated in the creation of the Cochrane Collaboration, which was committed to these principles and established to ensure that the reviews were kept up to date. In addition, they highlighted the benefits and weaknesses of the peer-review process: review articles written by a person generally considered to be an authority were usually only scrutinized by the editor and not reviewed by the writer's peers.

Failures of Peer Review

Peer reviewers fail to spot bias. For example, studies that have yielded relatively dramatic results are more likely to be cited in reports of subsequent similar studies than studies yielding unremarkable point estimates of effects. In a study of manufacturer-supported trials of non-steroidal anti-inflammatory drugs in the treatment of arthritis, Rochon and colleagues (1994) found that the data presented did not support the claims made about toxicity in about half the articles. Anyone managing or using scientific literature needs to understand the weaknesses of peer review.

Failure to Spot Poor Literature Retrieval

Recent research has shown that the very foundation of the scientific article—namely the review of the prior state of knowledge on which the research hypothesis was formulated, sometimes called the review of the literature—is all too often flawed. In a landmark article, Chalmers and Clarke (1998) examined reports of randomized controlled trials in a single month from the five major medical journals (Figure 7.1). Depressingly, they found no evidence that this position had improved four and eight years later (Clarke et al. 2002, 2007). This demonstrates that the research studies were based on an inaccurate estimate of the current state of knowledge and that they failed to add any results

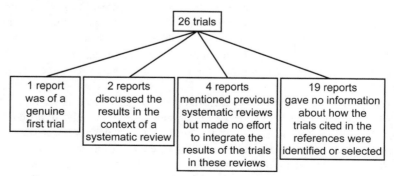

Figure 7.1   Discussion sections in reports of controlled trials published in general medical journals (Chalmers and Clarke 1998).

that emerged from the study to the existing knowledge base, thus making it very difficult for the reader to assess their implications.

Statistical Problems and Bias

Some problems in published reports of randomized controlled trials may be very difficult for the busy clinical reader to spot. This was demonstrated by statisticians in an analysis of 50 clinical trials during a three-month period in four top journals: *British Medical Journal, Journal of the American Medical Association, The Lancet,* and the *New England Journal of Medicine* (Assman et al. 2000). This analysis found that:

- about half the trials inappropriately used significance tests for baseline comparison;
- methods of randomization were often poorly described;
- two-thirds of the reports presented sub-group findings, but most without appropriate statistical tests for interaction;
- many reports put too much emphasis on sub-group analysis, which commonly lacked statistical power.

Another review (Moher et al. 2001) concluded that the CONSORT Statement, which recommended a standard approach to the reporting of clinical trials, had not yet produced a standardized approach to reporting. Moher et al. conclude that there are substantial risks of exaggerated claims of treatment effects arising from post-hoc emphasis across multiple analyses. Sub-group analyses are particularly prone to over-interpretation and one is tempted to suggest "don't do it" (or at least "don't believe it") for many trials.

Although it would be appropriate to appoint more statisticians to peer review papers, a preventive approach may be better. Research funders should follow the CONSORT principles and, based on tables in CONSORT, require research applicants to set out how they will report research results *before* funding is granted.

Unsystematic Systematic Reviews

Words and terms are tools. A word or term may initially perform helpful functions, defining and clarifying concepts or objects and providing new tools for people to use. However, as words and terms become more widespread in usage, their meaning often changes or is amplified. Potentially, a word or term may develop so many meanings that its mere use confuses more than clarifies.

A systematic review "synthesizes the results of an assembly of primary investigations using strategies that limit bias and random error" (CMSG 2010). It is useful when rigorously applied, but cannot always be accepted at face value as representing reliable evidence. Often, systematic reviews are not sufficiently systematic and thus are unreliable (Moher et al. 2007).

A critical evaluation of systematic reviews and meta-analyses on the treatment of asthma (Jadad et al. 2000) found that out of the 50 systematic reviews and meta-analyses included in the study:

- 12 reviews were published in the Cochrane Library,
- 38 were published in peer-reviewed journals,
- 40 of the reviews were judged to have "serious or extensive flaws,"
- all 6 reviews associated with industry had "serious or extensive flaws,"
- 7 out of the 10 most rigorous reviews were published in the Cochrane Library.

The critiques of review articles published in 1987 and 1988 have been repeated, and a team carrying out an analysis of "review articles" identified 158 review articles in 12 "core" medical journals, using the Science Citation Index to define the core journals (McAlister et al. 1999). Of the 158 review articles:

- only 2 satisfied all 10 methodological criteria of good quality,
- less than one-fourth described how evidence was identified, evaluated, or integrated,
- from the 111 reviews that made treatment recommendations, only 45% cited randomized controlled clinical trials to support their recommendations.

To improve this situation, the use of PRISMA guidelines is strongly recommended. PRISMA aims to help authors report a wide array of systematic reviews to assess the benefits and harms of a health care intervention (Moher et al. 2009; for further discussion, see Schünemann et al., this volume).

Duplicate Publications

Tramer et al. (1997) conducted a systematic search of full reports published on randomized controlled trials investigating ondansetron's effect on postoperative emesis and found that:

- 17% of published full reports of trials and 28% of patient data were duplicated,
- none of these reports cross-referenced the original source,
- covert publication can take place because articles submitted for publication are "masked" by change of authors or language or by adding extra data,
- duplication of data led to an overestimation of ondansetron's antiemetic efficacy by 23%,
- trials reporting greater treatment effects were significantly more likely to be duplicated.

Even the authors of systematic reviews may not spot duplication (von Elm et al. 2004).

Incomplete Reporting

Peer review often fails to identify incomplete reporting of research results, which is presented with significant bias. Bias is usually slanted toward the positive, namely to report positive results and not to report negative results. To alleviate this, both protocols and reports should be published (Chan and Altman 2005a, b).

Positive Bias

Overall, the flaws in the peer-review system tend to emphasize the positive effects of an intervention, thus leading the reader to overestimate the benefits and underestimate the harms of an intervention. This is further compounded by the tendency of authors to submit, and editors to publish, studies with positive results. The combined effect is known as positive publication bias; one estimate holds that this bias overstates the benefits of treatments by up to one-third (Schulz et al. 1995). The overall effect, or optimism bias (Chalmers and Matthews 2006), needs to be managed. Challenges for management include the increased proportion of trials funded by industry (Gøtzsche et al. 2006), combined with the fact that industry-sponsored trials often have constraints written into the support. For example, an analysis of research protocols found that constraints on the publication rights were found in 40 (91%) of the protocols from 1994 to 1995, and 22 noted that the sponsor either owned the data needed to improve the manuscript or both (Patsopoulos et al. 2006). On the positive side, the registration of controlled trials, according to standards being developed by the World Health Organization, will encourage completeness of reporting.

All of the problems described above, and more, contribute to what is known in Japanese as *muda*, a term used to signify any activity that does not add value to the outcome of a process. In medical literature, many factors have contributed to the production of waste (for an overview, see Chalmers and Glasziou 2009). However, instead of concentrating on this negative state of affairs, let us consider ways to impact a change.

Solutions

Any solution that is sought must fit to the reality and constraints of daily life. Not only does time and access constrain the ability of a reader to keep abreast of current literature, existing problems in reporting demand attention. The following actions can be taken, each of which focuses on a different part of the knowledge production line.

Better Review and Selection of Research Applications

As Jefferson and Godlee (1999) have pointed out, the process of peer review has failed not only in journal editing but also in research management. Steps are urgently needed to improve the review and selection of research applications. For this, research governance must improve the process of peer review, and, most importantly, insist that research applications are based on a comprehensive synthesis, systematic review, or previous work conducted in the field.

Better Research Conduct

Once the correct method has been chosen for a research application, particular attention must be given to its management. Steps must be taken to provide information for trial managers and all associated with the management of the research project.

Better Reporting of Research

Removal of Poor-quality Research Reports

A number of organizations have been created to assist clinicians and patients in gaining access to high-quality information (see Schünemann et al., this volume). PRISMA, for example, seeks to "purify" primary research evidence by identifying and removing those studies which, although they have been peer-reviewed, contain significant flaws in methodology so as to render them unfit to be included in the systematic review of the research evidence. "Pure" articles are published in secondary publication journals or made available as a filtrate of the research literature.

Maintenance and Availability of High-quality Research Reports

Whenever possible, results from high-quality studies should be combined using meta-analysis. Research conclusions should be written in a style that is accessible to clinicians and patient, and the evidence base must be kept current by identifying new studies for inclusion.

No matter how effective we may be in improving research reports, it is next to impossible for any one individual to keep up with current medical literature. Sackett et al. (1996) estimated that a general physician would need to read about 19 papers a day simply to stay current, but these 19 papers are but a small subset of the more than 1,500 indexed via MEDLINE each day. To address this problem, the American College of Physicians developed the ACP Journal Club which:

- developed explicit methods to scan the 100 top medical journals,
- selects journal articles based on strict and explicit quality criteria,

- selects a subset of these articles on the basis of their clinical relevance,
- prepared structured abstracts of the selected articles,
- invites a clinician with expertise in the topic to comment on the structured abstract, and
- prepares a "declarative title" summarizing the finding of the research study in a single sentence, which could be read in under fifteen seconds.

The ACP Journal Club has been widely copied and other secondary publications now exist: *Evidence-Based Medicine, Evidence-Based Mental Health, Evidence-Based Cardiovascular Medicine, Evidence-Based Oncology, Evidence-Based Nursing,* and *Evidence-Based Dentistry.*

These secondary publication journals distill the contents of over 300 journals and select only about 2% of the articles published originally in the primary journals; selection is based on quality and relevancy to the target readers. As such, secondary publication journals represent a new and important source of quality knowledge.

McKibbon et al. (2004) analyzed the work of the team tasked with filtering out poor-quality published articles and identifying those which were both of good methodological quality and high clinical relevance. They reviewed 60,352 articles in 170 journals in 2000 and of these only 3,059 original articles and 1,073 review articles met the criteria. Furthermore, the journals did not make an equal contribution to this total (Table 7.1).

Table 7.1   Contribution of articles from primary publications to evidence-based secondary journals, based on the analysis by McKibbon et al. (2004). For example, 4 journals contributed 56.5% of the articles selected by the ACP Journal Club, 28 journals contributed 43.5%, and among the remaining 55 journals no single article met the criteria for being included.

Number of Primary journals	Articles contributed (%)	Secondary publication
4	56.5	*ACP Journal Club*
28	43.5	(internal medicine)
55	0	
5	50.7	*Evidence-Based Medicine*
40	49.3	(general practice/primary care)
0	0	
7	51	*Evidence-Based Nursing*
34	49	
33	0	
9	53.2	*Evidence-Based Mental*
34	46.8	*Health*
8	0	

McKibbon et al. introduced a criteria of usefulness—the *number needed to read* (NNR); that is, the number of articles needed to be read before one of adequate quality and clinical relevancy could be identified. In those journals in which no article was found, NNR was infinity; however, for many journals, more than 100 articles needed to be appraised by a trained librarian and then assessed by a clinician to identify a single article of adequate quality and clinical relevancy. Top of the league was the Cochrane Database of Systematic Reviews.

Give Priority to Systematic Reviews

As highlighted by Mulrow (1987) and Oxman and Guyatt (1988), the National Perinatal Epidemiology Unit in Oxford prioritized:

- the search for all high-quality evidence available, both published and unpublished;
- the development of quality criteria to determine which evidence, published and unpublished, met explicit quality standards;
- the synthesis of those pieces of evidence which met this explicit criteria into a systematic review.

The systematic reviews which resulted covered both the field of antenatal and perinatal care. Based on this effort, the Director of the National Perinatal Epidemiology Unit, Iain Chalmers, proposed that the same method be used to cover the whole of health care. The National R&D Programme in England funded a center to promote this work, and the U.K. Cochrane Centre was created when Scotland, Wales, and Northern Ireland joined to support this work.

The U.K. Cochrane Centre was able to build on the work done by the National Perinatal Epidemiology Unit, based not only on the expertise accumulated in preparing systematic reviews but also on the dramatic developments that took place in the early 1990s in the Internet. Since then, the international Cochrane Collaboration has developed further and is committed to the production, maintenance, and dissemination of systematic reviews on the effects of health care.

A Cochrane Review needs to be kept up to date. It involves consumers at all stages in the process, and should be published, primarily in electronic form, in the Cochrane Library.

The evidence that a significant number of trials published in high-prestige journals were contradicted by subsequent articles emphasizes the point that readers should not change their practice on the basis of a single paper (von Elm et al. 2008). Although Cochrane Reviews are noted for their commitment to updating, all documents have to be explicitly and regularly updated. Unless they are clearly listed as such, documentation should be treated with caution.

Develop Skills of Critical Appraisal

Readers need to be suspicious of everything they read, regardless of the eminence of the author or venerability of its source. They must learn to appraise papers and all sources of medical information, including guidelines, advertisements, and articles in medical weeklies. They need to be able to appraise papers not only for their research quality and the quality of reporting but also for their contribution to the solution of the problems of the individual patient or population for which the professional is responsible. This often requires results to be rewritten to make them more usable; for example, by converting relative risk data into absolute risk data.

Be Aware of Certain Uncertainty

When a patient or professional first faces a problem, there may be uncertainty as to which action to take. This uncertainty is called "uncertain uncertainty"; namely, the decision maker does not know whether the knowledge that would help them make the decisions exists or not. By organizing knowledge properly, the person looking for knowledge can quickly find whether an answer exists or whether no one knows the answer, the latter being known as "certain uncertainty." To support the prioritization of future research, a database of uncertainties about the effects of treatments (DUETs) has been established (NHS 2010).

Support Journal Editors and Peer Reviewers

The improvement of research reporting is the primary responsibility of journal editors and publishers, and they are making progress. The Fourth International Congress on Peer Review and Biomedical Publication, held in Barcelona in September 2001, yielded impressive and encouraging results. The quality of reporting can be measured and reviewed systematically (Biondi-Zoccai et al. 2006). It is important for those who use evidence to contribute to these efforts and support education and research in this area.

Assist the Busy Reader

The gap between the amount of information available and the time available to process it is immense. Even if busy clinicians and patients were able to rely on peer-reviewed reports of primary research (given that all articles conformed perfectly to standards and reported without abbreviation), and the Internet was used to supplement conventional journal articles, not every reader is able to grasp the complexity of an issue. Good-quality systematic reviews are more reliable, but may also be difficult to read.

Busy readers benefit from synopses based on high-quality systematic reviews, but they also need to know when there is no reliable evidence on a particular topic. Journals have a valuable contribution to make in research, but they are not a source of knowledge support for clinicians and patients.

NHS Evidence is a service that provides easy access to high-quality clinical and nonclinical information about health and social care (NHS Evidence 2010). Although it can be accessed by anyone interested in health and social care making decisions, it is primarily designed for professionals and practitioners. A complementary service, NHS Choices, is available and may be more appropriate for patients and the general public (NHS Choices 2010).

Toward the Future: The Century of the Patient

Moving beyond our discussion of medical research and reporting, we need to consider the knowledge that is being created. A significant debate has transpired as to the type of information appropriate for patients versus clinicians. One approach views these as two separate groups, each with their own needs. Another perceives them as one population and allows individuals to seek out their own level.

Using the reporting of probabilities as an example, it is not difficult to find some patients who understand probabilities better than some clinicians. Even still, it can be argued that although patients understand probabilities, they lack an understanding of the pathology they face. However, it is not necessary to understand the physiology of, say, the gall bladder to weigh the risks and benefits of having a cholecystectomy.

Access to the Internet has made attempts to segregate knowledge intended for clinicians from patients futile. Thus, it may be more beneficial to focus on steps to personalize medicine. Personalized medicine can be thought of as relating the best, current evidence (i.e., which is mass-produced knowledge produced by teams in a way that no individual can match) to the unique needs and conditions of the individual (Figure 7.2). As such, it is a medical example of what industry terms mass customization.

Access to and understanding of evidence are only the beginning. Before decision making can be complete, evidence must be related to the needs and conditions of the individual patient. In turn, the patient must reflect on how these options relate to his/her personal values. Only then can an effective health care decision be achieved. In its absence, unnecessary treatment is often the result.

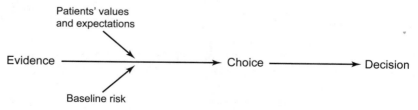

Figure 7.2   Scheme to mass customize medical decision making.

As society comes to grips with increasingly scarce financial resources, ways must be found to transform available resources more effectively. Knowledge is clearly one such resource; human ingenuity is another.

Equipping all members of society—patients and health care professionals alike—with the necessary skills in health literacy is the first step in understanding the available evidence. This, in turn, will increase the level of trust between everyone involved in health care (from industry, health care professionals, and patients) since everyone will have the tools to evaluate the information reported. Health care decisions can then be tailored to individual needs and preferences.

Just as knowledge drove the Industrial Revolution, so too can it transform health care. We must persevere in our efforts to improve research trials and the transparent reporting thereof, so that informed citizens can make optimal use of the results.

Overleaf (left to right, top to bottom):
Jack Wennberg, Gerd Gigerenzer, Marjukka Mäkelä
Al Mulley, Claudia Wild, Gerd Antes
Johann Steurer, Jay Schulkin, David Nelson
Holger Schünemann, Markus A. Feufel, Muir Gray

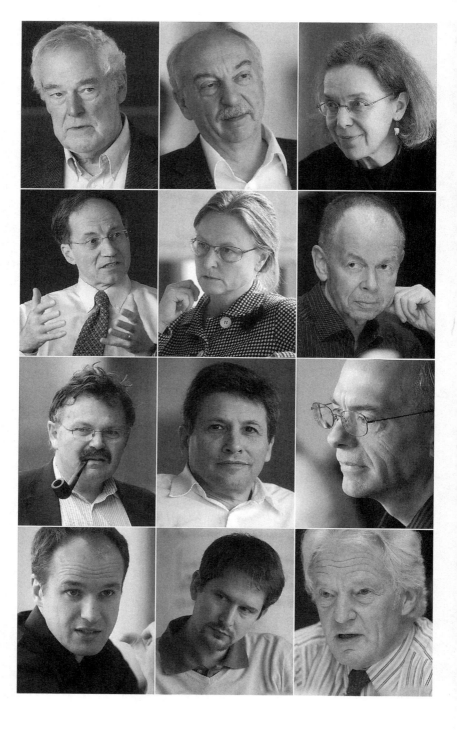

8

What Is Needed for Better Health Care: Better Systems, Better Patients or Both?

Markus A. Feufel, Gerd Antes, Johann Steurer,
Gerd Gigerenzer, J. A. Muir Gray, Marjukka Mäkelä,
Albert G. Mulley, Jr., David E. Nelson, Jay Schulkin,
Holger Schünemann, John E. Wennberg, and Claudia Wild

Abstract

Patients' health illiteracy is, in part, a consequence of how the health care system has been set up. Conversely, the flaws of the health care system and the interest groups it caters to can only exist to the degree that patients remain uninformed. Thus, to improve health care, two strategies are presented which aim to solve an interrelated problem from different angles. The first involves changing the health care system by introducing new, and enforcing existing, guidelines and procedures designed to reduce funding and reporting biases as well as financial conflicts of interests. If a health care system can be freed of these problems, patients, independent of their health literacy level, will be able to get good health care, simply by trusting their doctor and the information provided. The second requires educating the public to increase knowledge about how their health care system works (health system literacy). If patients become more health system literate, they will be able to identify if and why evidence is missing, incomplete, or unreliable and will get better health care because they are not easily misled by nonmedical interests acting within their health care system. Although it remains to be seen which of these approaches will be easier to implement, the association of the problems they target suggests that an effective intervention will need to incorporate both approaches.

Introduction

Research has shown that the communication of scientific evidence is often incomplete and/or nontransparent, thus reducing its usability (Gigerenzer et al. 2007). This compromises health literacy (i.e., the ability to understand

and use the current evidence base) of clinicians (Wegwarth and Gigerenzer, this volume), policy makers, as well as the general public (Gaissmaier and Gigerenzer, this volume). However, the issues that surround the problem of missing information and nontransparent communication constitute only one part of a larger, systemic health literacy problem. In this chapter, we review our group's discussions of this problem and provide initial suggestions as to how it can be addressed.

Over the past fifty years, a large infrastructure has been created to support research in basic science and the development of products and services for use in health care settings. In most health care systems, this infrastructure has supported and is currently funding research that is not based solely on the needs of patients and clinicians; instead it also caters to the diverging interests of stakeholders from industry (e.g., financial viability), politics (e.g., lobby interests), academia (e.g., career incentives, publication standards), and funding agencies (e.g., prioritization of certain types of research; Nelson, this volume). Moreover, when future research priorities are set or interventions identified to make care delivery safer and more efficient, previously generated data (Schünemann et al., this volume) and population-based databases (Mulley and Wennberg, this volume) are often underused or simply ignored. Thus, part of the available evidence used to make medical decisions may not (at least not directly) address questions that are pertinent to decision makers at the clinical or policy level. Finally, the sheer amount of research produced each year makes it difficult to discover which information may be relevant. In addition, one must know where to find it and be able to assess whether the information source is reliable. Together, these systemic problems hamper the quality of the available evidence and make it difficult for patients, clinicians, policy makers, and researchers to make evidence-based decisions.

To improve health care, we believe that patients' health literacy needs to be complemented by *health system literacy*; that is, people's understanding of how their health system works, including the reasons why and how it hampers theirs health literacy. Because patients with high health system literacy are able to identify if and why evidence is missing, incomplete, or unreliable, they are not easily misled by nonmedical interests acting within their health care system. Ultimately, they can use the available evidence and health care resources to address their needs in a more effective manner.

Tackling Low Health System Literacy

In a general sense, our goal is to raise awareness and inform the reader about the major problems and potential solutions that emerged from our discussions of health (system) literacy. To structure our discussions, we were guided by a process (Figure 8.1) which ranged from the selection of relevant research topics to the reporting and dissemination of obtained results, and medical decision

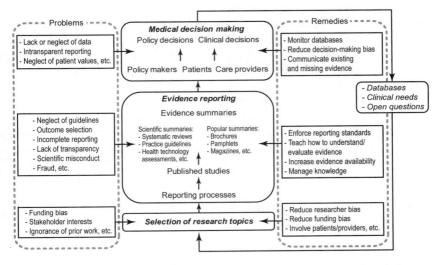

Figure 8.1 Tackling low health system literacy: Problems and remedies. Left: systemic problems that hamper good health care by biasing the selection of research topics, evidence reporting, and medical decision making. Right: remedies intended to improve health care by reducing systemic biases and increasing health system literacy of the stakeholders involved in the selection, reporting, and implementation of research.

making. As depicted in Figure 8.1 (left side), there are major problems and/or biases at each step in this process which may hamper patients' health literacy and evidence-based decision making. These problems are addressed in depth elsewhere in this volume: selection of research topics (Nelson, Chapter 5); the dissemination of evidence (Schünemann et al., Chapter 6; Gray, Chapter 7); and biases that undermine medical decision making (Gaissmaier and Gigerenzer, Chapter 2; Wegwarth and Gigerenzer, Chapter 9; Mulley and Wennberg, Chapter 3). Our discussions focused on identifying the mechanisms that could be implemented to remedy these problems or at least reduce their negative impact on informed and evidence-based decision making (Figure 8.1, right side).

Two different opinions or strategies emerged from our group: The first emphasized interventions that aim to raise levels of health system literacy by better *educating the public* as well as care providers. Here, the idea is that citizens with high health system literacy will be more health literate and able to make better decisions because they are aware of the biases that undermine evidence generation and dissemination. The second argued that uninformed medical decisions due to low levels of health (system) literacy could be circumvented if interventions are implemented to *change the health care system* so that a lack of information is no longer an impediment to good and sustainable decision making. For example, if the distorting influence of agendas, which reflect interests other than those related to good medical care, is reduced or eliminated, patients as well as providers will be able to make good medical decisions by simply trusting each other as well as the quality of the information they are given. In other words, the negative influence of systemic problems (Figure 8.1, left) on good health care can be reduced by (a) educating the public to increase health (system) literacy and (b) changing the health care system so that patients do not need to be health (system) literate to make good medical decisions.

On the surface, it seems easier to improve patient education and information than to change the current health care system. However, we could not agree which approach would ultimately yield more leverage, and therefore be more effective in bringing about the necessary changes. The interventions that we identified suggest that both approaches will be necessary to tackle the problem. To illustrate this, we describe examples of both classes of interventions with respect to the three major steps of the evidence generation process diplayed in Figure 8.1: selection of research topics, evidence reporting, and medical decision making.

Selection of Research Topics

Unlike basic research in most sciences, basic as well as applied health research must yield information that has the potential to improve care delivery and, ultimately, the functioning of the health care system. To do this, health research must ascertain knowledge gaps in clinical practice and ensure that practice-relevant questions receive adequate funding and attention using the best available scientific practice. The agenda-setting process for medical research often conforms, however, to other standards set by political, scientific, and financial interest groups (Nelson, this volume). The distorting influence that results from such interest groups hampers not only the value of research efforts for patients but also negatively impacts scientific quality. If the research community continues to set agendas for politically influential stakeholders, the data generated may be redundant (e.g., new placebo-tested drugs may not be better than already available competitors) or, worse, irrelevant to clinical practice. This is particularly detrimental in times of increasing financial bottlenecks, scarce resources, and aging populations with increasing needs for medical care. In this section, we discuss how the health care environment can be reshaped and the public involved in the selection of research topics, so that the evidence which results will be more beneficial to clinicians, patients, and policy makers.

Change the Health Care System

Reduce Researcher Bias

The first step toward change involves reducing researcher bias. The careers of medical researchers depend on how many of their articles get published in high-impact journals. Publication in these journals is more likely if the submitted manuscripts contain quantitative analyses of original data from clinical trials and report positive results (Gray, this volume). This, in turn, encourages individual scientists to "produce" such data to enhance their careers. To increase the number of publications, the same trial and patient data may get published several times by exploiting subgroup analyses. This has a detrimental effect as it limits a reader's ability to gauge the clinical implications of piecemeal results and inhibits an assessment of their validity. At the same time, a high number of publications gives the impression of continuous, even rapid, scientific progress and is generally fostered by the current research structures.

To circumvent researcher bias, journals must make a systematic (as opposed to selective) analysis of previous research a precondition for publication. Journals must also ensure that methodological "gold standards" have been considered during the research planning process. One example of this is a practice followed by *The Lancet*: researchers are guaranteed that their article will get reviewed if a trial protocol is submitted before the study is initiated. In addition, the (medical) science community must change its value systems and begin to consider the publication of both negative findings and evidence syntheses (as compared to original research) to be an integral part of what it means to be a good and successful researcher.

Reduce Funding Bias

The second step in changing the health care environment involves reducing bias associated with the funding of medical research. Here there are two fundamental yet related problems: selection is driven by the need to contribute to technological development as well as to basic science.

In the United States as well as in other Western countries (Shi and Singh 2008), the notion of "innovation" equates to high-tech knowledge and applications.[1] As a result, procedures which seem less high-tech may be disregarded because they are not as highly valued. Although they may yield inexpensive improvements to current clinical practices, they may be less likely to receive funding or be researched. Today, most Western health care systems are under considerable public pressure to finance projects that will yield high-end technologies to improve innovative products for clinical use and to reimburse the technologies once they are introduced into the health care market. To do this, health care systems must increasingly rely on industry, where research is conducted with the goal of successfully being able to sell the resulting technologies. As a result, approval and reimbursing agencies, health politicians, and

---

[1] For example, the 7th EU Framework Programme for Research and Technological Development is structured into nine "fields of cooperation." Six of these areas focus on various technologies; only two center on societal problems (health and public security). Although the areas are defined as fields of cooperation, the focus on specialized technologies limits interdisciplinary problem-solving activities.

health technology assessment (HTA) specialists are increasingly faced with new but often inefficient, or worse, clinically irrelevant medical products that are aggressively marketed by the developing companies.

To circumvent the problems associated with technology-driven funding, approval of health technologies should be based on "relative" or "comparative" effectiveness with respect to already available technologies (e.g., "head-to-head" trials comparing two actual products). To date the Food and Drug Administration (FDA) in the United States and the European Medicines Agency (EMA) approve medications on the basis of efficacy compared to a placebo group, not compared to competitors. Most surgical interventions and other medical interventions do not have to undergo a standardized approval process at all. Other approval criteria should include validated, patient-relevant outcomes rather than standard, surrogate outcomes (e.g., cognitive impairment has long been a neglected outcome of cardiac surgery).

To reduce funding bias further, we must stop searching for fields of application for new technologies and, instead, prioritize research agendas that aim to identify solutions to societal problems. To do so, we must also address the preference for basic rather than translational or evaluation research. To date, far more than half of R&D expenses in the United States are allocated for basic research, much less than for translational (e.g., health services) research, the monitoring of health systems performance (cf. Mulley and Wennberg, this volume), health literacy, or evaluation research (cf. Nelson, this volume). For medical research to be worthwhile and effective, scientists need to follow an innovation cycle by establishing a feedback loop between efforts that identify and monitor socially relevant problems, scientific theories and research, and translation and implementation efforts. A role model in this regard can be found in the United Kingdom, where the National Health Service (NHS) began to allocate resources for evaluation research about 15 years ago, including HTAs and research on patient-relevant outcomes (NIHR CCF 2010). The results of these efforts are used to generate new questions and problems to be solved through further basic research.

By paying greater attention to effectiveness considerations and making an effort to assess the impact of basic *and* translational research results, we will not only advance our knowledge but also come closer to solving major societal problems.

Educate the Public

Involve Patients and Providers in the Research Process

Involving people in the research process will ensure that useful evidence is generated. All citizens—clinicians, patients, and policy makers—have a vested interest when it comes to heath care, and all have a valuable contribution to make in providing information about clinical practice. Research grounded in the needs of those who will ultimately benefit has the potential of providing not only answers to pertinent clinical questions but being more readily implemented and accepted. Public involvement would also create bidirectional benefits: researchers would learn from patients and care providers, while patients and care providers would learn about research methods and results, thereby contributing to their health (system) literacy. This approach has the potential of yielding research findings that matter and deliver better evidence-based care.

One way to increase the selection of clinically relevant research topics is to conduct research on patient-relevant outcomes. In the United Kingdom, for example, the National Institute for Health Research (NIHR) strives to increase the involvement of patients or, more generally, members of the public in the research development process (NIHR Awareness 2010). To identify research topics that address patients' needs, NIHR attempts to involve patients at all stages of the research process: from the development of research priorities, to helping scientists decide what goals research should achieve, recruiting participants, choosing research methods, and publicizing evidence that is easy to comprehend and can be applied during care delivery. However, the extent to which patients can or want to be involved in all stages of the research process is unclear.

Some in our group suggested that it may not be necessary to involve patients or even health care providers in all methodological or analytic decisions, as they are unlikely to understand them. We agreed, however, that patients can and should be involved in developing and funding research studies as well as in the presentation, interpretation, and dissemination of findings.

Another way to increase the selection of clinically relevant research topics is to involve health care providers in the research selection process. Take, for example, the Managed Uptake of Medical Methods (MUMM) program developed by the Finnish hospital districts in association with the Finnish Office for Health Technology Assessment (Finohta).[2] Under MUMM, hospitals themselves propose and select which new medical technologies should be evaluated by Finohta.

In 2008, for example, the hospital districts in Finland proposed that an HTA be done on bariatric surgery, and Finohta agreed to perform the HTA (cf. Ikonen et al. 2009). The Finnish Social Insurance Institution (SII) postponed its decision to fund bariatric surgery in the private sector until the HTA was 18 months underway. HTA results suggest that, given the estimated number of operations per year (1,300–2,600), centralizing operations to no more than ten hospitals was acceptable in terms of safety standards and that, over a period of ten years, this centralization would likely save the health care system up to 13,000 Euros per operation (cf. Mäkelä and Roine 2009). The Finnish Ministry

---

[2] Finohta is a unit working within the National Institute for Health and Welfare that in Finland evaluates the effectiveness, harms, and cost of health technologies as well as their social, ethical, organizational, and legal consequences.

of Health, the hospital districts, and the SII are currently discussing how to implement these findings.

The MUMM program demonstrates clearly how cooperation between knowledge customers and HTA researchers (e.g., with respect to the chosen topic, the time frame, and the level of detail of an HTA) can lead to the identification of clinically relevant topics, timely research efforts, and facilitation of implementation once evidence is obtained.

Evidence Reporting

In addition to the lack of relevant research, low levels of health literacy are exacerbated by nontransparent reporting of evidence (which compromises its usability) and the difficulty one encounters in accessing existing evidence. The absence of complete and transparent evidence is primarily due to the following:

1. Existing research and reporting standards are not adhered to nor are they enforced (cf. Schünemann et al. and Gray, both this volume).
2. Nonmedical agendas adversely influence reporting.
3. Researchers and physicians lack knowledge about the well-established principles of effective risk communication (cf. Gigerenzer et al. 2007).

In line with our overall strategies for interventions, we present ways in which available evidence can be reported optimally by affecting changes in the health care system and through educating the public.

Change the Health Care System

Selective publication of original research has been the topic of intense debate over the last decades, but thus far little has improved. Many researchers still publish their studies selectively (the "file drawer" problem). Evaluation research performed in various countries has consistently shown that only about 50% of the trials approved by ethics boards are actually published within ten years after completion (Blümle et al. 2008). One contributing factor to the "file drawer" problem may be that about one-third of the trials published in the *British Medical Journal* (BMJ) and about two-thirds of the articles published in the major North American journals are funded by the pharmaceutical industry, which has a vested interest in presenting positive results (Egger et al. 2001). In fact, those studies that are published often suffer from selective, result-driven reporting of what actually transpired during the research process. Often, primary patient-relevant outcomes are dropped and secondary (surrogate) outcomes are reported instead; other characteristics are changed to avoid unfavorable (i.e., nonsignificant), and therefore "difficult to sell" results (Wild and Piso 2010). Because studies that yield positive results tend to be published more quickly and frequently, positive outcomes appear in publications, usually without acknowledgment of their serendipitous origin.

Adding to publication bias on the researchers' side is the fact that most medical journals do not enforce existing reporting guidelines, let alone transparent formatting of the reported evidence (cf. Schünemann et al., this volume; Hopewell et al. 2010). One likely reason is that journal editors must balance scientific with financial interests. Richard Smith (2005), former editor of the *BMJ* and former chief executive officer of the BMJ Publishing Group, explains the dependency between medical journals and the pharmaceutical industry this way:

> The most conspicuous example of medical journals' dependence on the pharmaceutical industry is the substantial income from advertising, but this is, I suggest, the least corrupting form of dependence....For a drug company, a favorable trial is worth thousands of pages of advertising....Publishers know that pharmaceutical companies will often purchase thousands of dollars worth of reprints, and the profit margin on reprints is likely to be 70%. Editors, too, know that publishing such studies is highly profitable, and editors are increasingly responsible for the budgets of their journals and for producing a profit for the owners....An editor may thus face a frighteningly stark conflict of interest: publish a trial that will bring US$100,000 of profit or meet the end-of-year budget by firing an editor.

It is in the very interest of pharmaceutical companies to present the results in a way that is most likely to impress the readers and, particularly, the doctors who receive the reprints (e.g., by reporting relative instead of absolute risk reductions). Most clinicians are likely to be unaware of the biases inherent in the production, publication, and formatting of the reported evidence, thus demonstrating another example of deficient health system literacy. Thus, positive study results may receive increased attention and gain credibility simply because they have been pushed through various media.

Selective reporting depletes health literacy levels of all stakeholders in the health care system and may cause serious errors in the assessment of interventions, in the planning of further research, and in the work of ethics boards. Specifically, systematic reviews which summarize the results from multiple trials give, on average, an overoptimistic impression of the effectiveness of a treatment because negative trials have not been included. Ethics boards may approve trials that have been run before, with negative results, or have even been cancelled or stopped because of serious side effects. As a result, patients may be exposed to adverse effects that went unreported in similar previous trials; this is not only unethical but has potentially harmful effects.

Complete and transparent reporting of all (i.e., positive and negative) research results is therefore a crucial prerequisite for health literacy and the realization of good evidence-based health care.

Enforce Existing and Implement New Reporting Standards

To reduce bias in evidence dissemination, several issues must be addressed. First, mechanisms that are already in place (see reporting guidelines in EQUATOR Network 2010) must be adhered to and enforced, so that their potential impact can be realized. Concurrently, these mechanisms must be evaluated for flaws in implementation or intent. Once the use of guidelines becomes common, it will then be possible and necessary to assess their impact; that is, whether they have yielded benefits in terms of increased quality of the reported evidence and, ultimately, better health outcomes.

Second, new procedures currently under discussion must be introduced. To date, this has been possible in only a few countries, such as the United States. Some of these procedures focus on pre-research activities and include prospective trial registration and, more generally, scientific guidelines for good research and reporting. Another group focuses on post-research activities and consists of mechanisms such as result registration (in trial registers), quality assessment of research results, and new requirements for the publication process such as open access databases and a legal basis for mandatory disclosure of trial results for drugs and medical devices. So far, these procedures have been implemented in only a few countries, such as the United States.

To date, Richard Smith and Ian Roberts (2006) have put forth the most radical proposal to circumvent reporting biases (e.g., the fact that authors' interpretations of data are more closely correlated with their beliefs and expectations than with the data). Details of their proposal are summarized in Table 8.1. In essence, they propose to eliminate subjective elements by making study and data analysis plans public before, during, and after a study. Their most drastic suggestion is to eliminate any kind of data interpretation by investigators.

Table 8.1 Overview of a new research and reporting system, as proposed by Smith and Roberts (2006).

1.	A systematic review is posted on the Web.
2.	If a new trial is needed, it is registered; a full protocol is devised in light of the systematic review and posted on the Web.
3.	Anybody can comment online on the interpretation of the systematic review data, the importance of the trial question, or the reliability of its methods.
4.	The statistical analysis would be prespecified and preprogrammed.
5.	Once data collection is complete, the entire data set would be uploaded and the analyses run.
6.	There would be no investigator commentary on the trial data.
7.	The systematic review would be updated to include the new trial.
8.	Journals would not publish trials but rather commentaries and reports on systematic reviews.

Instead, everybody should have the opportunity to comment on the study design and the relevance of the results.

Although the proposal by Smith and Roberts strives to eliminate investigator-driven, potentially biased post hoc analyses and biased interpretations in discussion sections, it is unclear to what degree this radical approach can actually eliminate biases. Despite seemingly democratic data management and interpretation procedures, there are currently few people who can actually understand, and therefore evaluate and comment on, the reported results. In other words, methodologists and researchers still hold the power over the data, and their biases would go unnoticed by those less experienced with study design, data analyses, and interpretation. Therefore, to increase health (system) literacy and the quality of medical decision making, another complementary leverage point is vital: clinicians, policy makers, and the general public must be better informed and educated.

Educate the Public

Teach How to Understand and Evaluate Evidence

An important factor for achieving better health care is patients' initiative and involvement in their own treatment process. The general public is by and large unaware of scientific evidence that is relevant to most medical decisions. Even if they are aware of such evidence, most people, including physicians, find it difficult to understand (cf. Gaissmaier and Gigerenzer; Wegwarth and Gigerenzer, both this volume); it is often perceived as counterintuitive, abstract, or even a nuisance. In short, it interferes with their usual way of thinking and conflicts with what they would like to achieve. Thus, to enable health literacy, health system literacy, and statistical literacy, patients, doctors, and policy makers need specific training in how to evaluate and understand the evidence presented to them as well as the process of communicating evidence to others.

As a society, we are most likely to impact a person's level of statistical literacy in health by including the mathematics of uncertainty in the educational curriculum of children and adolescents (for methods, see Martignon and Krauss 2009). To increase people's health (system) literacy and their ability to evaluate the quality of the obtained evidence, it will be necessary to inform people about publication biases, biases of journal editors, as well as the interest groups and personal agendas that underlie these biases. Whereas researchers and some skeptical citizens may be aware of these problems, most are unaware that research results may not be as objective as they are often portrayed. Merely pointing out biases (as we are doing here) does not suffice, however. Clinicians and patients also need to know where they can obtain quality evidence when they need it.

Make Evidence Widely Available

At present, existing evidence suffers not only from biases but is also disorganized and therefore difficult to access. To improve this situation, evidence should be collected globally and its quality assessed, summarized, and communicated in a transparent format. Over the last 15–20 years, different types of formats have been developed and implemented. These may roughly be categorized as evidence reports, clinical guidelines, HTA reports, patient information texts, and other less common, or less standardized, formats. Although these formats are generally available (e.g., in Cochrane Reviews), there is great variability with respect to the ease of access to these sources, between countries as well as between cities and institutions. Reasons for these inequalities include logistic, language, and financial barriers. For example, even in a G8 country such as Germany, it is not uncommon to find a nonuniversity teaching hospital that lacks a library or access to relevant journals. Doctors at these institutions often have no, or only limited, access to the Internet or other electronic information sources. Thus, even the basic preconditions for evidence-based practice are not always given.

Another limiting factor is language. High-quality evidence is currently published almost entirely in English, in scientific journals that are not openly available (i.e., access is managed through subscriptions). This situation can only be circumvented with adequate funding and knowledge management. For example, Cochrane Reviews provide quality evidence to both lay and expert audiences, and are translated into several languages. However, except for abstracts, studies prepared by the Cochrane Collaboration are currently not freely available. Access to the Cochrane Library must be purchased and costs approximately US$0.018 per citizen per year for national provisions, allowing barrier-free access throughout the entire country. This financial barrier greatly hinders the availability of transparent, easy-to-use evidence for patients, clinicians, and policy makers. While some European countries and Canada invest in the health literacy of their citizens and provide them free access to the Cochrane Library, G8 countries such as the United States and Germany currently do not. Also, in Germany, there appears to be little awareness of the very existence of the Cochrane Collaboration among politicians, physicians, and patients.

Increase Efforts at Knowledge Management

Finally, access to current knowledge requires continuous efforts to update reviews of already available evidence, and the prerequisite funds to accomplish so-called cumulative meta-analyses and evidence summaries. The Cochrane Collaboration is currently the only major organization that continuously updates the systematic reviews contained in its library. In light of the ever-increasing flood of new research studies, all of which are subject to the biases mentioned above, lack of funding for knowledge management is dangerous, leading to outdated data sources and, ultimately, inferior information for those who have to apply the evidence on a daily basis.

Medical Decision Making

Ideally, relevant evidence is available before a decision is made and taken into consideration during the decision-making process. Unfortunately, this rarely happens. In the absence of relevant evidence, clinical decisions have to be made under considerable uncertainty. In other situations, evidence exists but people have no access or simply ignore its implications. As described by Gigerenzer and Gray (this volume) a common but costly, and sometimes dangerous, medical problem is blood stream infection due to the insertion of central vein catheters. Research based on data from more than 100 intensive care units (ICUs) has shown that the rate of infection can be reliably reduced from 2.7 to close to 0 infections per 1,000 catheter-days by following a simple checklist procedure that outlines how to insert central vein catheters safely (Pronovost et al. 2006). Although this checklist is simple and based on solid evidence, it has not been widely implemented. Why has this fairly inexpensive but effective approach not been adopted? More generally, what can be done to exact a more efficient use of available evidence when it comes to making medical decisions?

Change the Health Care System

Monitor System Performance through Population-based Databases

Many health care interventions lack sufficient evidence to assess their benefits and harms reliably. A simple solution would be to perform more valid trials and studies. While this is, in principle, possible, it is time-intensive and costly. Much research money and efforts could be saved if existing evidence was utilized more effectively; namely, data that is stored in population-based databases. Most of this data are currently "locked up" in file drawers of hospital administrations, sickness funds, and clearing houses of pharmacies or other institutions, which routinely store data about medical resource usage. We believe that it is inefficient, and in some cases unethical, to store such information without installing mechanisms to allow access and publication in appropriate and useful ways. This data could provide the rationale for focused interventions and play an important role in clinical and policy decision making, particularly at a time when worldwide financial constraints are forcing cutbacks in public funding of health care.

Routine databases could be exploited, for example, to manage more effectively the problem of "supply-sensitive" care, for which the frequency of treatment depends on the resources that are locally available (e.g., the number of medical specialists or hospital beds per person). In certain regions of the United States, for instance, there is evidence that supply-sensitive care is over-used in treating patients with chronic illness. Clinical decision making seems geared to the assumption that more is better, and this leads to resource exhaustion, no matter how many resources are available. However, patients living in such high-intensity regions do not enjoy better (and indeed sometimes worse) outcomes than those who live in low-intensity regions, in terms of survival rates, relative advantage in functional status, and patient satisfaction with hospital experiences (see Wennberg et al. 2008).

Based on data from 306 hospital referral regions in the United States, Table 8.2 shows that the Medicare program paid $22,500 more for a chronically

Table 8.2 Practice patterns in managing chronic illness of Medicare patients who died between 2001 and 2005 according to U.S. referral regions that ranked highest and lowest on hospital care intensity. The hospital care intensity (HCI) index for the last two years of life is based on patient days spent in hospital and number of inpatient visits. The low and high quintiles contain approximately equal numbers of patients (after Wennberg et al. 2008).

	HCI Quintile		
	Lowest	Highest	Ratio
HCI index score	0.67	1.46	2.17
Resource inputs during the last 2 years of life:			
Medicare spending per patient	$38,300	$60,800	1.59
Physician labor inputs per 1,000 patients[a]			
All physicians	16.6	29.5	1.78
Medical specialists	5.6	13.1	2.35
Primary care physicians	7.4	11.5	1.55
Ratio primary care physicians to medical specialists	1.34	0.88	0.66
Hospital bed inputs per 1,000 patients	40.0	70.8	1.77
Terminal care:			
Patient days per patient last 6 months of life	8.5	15.6	1.83
Inpatient visits per patient last 6 months of life	12.9	36.3	2.82
Percent who see 10 or more doctors last 6 months of life	20.2	43.7	2.16
Percent of deaths with ICU admission	14.3	23.2	1.63
Percent enrolled in hospice	30.1	30.2	1.00

[a] To develop measures of physician labor input, Wennberg and colleagues used data from a national study of physician productivity to obtain estimates of the average annual number of work relative value units (W-RVUs) produced per physician on a specialty-specific basis. Using Medicare Part B data, they then calculated the specialty-specific sum of W-RVUs provided to a cohort over a given period. Finally, the sum of W-RVUs was divided by the average annual number of W-RVUs per physician to estimate the "standardized full-time-equivalent (FTE) physician labor input" per 1,000 cohort members.

ill patient living in a high-intensity region ($60,800) compared to those who live in low-intensity regions ($38,300). Moreover, providers in high- as compared to low-intensity regions used 2.35 times more medical specialists (13.1 compared to 5.6 expert physician labor inputs per 1,000 patients) and 77% more hospital beds when providing care (70.8 as compared to 40.0 hospital bed inputs per 1,000 patients). In high-intensity regions, 23% of the patients experience a "high-tech" death (e.g., in the ICU) compared to 14.3% of the patients who live in low-intensity regions. Overall, care intensity during the last two years of a person's life "explains" the 70% variation in overall Medicare spending. This reason alone makes a strong argument for exploiting routine databases to improve medical decision making, as it would reduce unwarranted practice variation and inefficient use of resources.

The opportunities for using large databases will differ, of course, from country to country depending on how the health services and health insurance systems are organized. However, all Western health economies have many, if not all, of the essential data elements for monitoring health systems performance. Information about how the health care system actually works will help improve people's health system literacy and, ultimately, health care.

Reduce Decision-making Bias

As demonstrated above with the simple checklist procedure (Pronovost et al. 2006), good evidence, even if available and easy to implement, may simply be ignored. The degree of "evidence neglect" that occurs is specific to the medical domain; it is not found to a similar extent in other safety critical domains, such as commercial aviation. Potential reasons are manifold. It may be that medicine lacks a safety culture, preferring to place blame on "negligent" individuals instead of faulty organizational procedures (e.g., Wilf-Miron et al. 2003). In addition, medical failures are frequent and do not usually cause a lot of media attention; medical innovations are also associated with high-tech solutions, not simple checklists (cf. Shi and Singh 2008). Thus, there is no interest on the part of pharmaceutical or medical device companies to develop and implement simple interventions, especially if monetary gain is limited. Another reason might be physicians' beliefs that simpler interventions (e.g., a checklist) undermine their claims to expertise or their therapeutic freedom. Alternatively, some physicians—especially those that are reimbursed fee-for-service—may hope that simple interventions are not assessed to be effective, and are thus not officially implemented, because if they were, coverage by health insurance companies would equate to lower payment fees. Without coverage, an intervention may be used despite the lack of evidence of benefits; they can be prescribed without having to consider cost limits imposed by health insurances; and patients will pay for the (presumably) necessary medication out of their own pocket. To make things worse, patient information materials are often sponsored, if not entirely designed, by biomedical companies and their marketing departments.

A promising trend toward reducing the impact of financial interests on health care providers can be found in private initiatives by physicians: the "No Free Lunch" (2010) initiative in the United States or the "Mein Essen zahl ich selbst" (MEZIS 2010) in Germany and Austria. The physicians involved in these initiatives fight against corruption in the health care sector and biased advertising for medications. Their goal is to decrease (financial) dependencies between stakeholders in the system and generate transparent structures to support their interrelationships and communication patterns. Measures include continuing education opportunities for physicians that are financially and organizationally independent of the pharmacological industry. For example, e-learning applications can spread knowledge effectively to a potentially unlimited pool of participants and can be implemented without financial assistance from pharmaceutical companies.

Subject matter experts (e.g., those who serve on commissions for or against the recommendation of particular vaccinations or medications) often work as volunteers, without monetary compensation. Some members of our group felt that to reduce dependencies and opportunities for corruption, experts who serve on national health committees should be financially compensated. Others, in contrast, strongly opposed this proposal as being incompatible with the ideal of independent science. This group suggested that other incentives ("the honor to be considered a national expert") or sanctions ("undeclared conflict of interests will result in exclusion from any national expert committee") might have the same or even more sustainable effects.

Educate the Public

Communicate Existing and Missing Evidence

Transparent reporting implies more than properly formatting the available information. Those who report medical risks must acknowledge when scientific evidence is lacking and that medical decisions have to be made despite considerable uncertainty. Even with advanced technologies, society will never be able to anticipate and be fully prepared to react to epidemic threats such as the H1N1 (swine flu) virus. Instead of arguing for or against particular reactions to an uncertain health threat (e.g., to get vaccinated or not), we believe that patients benefit from an open discussion about reliable evidence and unknowns at the time. In Germany, for example, the *Ständige Impfkommission*, a permanent commission in charge of preventing infectious diseases, recommended vaccination against the H1N1 virus. At the time of recommendation (October, 2010) little was known about the potential threat to national health or the potential risks of vaccination. What was known, however, was not openly communicated (for details, see Feufel et al. 2010):

1. The swine flu virus had caused about 180,000 infections and 60 deaths in Germany. In contrast, seasonal flu results annually in 760,000–1,630,000 additional doctor's visits and approximately 8,000–11,000 deaths (Robert Koch Institute 2009).
2. The majority of citizens who died from H1N1 had serious preconditions, which amplified disease severity.
3. The development of the viral disease during the following winter was unclear but disease severity had not increased considerably during the winter season, which had just ended in the southern hemisphere.
4. The adjuvants added to increase the effectiveness of the vaccination serum had not been sufficiently tested prior to the implementation of the vaccination.
5. There were effective alternative prevention measures, such as using disinfectants and washing hands frequently.

Often, it is thought that contradicting facts and uncertainty might confuse people and make decisions more difficult. However, paternalistic campaigns that suggest "what to do" based on selective reporting and insufficient data only create false certainty, damage trust within a society, and render informed decision making fictional. We believe that the transparent reporting of both available as well as missing evidence is integral to a responsible management of uncertainty; it is an integral part of any democratic decision process, particularly when it comes to decisions about an individual's health and well-being. The future of health care in 2020 requires more transparent and democratic approaches to information management, so that care providers and patients will be able to work together more effectively to realize good and sustainable medical care. It is time to invest trust in patients, physicians, and policy makers: if informed about what is known and what is unknown, people will be able to make responsible decisions.

In summary, to improve the quality of medical decision making through increased health (system) literacy, we need to take advantage of data that already exists in public data repositories. Moreover, whether evidence is available or not, we must not let financial interests and sloppy information policies get in our way when it comes to informing patients and delivering good medical care. The future of health care in 2020 requires more transparent and democratic approaches to information management, so that care providers and patients will be able to work together more effectively to realize good and sustainable medical care.

Conclusions

The general public as well as many clinicians and policy makers are not well equipped to make evidence-based medical decisions that reliably and sustainably meet their needs. Because they cannot understand and use the evidence offered, they are said to have low health literacy. This is not due to people's inherent inability to understand and process medical evidence but is rooted in the obstacles and biases undermining the processes of evidence generation, reporting, and medical decision making. Without knowledge of the root causes underlying health system functioning, patients and clinicians—often without being aware of it—do not know where to find relevant and transparent information to address their concerns, and are at a loss when it comes to assessing the trustworthiness of the evidence offered. This suggests that health system literacy is a precondition for health literacy, and, ultimately, effective medical decision making. To circumvent the problems related to low health system literacy, we discussed two solutions:

1. Change the health care system so that patients can get good health care, simply by trusting their doctors and the information given. Specifically, we suggested several interventions to reduce the detrimental effect of non-medical agendas on the selection of research topics, evidence reporting, and medical decision making, including the enforcement of existing and new reporting standards, as well as the monitoring of system performance through the use of population-based databases.

2. Educate the public to increase health system literacy in addition to health and statistical literacy in patients and doctors alike. In particular, we discussed interventions to increase health (system) literacy by involving patients and providers in the research selection process, communicating both existing and missing evidence transparently and completely, as well as informing the public how to understand and evaluate the evidence they are offered. To make this work, we also identified the need to increase efforts at knowledge management and make the ensuing results more widely available.

It remains to be seen which of these approaches will be easier to implement. Given the multifaceted nature of the problem, we feel that an effective intervention will most likely need to incorporate both approaches.

Health Illiteracy: Spread to the Public

9

Statistical Illiteracy in Doctors

Odette Wegwarth and Gerd Gigerenzer

Abstract

In most psychological, legal, and medical research, patients are assumed to have difficulties with health statistics but clinicians not. Doctors may be said to pay insufficient attention to their patients' feelings, not listen carefully to their complaints, take only an average of five minutes time for consultations, or withhold information; yet rarely is it considered that they might also be statistically illiterate. However, studies indicate that most doctors have problems in understanding health statistics, including those from their own area of specialty. Such statistical illiteracy makes informed shared decision making impossible. The reasons for these disconcerting findings appear to be less rooted in doctors' cognitive limitations but rather in medical schools that ignore the importance of teaching risk communication. Doctors could be taught, with little effort, the simple techniques of risk communication, which would eliminate most of their statistical confusion.

Introduction

In 1996, results of four randomized trials on mammography screening, which included approximately 280,000 women (Nyström et al. 1996), showed that out of every 1,000 women who participated in screening over ten years, 3 women died of breast cancer; for every 1,000 women who did not participate in screening over a 10-year period, 4 women died of breast cancer. Further analysis showed similar effects: breast cancer mortality was 4 out of every 1,000 women who attended mammography screening over a course of ten years, compared to 5 out of every 1,000 who did not (Nyström et al. 2002). In 2006, a subsequent Cochrane Review of these and further randomized trials involving approximately 500,000 women found the absolute risk reduction to be even smaller: it was estimated that mammography screening would save 1 woman out of every 2,000 from dying of breast cancer (Gøtzsche and Nielsen 2006). In addition, the authors emphasized that for every woman who does not die of breast cancer, 10 women receive overtreatment as a result of screening participation. Gøtzsche and Nielsen thus concluded that it is unclear whether the benefits from screening override the inherent harms.

In 2008, we conducted a study that focused on gynecologists' knowledge of the benefits and harms of mammography (Wegwarth and Gigerenzer 2010a). This study was conducted nearly two years after the publication of the comprehensive Cochrane Review about the benefits and harms of mammography (Gøtzsche and Nielsen 2006). One of us called gynecologists who were practicing in different cities across Germany and told them the following story:

> My mother recently received an invitation to attend mammography screening. She is 55 years old, has no history of breast cancer in her family, and also no symptoms pointing toward breast cancer. Thus she doubts whether the screening would be effective for her. I, however, think that it might be advisable to get a mammogram at her age and would like to learn about the benefits and harms of the mammography.

Of the 20 gynecologists who were willing to talk to us, 17 gynecologists strongly recommended mammography, emphasizing that it is a safe and scientifically well-grounded intervention. Only 7 of these were able to provide numbers on the requested benefit, which ranged from 20% to 50%. While the estimate of "50%" is not supported by studies on mammography, "20%" is the relative risk reduction that corresponds to the absolute reduction of breast cancer mortality from 5 to 4 out of 1,000 women (Nyström et al. 2002). When the gynecologists were asked about the harms, the picture looked even more discouraging: None of them mentioned the risk of receiving an overdiagnosis and overtreatment due to mammography screening. Instead, the majority described mammography and its potential harms as "negligible." Only 3 out of the 20 gynecologists provided numbers for specific harms and the information provided by two of them were wrong.

This lack of knowledge on the part of doctors directly impairs patients' knowledge, as substantiated by a study held in nine European countries, including Germany (Gigerenzer et al. 2009). On average across these countries, frequent consultation by physicians was not associated with a patient's better understanding of the benefit of screening, but rather with a slightly higher overestimation of its benefit.

Do Doctors Know the Benefits and Harms of Screening?

The above example indicates clearly that many gynecologists know little about the benefits and harms of mammography. Is this situation unique to gynecologists alone?

Let us turn to PSA screening. In 2004, *Stiftung Warentest*—the German equivalent of the *U.S. Consumer Reports*—tested the quality of urologists' counseling. In a study, a 60-year-old man (a physician) made undercover visits to 20 urologists in Berlin, drawn randomly from a total of 135, and asked for advice on PSA screening (Stiftung Warentest 2004). Medical society guidelines require thorough and systematic counseling before the first PSA test is conducted. For instance, counselors should explain that the PSA test can miss cancers and cause false alarms. The patient should also be informed that, even in the event of a true positive result, not every cancer needs to be treated (i.e., that nonprogressive cancers exist) and that treatment may lead to harms, such as incontinence and impotence. Moreover, patients should learn how large the expected benefits and harms are. PSA screening prevents 0–0.7 prostate cancer deaths out of every 1,000 men (Andriole et al. 2009; Schröder et al. 2009). In terms of overall cancer mortality, PSA screening does not save a single life, as reported in the U.S. trial (Andriole et al. 2009). However, PSA screening can lead to harms. A European trial (Schröder et al. 2009) found that out of 1,000 screened men, approximately 30 will be treated for a nonprogressive cancer that otherwise would not have presented any symptoms during the man's lifetime or resulted in death, and which would never have been detected had the man not undergone screening. Only 2 of the 20 urologists knew the relevant information and were able to answer the patient's questions. Four others knew some of the information. However, the majority of 14 urologists could not answer most of the patient's questions, wrongly argued that it was scientifically proven that PSA screening prolongs life, and were not aware of any disadvantages.

Do Doctors Understand 5-Year Survival Rates?

Screening benefits are often framed as a change in 5-year survival rates, either over time or between groups. A higher survival rate does not necessarily mean, however, that a patient will live longer, as changes in 5-year survival rates are uncorrelated (r = 0.0) with changes in mortality rates (Welch et al. 2000). This lack of correlation is due to two biases. First, screening increases the time between detection and death by establishing an early diagnosis without necessarily affecting the time of death (lead-time bias). Second, screening detects cases of nonprogressive cancer, which inflates the survival rates because, by definition, these people do not die of the diagnosed cancer (overdiagnosis bias). How do doctors interpret the misleading information from changes in 5-year survival rates?

In a recent study (Wegwarth, Gaissmaier, and Gigerenzer, submitted), 65 physicians in internal medicine and its subspecialties in Germany were presented data on 5-year survival rates and the corresponding disease-specific mortality rates, from the Surveillance, Epidemiology and End Result (SEER) program for prostate cancer. Upon reviewing changes in 5-year survival rates, 66% felt that screening was warranted and should be recommended to patients in the future; 79% judged it to be effective. When presented with mortality rates, however, only 8% of the same physicians recommended screening and 5% judged it to be effective. Physicians were also asked to estimate how many deaths would be prevented in every 1,000 men if screened regularly. When presented with 5-year survival rates, their mean estimate was 150 prevented deaths; however, the SEER mortality reduction is zero. When mortality rates were shown, all physicians except one understood that no life is saved. Finally, only two physicians understood the concept of lead-time bias, and no one understood overdiagnosis bias.

This study demonstrates that 5-year survival rates mislead physicians about the benefit of cancer screening and that mortality rates are more instructive. Another example can be found in the use of relative risks versus absolute risks.

Do Doctors Understand Relative Risk Reduction?

There are many ways to express a benefit: as a relative risk reduction (RRR), an absolute risk reduction (ARR), or as the number of people needed to be treated (NNT) (or screened) to prevent 1 death from cancer (which is 1/ARR). Consider the drug Lipitor® (Gigerenzer et al. 2007), which aims at reducing people's risk of suffering a stroke. The benefit of taking the drug on a regular basis over four years can be expressed in the following ways:

- RRR: Lipitor® reduces the chances of suffering a stroke by around 48%.
- ARR: Lipitor® reduces the chances of suffering a stroke from around 28 in 1,000 to around 15 in 1,000 (i.e., 13 in 1,000 or 1.3%).
- NNT: To prevent 1 stroke, 77 people need to take Lipitor®.

Whereas ARRs and NNTs are typically small numbers, the corresponding relative changes appear large, particularly when the base rate is low. As a consequence, the format of RRR leads laypeople as well as doctors to overestimate the benefit of medical interventions.

Let us consider diabetes prevention. At various European diabetes conferences, Mühlhauser, Kasper, and Meyer (2006) presented results from three diabetes prevention studies to 160 nurse educators, 112 physicians, and 27 other professionals. When the results were presented as RRRs, 87% of the health professionals evaluated the effect of the preventive intervention as important or very important. However, when the same results were presented by giving the corresponding fasting plasma glucose values, only 39% of the health professionals evaluated the effect similarly.

Take another example: this time mammography. In a study conducted in a Swiss hospital, 15 gynecologists were asked what the widely publicized 25% risk reduction (from 4 to 3 in 1,000 women) by mammography really means (Schüssler 2005). This number corresponds to the first review released in 1996 (Nyström et al. 1996) on the effects of mammography attendance, where the risk of dying from breast cancer was reduced from 4 to 3 (or 25%) women out of 1,000. Asked how many fewer women die of breast cancer given the RRR of 25%, one physician thought that 25% meant 2.5 out of 1,000, another 25 out of 1,000; the total range of the answers varied between 1 and 750 out of 1,000 women. Another group of 150 German gynecologists who took a course in risk communication as part of their continuing education were asked to explain the meaning of the 25% risk figure (Gigerenzer et al. 2007). Using an interactive voting system, the physicians were presented with the following and asked to choose between four alternatives:

> Mammography screening reduces mortality from breast cancer by about 25%. Assume that 1,000 women aged 40 and over participate in mammography screening. How many fewer women are likely to die of breast cancer?

1	[66%]
25	[16%]
100	[3%]
250	[15%]

The bracketed numbers show the percentage of gynecologists who gave the respective answer. Two-thirds understood that the best answer was 1 in 1,000. However, 16% believed that the correct answer was 25 in 1,000, and 15% responded that 250 fewer women in 1,000 would die of breast cancer. Several other studies indicate that when benefits are presented in terms of RRRs, health care providers and managers are often misled to overestimate benefits. Naylor et al. (1992) found that physicians rated the effectiveness of a treatment higher when benefits were described as RRRs (a medical intervention results in a 34% decrease in the incidence of fatal and nonfatal myocardial infarction) rather than as ARRs (a medical intervention results in a 1.4% decrease in the incidence of fatal and nonfatal myocardial infarction: 2.5% vs. 3.9%) or NNTs (77 persons must be treated for an average of just over five years to prevent 1 fatal or nonfatal myocardial infarction). British researchers submitted four identical proposals for the funding of a breast cancer screening program and a cardiac rehabilitation program—identical except that benefits were presented differently in the proposals as RRRs, ARRs, the absolute values from which the ARR is computed, or NNTs (Fahey et al. 1995). Only 3 out of the 140 reviewers (members of the Anglia and Oxford health authorities) noticed that the four proposals were equivalent. When the benefits of a breast cancer screening program and a cardiac rehabilitation program were described in terms of RRR, 76% and 79%, respectively, of these programs received approval for funding from the authorities, compared to 56% and 38%, respectively, when the benefits were expressed as ARR. Similar low percentages were observed when absolute values or NNTs were used, which are also transparent ways of framing evidence. These studies indicate that many health care professionals overestimate the benefit of treatments when information is framed in terms of relative risk as opposed to absolute risks or NNT.

Are Doctors Confused by Sensitivities and Specificities of a Test?

A doctor's understanding of positive and negative test results is essential to the patient who has taken a test. Not knowing the meaning of a positive result can lead to overdiagnosis, overtreatment, unnecessary fear, or, in the case of HIV tests, even suicide (Gigerenzer 2002).

Consider a woman who has just received a positive screening mammogram and asks her doctor whether she has breast cancer for certain and, if not, what the chances are that she does (the positive predictive value). One would assume that every physician knows the answer. However, does this assumption hold true? At the beginning of one continuing education session, 160 gynecologists were provided with the relevant health statistics needed to derive the answer to this question in the form of conditional probabilities, which is the form in which medical studies usually report test statistics (Gigerenzer et al. 2007):

> Assume that you conduct breast cancer screening using mammography in a certain region. You know the following information about the women in this region:
>
> - The probability that a woman has breast cancer is 1% (prevalence).
> - If a woman has breast cancer, the probability that she tests positive is 90% (sensitivity).
> - If a woman does not have breast cancer, the probability that she nevertheless tests positive is 9% (false positive rate).
>
> A woman tests positive. She wants to know from you whether this means that she has breast cancer for sure, or what the chances are. What is the best answer?
>
> (A) The probability that she has breast cancer is about 81%.
> (B) Out of 10 women with a positive mammogram, about 9 have breast cancer.
> (C) Out of 10 women with a positive mammogram, about 1 has breast cancer.
> (D) The probability that she has breast cancer is about 1%.

Gynecologists could either derive the answer from the health statistics provided or simply recall what they should have known anyway. In either case, the best answer is (C); that is, only about 1 out of every 10 women who tests positive in screening actually has breast cancer. The other 9 are falsely alarmed; that is, they receive a positive test result although they do not have breast cancer. Only 21% of the gynecologists found the best answer; the majority (60%) disconcertingly chose "9 out of 10" or "81%," thus grossly overestimating the probability of cancer. Another troubling result was the high variability in physicians' estimates, which ranged between a 1% and 90% chance of cancer.

In another case involving fecal occult blood test (FOBT) screening, Hoffrage and Gigerenzer (1998) tested 48 physicians with an average professional experience of 14 years, including radiologists, internists, surgeons, urologists, and gynecologists. The sample had physicians from teaching hospitals slightly overrepresented and included heads of medical departments. They were given four problems, one of which concerned screening for colorectal cancer with FOBT. Half of the physicians were given the relevant information in conditional probabilities: a sensitivity of 50%, a false positive rate of 3%, and a prevalence of 0.3%. They were then asked to estimate the probability of colorectal cancer given a positive test result. Their estimates ranged from a 1–99% chance of cancer. The modal answer was 50% (the sensitivity), and 4 physicians deducted the false positive rate from the sensitivity (arriving at 47%). When interviewed about how they arrived at their answers, several physicians claimed to be innumerate and in their embarrassment felt compelled to hide this fact from patients by avoiding any mention of numbers.

Few doctors appear to be able to judge the positive predictive value of a test. In a study from 1978, only 18% of the physicians and medical staff who participated could infer the positive predictive value from probability information (Casscells et al. 1978). Eddy (1982) reported that 95 out of 100 physicians overestimated the probability of cancer after a positive screening mammogram by an order of magnitude. Similarly, Bramwell, West, and Salmon (2006) found that only 1 out of 21 obstetricians was able to estimate the probability of an unborn child actually having Down syndrome given a positive test, with those giving incorrect responses being fairly confident in their estimates. In one Australian study, 13 out of 50 physicians claimed they could describe the positive predictive value, but when directly interviewed, only one was able to do so (Young et al. 2002). Similar effects were reported for members of the U.S. National Academy of Neuropsychology (Labarge et al. 2003). Ghosh and Ghosh (2005) reviewed further studies which showed that few physicians were able to estimate the positive predictive value from the relevant health statistics.

Do Doctors Produce the Illusion of Certainty?

Some test results are more threatening than others and need to be handled with particular care. One such example is a positive HIV test result. At a conference on AIDS held in 1987, former Senator Lawton Chiles of Florida reported that out of 22 blood donors in Florida who had been notified that they had tested positive with the ELISA test, 7 committed suicide. Others with false positive results lost their jobs and/or families and suffered extreme emotional damage. Yet the chances of an individual being infected can be as low as 50–50, even if the results of both AIDS tests—the ELISA and Western blot (WB)—are positive (Stine 1999:367). This holds for people with low-risk behavior. Indeed, the test (consisting of one or two ELISA tests and a WB test, one blood sample) has an extremely high sensitivity of about 99.9% and a specificity of about 99.99%. Nonetheless, due to a very low base rate, on the order of one in 10,000 among heterosexual men with low-risk behavior, the chance of infection is as low as 50% when a man tests positive in screening. This striking result becomes clearer when translating these percentages into natural frequencies (Figure 9.1): Out of every 10,000 men at low risk, it is expected that 1 will

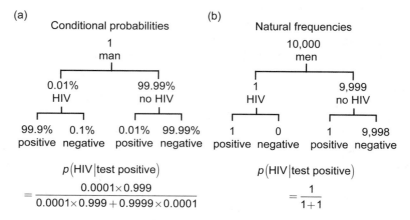

Figure 9.1 How natural frequencies facilitate Bayesian computations. A heterosexual man with low-risk behavior gets a positive HIV test result (positive ELISA test and positive Western blot test) in a routine examination. What are the chances that he is actually infected with HIV? The information in (a) is expressed in terms of conditional probabilities. The formula is known as Bayes's rule. The information in (b) is expressed in terms of natural frequencies, which simplify the computation and foster insight (adapted from Gigerenzer 2002)

be infected and will test positive with high probability; from the other, noninfected men, it is expected that 1 will also test positive (the complement to the specificity of 99.99%). Thus, 2 men test positive, and 1 of these is infected. This information needs to be properly communicated by AIDS counselors to everyone who takes the test.

To learn more about the quality of counseling of heterosexual men with low-risk behavior, an undercover patient visited twenty public health centers in Germany, taking an HIV test each time (Gigerenzer et al. 1998). The patient was explicit about the fact that he belonged to the low-risk group. In the mandatory pretest counseling session, the patient asked if there was a chance of testing positive even without the virus and, if so, how often this might happen. He also asked if there was a possibility of testing negative even if he had the virus. Sixteen counselors claimed that false positive test results never happen, although three of them retracted their statements when the patient asked whether they were absolutely certain of their responses. Only three counselors told the client that false positives can occur because the specificity is not perfect, albeit very high. One counselor provided no concrete information but insisted on mere trust. Note that if no false positives occur, a positive test would imply a HIV infection with certainty.

The illusion of certainty and the inability of medical professionals to understand health statistics is obviously alarming. But why are so many of them statistically illiterate?

Causes

Basic Numeracy

An elementary skill for critically assessing the findings of studies on particular medical interventions in the relevant medical literature is called *basic numeracy*. Schwartz and Woloshin (2000, unpublished data) tested physicians at Dartmouth Hitchcock Medical Center on basic numeracy using a simple three-question scale (Schwartz et al. 1997). The first question tests a respondent's ability to convert a percentage to a concrete number of people (out of 1,000); the second measures the ability to translate in the other direction; and the third tests basic familiarity with chance outcomes (see Gassmaier and Gigerenzer, this volume).

Only 72% of the physicians could answer all three questions correctly. The most difficult operation was to convert 1 in 1,000 into a percentage. One out of four physicians got it wrong. Similar results were obtained by Estrada, Barnes, Collins, and Byrd (1999), who reported that only 60% of medical staff answered all three questions correctly. Such results are a cause for concern. Doctors who are not able to assess medical statistics critically are doomed to rely on hearsay or on potentially misleading information provided by medical journals and the pharmaceutical industry.

Medical Journals and Doctors' Leaflets

When medical journals report on studies, nontransparent health statistics such as RRR are the rule rather than the exception. Nuovo, Melnikow, and Chang (2002) analyzed 359 articles that reported on randomized trials conducted in 1989, 1992, 1995, and 1998, published in *Annals of Internal Medicine, British Medical Journal (BMJ), Journal of the American Medical Association (JAMA), The Lancet,* and the *New England Journal of Medicine.* Only 25 articles reported the ARR, and 14 of these 25 also included the NNT, which is simply the inverse of the ARR. That is, only about 7% of the articles reported the results in a transparent way. The same journals along with the *Journal of the National Cancer Institute* were analyzed again in 2003 and 2004 (Schwartz et al. 2006). Out of 222 articles, 68% failed to report the absolute risks for the first ratio measure (such as relative risks) in the abstract; about half of these did report the underlying absolute risks elsewhere in the article, but the other half did not. An analysis of *BMJ, JAMA,* and *The Lancet* from 2004–2006 found that in about half of the articles, absolute risks or other transparent frequency data were not reported (Sedrakyan and Shih 2007). These analyses indicate that one reason why physicians, patients, and journalists use RRRs is because the original studies regularly provide information in this form.

Furthermore, readers are misled by *mismatched framing.* Benefits and harms of treatments are reported in different currencies: benefits in big numbers

(RRR), but harms in small numbers (absolute risk increases). For instance, the Report of the U.S. Preventive Services Task Force (2002:93) states the RRR (not the ARR) when describing the benefits of screening: "Sigmoidoscopy screening reduced the risk of death by 59% for cancers within reach of the sigmoidoscope." However, when the harms associated with the procedure are described, they are reported in absolute risks: "Perforations are reported to occur in approximately 1 of 1,000–10,000 rigid sigmoidoscopic examinations' (US Preventive Services Task Force 2002:94). An analysis of three major medical journals, *BMJ, JAMA*, and *The Lancet*, from 2004 to 2006 revealed that when both benefits and harms of therapeutic interventions were reported, one in three studies used mismatched framing. In most cases, relative risks were reported for benefits and absolute frequencies for harms (Sedrakyan and Shih 2007).

Pharmaceutical leaflets distributed to physicians show similar serious flaws. Researchers from the German Institute IQWiG (Institute for Quality and Efficiency in Health Care) compared the summaries in 175 leaflets with the original studies (Kaiser et al. 2004). In only 8% of the cases could summaries be verified. In the remaining 92%, key results of the original study were systematically distorted, important details omitted, or the original studies were not cited or impossible to find. For instance, one pamphlet from Bayer stated that their potency drug Levitra® (vardenafil) works up to five hours—without mentioning that this statistic was based on studies with numbed hares. In general, leaflets exaggerated base line risks and risk reduction, enlarged the period in which medication could safely be taken, or did not reveal severe side effects of medication pointed out in the original publications.

Medical Education

One may wonder why the training and continuing education of doctors does not prepare them adequately to understand health statistics. Lisa Schwartz and Steven Woloshin contacted the Association of American Medical Colleges (AAMC), the national association that accredits U.S. medical schools, and asked if there were any ongoing AAMC initiatives addressing statistical literacy in medical school education (Gigerenzer et al. 2007). The answer was no.

Further, one of us (OW) contacted 135 medical schools in the United States as well as the American Board of Internal Medicine (ABIM) by e-mail and asked to what extent they require courses and exams on medical statistics and risk communication. The ABIM stated that their certification represents the highest standard in internal medicine and its twenty subspecialties, and the awarding thereof means that internists have amply demonstrated the clinical judgment, skills, and attitudes essential for the delivery of excellent patient care. Apparently, however, the ABIM does not consider statistics and risk communication an essential part of excellent patient care: Only 3% of the questions asked within the certification exam cover medical statistics (clinical epidemiology), and risk communication is not a topic at all. Of the 135 medical schools contacted, only 12 responded to our question. In the best cases, biostatistics and clinical epidemiology did not exceed the benchmark of 3% either, nor was transparent risk communication part of any curricula. Some medical schools seemed aware of the fact that this does not meet the requirements of a medical world in which evidence-based medicine is slowly becoming standard. For instance, the medical school at the University of Minnesota responded that they are in the process of a large curriculum change for 2010/2011, which will include a greater emphasis on biostatistics and risk management.

Similarly, at Germany's medical schools, teaching medical statistics (clinical epidemiology) is represented in only a tiny proportion of the curricula, and transparent risk communication is only beginning to be taught (e.g., at the Charité in Berlin). Alarmed by the evidence on the lack of understanding health statistics by gynecologists (Gigerenzer et al. 2007), the gynecologist who conducted the *Stiftung Warentest* study offered to conduct a course on risk communication as part of the CME program of the Deutsche Fachgesellschaft für Gynäkologie und Geburtshilfe (German Society of Gynecology and Obstetrics). The society declined the offer: they did not perceive that there was a problem nor did they see a need for training on that topic.

In Germany, the course on risk communication for gynecologists conducted in 2006 and 2007 by one of us (GG) still appears to be the only one ever offered. Despite the fact that the attending 1000 physicians rated it as the most informative course within the CME program, the sponsor (Bayer-Schering) discontinued the course.

Remedies

Nontransparent statistics in medical journals, misleading information in leaflets for doctors, and a lack of training in medical statistics and risk communication at medical schools and during continuing medical training are major causes of statistical illiteracy in doctors. The good news, however, is that statistical illiteracy is largely a product of doctors' environment and thus can be addressed. Once doctors are fully able to assess medical statistics critically in any written form and to communicate this information transparently to their patients, informed shared decision making can become a reality.

Teach Medical Students and Doctors to Understand Health Statistics

Teaching statistical thinking to doctors during their medical training would eliminate much of the statistical illiteracy problem. However, good statistical education in medicine entails more than just teaching specific statistical techniques, such as multiple regression for clinical practice (Appleton 1990). Courses in medical statistics need to make doctors appreciate the connection between statistics at medical school and real events in practice. Motivation can be increased by introducing relevant problems and teaching statistics as a problem-solving method. For instance, when teaching students how to understand the sensitivity and specificity of a test, one could introduce a realistic story about a woman who has just received a positive mammogram or a low-risk man who has just received a positive HIV test (Gigerenzer 2002). After hearing such an example, the students are given the relevant information in the form of a natural frequency tree, which enables them to easily compute how likely it is, for instance, that the woman actually has breast cancer, given the positive result. In this way, students are taken from a gripping practical example to statistical thinking. As a next step, they can learn where to find the relevant information themselves and ask questions about the assumptions for applying statistical principles to the real world. This form of teaching is also referred to as *integrated teaching*. A systematic review (Coomarasamy and Khan 2004) found that integrated teaching is superior to the commonly offered stand-alone courses. Both stand-alone courses and integrated teaching improve knowledge, for example, by defining and understanding the meaning of different health statistics. Yet only integrated teaching provides students with the skills to know immediately which information is required and where to locate it, as well as how to apply that knowledge accurately to a given problem. Thus, learning by doing, not by rote, is necessary. In its best form, integrated teaching requires medical students to pose a clinical question, answer it, and then present the critically appraised topic to their teachers and peer group for grading. Currently, integrated teaching is offered at the medical schools of the University of Sydney (PEARLS program) and University of Manchester (BestBets). This alone, however, may not be enough to prepare doctors for all the potential pitfalls medical statistics has to offer. An understanding of the difference between transparent and nontransparent risk communication is essential for every doctor (Kurzenhäuser and Hoffrage 2002; Hoffrage et al. 2002).

Teach Medical Students and Doctors the Techniques of Risk Communication

Every bit of medical information can be framed in two ways: one that is misleading for many doctors and patients; the other which is transparent and easily understood. Using examples that have practical relevance is not enough; probabilistic information must be presented in a form that is easy for the human mind to grasp. For instance, absolute risks, natural frequencies, and frequency statements are transparent while relative risks, conditional probabilities, and single-event probabilities confuse many physicians.

Absolute Risks versus Relative Risks

There are several reviews of studies comparing relative risks with absolute risks (Edwards et al. 2001; Gigerenzer et al. 2007; Covey 2007; McGettigan et al. 1999; Moxey et al. 2003). As mentioned, the common finding is that RRRs lead medical students and doctors to overestimate systematically treatment effects because they are mute about the baseline risks (e.g., Lipitor® reduces the frequency of strokes: from 28 to 15 in 1,000 people) and the absolute effect size (13 in 1,000 people). When people hear about the 48% risk reduction of Lipitor®, they are likely to think that this percentage means that 480 strokes are prevented in every 1,000 people who take Lipitor®. In fact, it refers to the baseline of people who do not take the drug and suffer a stroke. Similarly, NNT (which is the inverse of ARR) is a transparent way of communicating benefits or harms. Thus, to avoid being misled, every doctor and medical student should know the difference between absolute risks and relative risks.

Natural Frequencies versus Conditional Probabilities

Estimating the probability of a disease given a positive test is much easier with natural frequencies than with conditional probabilities (sensitivities and specificities). Recall the test discussed earlier, where doctors were presented with four problems, one of which concerned screening for colorectal cancer with FOBT. Half of the physicians were given the relevant information in *conditional probabilities* (a sensitivity of 50%, a false positive rate of 3%, and a prevalence of 0.3%). Asked for the probability of colorectal cancer given a positive test result, the estimates of these doctors ranged from a 1% to 99% chance of cancer. The other half of the physicians received the relevant information in *natural frequencies*: 30 out of every 10,000 people have colorectal cancer. Of these 30, 15 will have a positive FOBT result. Of the remaining people without cancer, we expect that 299 will nonetheless test positive. Given that information, 13 out of 24 physicians estimated the positive predictive value correctly (4 to 5 in 100); the rest were close. This example demonstrates that the problem lies largely in an inadequate external representation of information rather than in a doctor's mental abilitites.

Figure 9.2 explains why natural frequencies are more useful in expressing positive predictive value: they reduce the necessary calculations. The left side shows the calculation with conditional probabilities, while the right side uses natural frequencies. The four probabilities at the bottom of the left tree are conditional probabilities and are normalized relative to base rates of having colon cancer and not having colon cancer. To infer a patient's likelihood of having colon cancer given a positive test, a doctor would need a formula called Bayes's rule. Here, the doctor would insert as a numerator the probability of cancer multiplied by the likelihood of testing positive given the cancer, and in the denominator the same term plus the probability of no cancer multiplied by the likelihood of testing positive given no cancer. In contrast, the right side of Figure 9.2 shows how natural frequencies simplify the calculation. Unlike conditional probabilities, all four natural frequencies at the bottom of the right tree are simple counts that are not normalized with respect to base rates (Gigerenzer

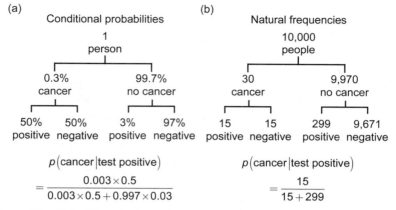

Figure 9.2   Probability of colorectal cancer given a positive FOBT result. The left side illustrates the calculation with conditional probabilities expressed as percentages; the right side shows how natural frequencies simplify the calculation. Note that relative frequencies, which are numerically identical to conditional probabilities, do not facilitate the calculation (Gigerenzer and Hoffrage 1995, 1999).

and Hoffrage 1995), which makes it easy to see how likely a positive test result actually reflects having the disease.

Frequency Statements versus Single-event Probabilities

Another nontransparent representation is a single-event probability statement, which refers to a singular person or event rather than to a class. Doctors often use single-event probabilities to inform their patients about potential side effects of drugs. For instance, if a physician tells a patient, "If you take Prozac®, you will have a 30–50% chance of developing a sexual problem, such as impotence or loss of interest," this single-event statement invites misunderstanding. The problem is that the reference class of the 30–50% is unclear. Many patients are frightened by such a statement, because they believe that something will go awry in 30–50% of their own sexual encounters (Gigerenzer 2002). However, if they are instead told that "out of every 10 patients who take Prozac®, 3–5 experience a sexual problem," patients are likely to understand their real risk better and be less concerned about taking the medication. These and other transparent techniques can easily be taught. Our experience has shown that doctors can be trained to understand statistics and use them confidently, as evidenced by the feedback at the end of our courses.

Statistical Literacy in Health: A Democratic Ideal

The revolutionary spread of statistical thinking to various branches of science such as physics and biology has yet to reach all doctors. Many medical organizations, physicians, and students continue to see statistics as inherently mathematical and clinically irrelevant to the individual patient (Altman and Bland 1991; Gigerenzer 2002). Their attitude is reinforced by medical school curricula, which rarely recognize statistical literacy—let alone transparent risk communication—as an essential part of medical training.

Doctors' illiteracy is primarily due to their environment, not their minds. This health care system is a major obstacle to the ideal of shared decision making and needs to be changed if doctors do not want to lose their patients' trust in the long run. As we have illustrated throughout this chapter, one key means of changing the extent of statistical illiteracy among doctors is to develop and implement efficient and transparent representations of health statistics.

The dream of statistical literacy is fundamental not only to a functioning patient–doctor communication but also to a functioning democracy. It embodies the Enlightenment's ideal of people's emergence from their self-imposed immaturity: the ideal of daring to know (Kant 1784). The "empire of chance" (Gigerenzer et al. 1989) has conquered and changed almost everything it has touched, from physics to insurance to baseball statistics. We hope that it will eventually prevail over doctors' statistical illiteracy as well.

10

Statistical Illiteracy in Journalism

Are Its Days Numbered?

Bruce Bower

Abstract

At a time when financial pressures and a digital revolution threaten the survival of many media outlets, a focus on statistical literacy can improve health and medical reporting and perhaps foster survival-enhancing changes in how the media cover these topics. Journalists often lack knowledge about statistical thinking. First reports of scientific findings, advances in "hot" research fields, and results that contradict previous assumptions draw special attention from the media, but underlying statistical problems and uncertainties in such studies are rarely mentioned in news stories. Clinical trials, significance testing, and meta-analyses create particular confusion for journalists. Possible ways to remedy this problem include early statistical education, professional development courses, online assistance sites, and efforts to use personal stories to illuminate the predictive value of medical tests.

Introduction

Journalists have been thrust into an uncertain world over the past decade. Like antelope crossing a dry stretch of savanna, herds of news gatherers nervously crane their necks and sniff the wind, checking to see who succumbs next to the pitiless lions of the Computer Age. Newspaper reporters, magazine writers, television news producers, and a gaggle of assorted media types just want to reach the next water hole in one piece.

It is especially ironic that journalists trying to navigate through this hazardous habitat understand so little about statistical risks. Media reports routinely misrepresent and sensationalize the implications of health and medical findings that hinge on statistical analyses.

Even more troubling, it's often not clear whether anyone in the journalistic chain of command cares about accurately deciphering what health studies really mean. Media stories that make bold, frightening claims about medical treatments regularly trump sober analysis. The satisfaction of ensuring a well-informed public pales in comparison to a desperate need for more paid subscriptions, higher advertising revenue, and a greater number of web-site hits.

A chaotic, perilous situation such as this can, however, set the stage for a dramatic change which otherwise would not have been taken. Of course, daring exploits can fall flat. But if properly thought out and executed, a new emphasis on statistical thinking could help harried news gatherers fend off the hungry lions.

A focus on statistical literacy would alter not only how journalists evaluate scientific studies but what they opt to cover in the first place. The rules of competition in the media world—from science writers and general assignment reporters to bloggers and podcasters—just might shift.

Journalists would have at least one incentive to get the scoop on the pros and cons of each new research paper and press release. Reporters determined to demonstrate their statistical competence would lead the way, racing to debunk sensationalized health and medical claims made by rival news outlets. Health and medical reporting would still be far from perfect, especially given tight deadlines and pressures to attract a wide audience. But a competition could develop between media sources which do and don't present the statistical implications of new studies in accurate and understandable formats.

Risk Aversion

My introduction to newspaper reporting came in 1979 when I entered a graduate program in journalism at a university in the United States. As a reporter on a newspaper published by the journalism school, I covered the university's medical center.

My first big break involved a story about a psychiatrist who had conducted a study suggesting that hallucinations and other symptoms of schizophrenia could be eased by hooking patients up to dialysis machines. Dialysis removes impurities from the blood and is typically used to treat people with kidney failure.

The newspaper's editor, who had formerly run a big-city daily newspaper, wanted to put the story on the front page. He wasn't interested in the study's sample size or the nature of any control groups. He didn't want to see if any other evidence had been published indicating that dialysis could effectively treat such a severe psychiatric disorder. He certainly didn't want to be bothered with statistics about the proportion of patients who showed improvement on dialysis and the extent to which various symptoms diminished over a relatively short treatment period.

It was good enough, for the editor and for me, that the local psychiatrist regarded his findings as "encouraging" and that they were about to be published in a scientific journal. I got my first front-page byline. Within the next several years, independent investigations confirmed that dialysis has no effect on schizophrenia's severity. At that point, I realized that my misleading front-page story contained an important lesson: Pay attention to the methodological and statistical details of scientific studies, especially those trumpeting provocative findings. My school experience also illuminated the lack of interest in and understanding of statistics among reporters and editors dedicated to digging up the "truth."

Numbers Get No Respect

Nearly thirty years later, journalism schools—at least in the United States—largely remain number-free zones. Budding journalists hope to investigate politicians' back-room deals and a slew of social injustices, not the assumptions and statistical methods that underlie influential scientific studies.

A survey of health reporters working at daily newspapers in five Midwestern states found that at least four out of five had no training in covering medical news or in deciphering health statistics (Voss 2002). Despite their statistical ignorance, most U.S. journalists get no on-the-job training in how to understand and explain health research (Kees 2002).

News media stories about scientific findings regarding medications for major diseases often contain misleading or incomplete information about the risks, benefits, and costs of the drugs (Moynihan et al. 2000). Financial ties between scientists and pharmaceutical companies making drugs being studied also frequently go unreported.

Several other problems with media reports about studies of new medications and other interventions have been noted (Gigerenzer et al. 2007). First, quantitative data on how well newly approved prescription medications work often do not get presented. Instead, news stories frequently include anecdotes in which patients describe astounding benefits of a new drug. Side effects of new medications, and data on the types and proportions of patients likely to develop drug-induced complications, appear only in a minority of media reports.

When numbers are included in news about a medication's benefits, reductions in relative risk get emphasized without describing baseline risks or the absolute effect size. The public hears, say, that a medical screening technique reduces the risk of death by 20%. This effect seems larger than it actually is if the media report does not clarify, for example, that the death risk falls by 1 in 1,000, from 5 in 1,000 who do not get screened to 4 in 1,000 patients who do get screened.

Media coverage of research at major scientific meetings also frequently fails to note that uncontrolled studies of new medical treatments, in which patients who receive the new treatment are not compared to other patients who get no treatment or an inactive placebo treatment, cannot determine whether those treatments are related to any observed health improvements.

To make matters worse, journalists often write health and medical stories based on press releases that suffer from the same sorts of statistical shortcomings characteristic of the media in general. In particular, press releases from medical journals and other sources frequently include no descriptions of study limitations.

A string of highly publicized drug recalls over the past decade has encouraged both incisive investigative journalism about clinical drug trials and sensationalized coverage about alleged dangers of commonly used medications (Dentzer 2009).

Outbreak of Confusion

Journalists have a long history of misreporting science and statistics. Consider the parrot fever panic of 1930 (Lepore 2009). At the time, newspaper reports had just appeared about a disease called parrot fever, or psittacosis, which had spread through South America and Europe. Little was known about the condition except that it typically proved fatal.

When three people fell seriously ill in Baltimore, Maryland, after exposure to a parrot purchased from a local pet shop, reports quickly spread in U.S. newspapers of a possible parrot-fever pandemic. Descriptions of parrot fever in the press ranged from "highly contagious" to "not contagious in man." Newspaper and magazine articles about new cases of possible parrot fever appeared in different parts of the country.

Autopsies and blood tests of suspected parrot-fever cases that came out negative for psittacosis received little or no coverage. Newspaper publishers knew that stories about a plague lurking in people's homes would sell their product and attract advertising.

Although presented as a dangerous and baffling disease, much was already known about parrot fever. The disease infects parrots and related birds, and it is only possible to catch psittacosis from an infected bird. Few infected birds had been brought to the United States. In 1930, 1 in 5 people infected with parrot fever died. Only those who had been in contact with certain tropical birds recently imported from South America had reason to worry about getting infected.

After a couple weeks of national panic stoked by dramatic press reports, a backlash occurred. News stories and public opinion suddenly reversed course and insisted that parrot fever did not exist and had been a silly diversion.

Vaccinated against Risk

Much has changed in the media world since the parrot fever panic, but communication problems regarding scientific findings persist. Witness the ongoing debate between scientists and the general public over the idea that vaccines cause autism. Autism belongs to a set of related conditions characterized by repetitive behaviors and difficulties with communication and social interaction.

Scientific evidence indicates that no link exists between early vaccinations and autism. However in the United States and England, many parents—especially those with children diagnosed with autism or related developmental disorders—do not believe it.

Anthropologist Sharon Kaufman of the University of California, San Francisco, finds that parents of children with autism frequently mistrust scientific and medical authorities (Gross 2009). These parents feel betrayed by experts who could not provide protection against the risk of conceiving a child with autism. They feel the need to take personal responsibility for finding out what really causes autism, often by consulting web sites and popular books that present anecdotes consistent with a vaccine-autism link.

Anti-vaccination web sites typically masquerade as sources of reliable scientific information. Nearly all of these sites portray physicians and scientists as conspirators in a money-making scheme with the pharmaceutical industry or as pawns of an underground movement dedicated to the spread of vaccines.

In this volatile atmosphere, media reports have offered a mixed bag of information. Science writers and mainstream media outlets have frequently reported on studies that find no association between childhood vaccinations for infectious diseases and autism. Media stories have tried to strike a balance between opposing sides of the issue without explaining that scientific findings support only one side. Television interview shows have provided platforms to those who claim that vaccines cause autism, without giving equal time to scientists capable of explaining why research does not support that claim.

As in the parrot-fever panic, fears about vaccines causing autism have been stoked by a lack of public understanding about risk that the media have done little to address. News reports rarely explain that fewer than 1 in one million people who get the measles, mumps, rubella (MMR) vaccine—the target of most parental concerns regarding autism—develop a serious allergic reaction. The risks of not vaccinating children against common infections are far greater but get even less attention from the media. Of particular concern to public health officials, low vaccination rates create conditions for the rapid spread of various diseases among unprotected individuals.

Parents concerned that environmental factors have led to rising autism rates have noted that infants now get 14 vaccinations by age two, versus 7 in 1983. For them, this correlation between rising numbers of vaccinations and rising autism rates amounts to causation.

Media stories routinely ignore this concern and remain silent about the distinction between correlation and causation, which is critical to understanding health and medical studies of all kinds.

Roots of the Problem

Like most people, journalists grow up learning little or nothing about statistical thinking. To make matters worse, journalists rarely receive continuing education in statistics and scientific methods. However, the media's problem in reporting health and medical findings goes deeper than that.

Tom Siegfried, editor of *Science News* magazine, explained this predicament in a public lecture at the University of Tennessee (published later in Siegfried 2010). Statistical methods often get misused in research, and the worst scientific offenders are most likely to attract news coverage of their journal papers.

"Even when journalists get the story right, what you read is likely to be wrong," Siegfried said. "In other words, even if the reporter quotes the scientist correctly and in context, faithfully presents the conclusions of the scientific paper and represents the meaning of the findings for science just as the scientists do, odds still are that it's wrong."

This happens because journalists most want to write about a scientific paper when it is the first report of a particular finding, when it describes an advance in a hot research field that is of wide interest, and when it contradicts a previous finding or belief. These are the papers most likely to be wrong.

False Leads

Problems with statistical methodology afflict many scientific fields and have created a situation in which most published research findings are more likely to be false than true (Ioannidis 2005). A piece of research is especially likely to be false when the studies conducted in a field generally consist of small samples; when effect sizes are small; when there are many tested relationships that have not been preselected as likely to be fruitful; when there is great flexibility in designs, definitions, outcomes and analytical techniques; when there are financial and other interests that create conflicts for scientists; and when many competing teams are simultaneously involved in a chase for statistical significance.

Into this complex arena stride journalists, each trying to find first reports of surprising or potentially important findings. Yet initial reports that display any or all of the above warning signs are likely to be wrong or to overstate the magnitude of any actual effects. In addition, journalists frequently do not realize that a novel finding may simply be due to chance.

Genetic association studies illustrate these dangers. Initial reports have often overestimated the extent of associations between particular gene variants and complex disorders, such as schizophrenia. Many genes make weak to moderate contributions to such disorders. It is hard to know at first whether any measured genetic associations reflect actual genetic effects or chance effects. Publication practices contribute to this problem, since rare positive findings are more likely to appear in print than greater numbers of negative findings.

Genetics is also a hot research field. Laboratories around the world are all trying to generate new discoveries about genes involved in various diseases. Publication practices mislead journalists from the start, since rare positive findings are more likely to appear in print than greater numbers of negative findings. There is no reason to accept any journal paper reporting a new genetic association to a particular ailment as valid until other published studies confirm the linkage and clarify the reasons for negative findings.

The final journalistic misstep occurs upon seeing any report or press release that begins with the claim, "contrary to previous scientific belief." A novel finding that clashes with a prior body of evidence is more likely to be due to chance than to a major advance in knowledge. As Tom Siegfried told his lecture audience, "Ordinarily, 'contrary to previous belief' should be a warning flag that the result being reported is likely to be wrong. Instead, it is usually a green light to go with the story."

Fooled by Significance

A journalist aware of these news-gathering pitfalls might reason that at least a study with "statistically significant" results accepted by a peer-reviewed journal is newsworthy. But again, this assumption is false. It not only encourages misleading coverage of health and medical news but discourages reporters from taking the time to understand statistical methods used by scientists.

Journalists typically do not realize that a statistically significant effect does not equal a significant effect, in the everyday usage of the word "significant." For instance, in a study with a large sample size, small effects will show up as statistically significant. A new drug may meet statistically significant criteria for producing more cures for a disease than an old drug, but that may mean that for every thousand people prescribed the new drug, two additional people get better. In this case, statistical significance does not translate into clinical significance, even if the new drug changes the lives of two extra people for every thousand treated.

Neither do most journalists know that a lack of statistical significance does not mean that no effect exists. A study may find that a new drug cures 15 out of 20 individuals with a skin infection, versus 10 out of 20 infected individuals treated with an old drug, but that difference still falls short of statistical significance because of the study's small sample size.

There is also little awareness in the media that a high level of statistical significance says nothing about the likelihood of any proposed explanation for that level of statistical significance or the veracity of null hypotheses—predictions that key experimental variables bear no relationship to one another (Bower 1997).

Scientific critics of the ritualistic use of this methodology have argued that it should be replaced by the development of theories that make precise predictions and call for the creative use of statistical methods (Gigerenzer 2004).

Finally, journalists entranced by statistical significance usually fail to grasp that this technique assesses relationships among only a few measures, which respond to many other influences that are not tested for and may not be known. Group averages measured in significance testing also mathematically obscure critical differences among individuals.

Clinical Trials and Errors

When significance testing gets applied to clinical trials, media misinterpretation of the results becomes especially worrisome. Double-blind, randomized, controlled clinical trials are considered essential for establishing whether new medications work as intended so that they can be approved for use and prescribed by physicians.

That does not ensure infallibility—far from it. Clinical trials typically use significance testing to examine average differences between groups administered either a new medication or a placebo substance with no active ingredients. Individual differences in responses to the medication and the placebo are left unexamined.

Consider clinical trials that have consistently found that antidepressants work about as well as placebos at treating depression. Dozens of these trials show that taking antidepressants for a few weeks or months lowers average scores on a self-report depression questionnaire only slightly more than taking placebo pills for the same amount of time. Some researchers have taken this data to mean that antidepressants have no clinical significance. But physiological and psychological differences among individuals, as well as clinicians' observations, suggest that some depressed people will respond to one drug but not to others. By averaging the results of clinical trials, large responses of some patients to certain antidepressants may be mathematically hidden by small or no antidepressant responses of other patients.

This situation recalls an old joke about a statistician who puts his head in the freezer and his feet in the oven and exclaims, "On average, I feel fine."

Journalists get a false feeling of security about clinical trials not only because they present impressive-looking averaged results but because they are randomized. Patients with the same disorder who share any number of other characteristics, such as race or age, are assigned at random to receive either a new drug or a placebo.

However, randomized trials cannot control for the many possible, and often unknown, variables that can affect patients' drug and placebo responses. As Tom Siegfried noted (Siegfried 2010), there are three million places where individuals vary by one of the letters in the genetic catalog, or genome. If only 1% of them matter for any given drug or disease, that is 30,000 genetic differences to randomize. If only 0.1% matter, that still leaves 3,000 genetic differences to randomize. In short, there is no way to know what critical variables—genetic or otherwise—did not get randomized or which trials randomized the correct variables and which did not.

In addition, subjects entering a clinical trial rarely constitute a random sample of individuals from a well-defined population. Thus, results collected from different centers in a clinical trial can vary in unknown ways.

Combining the Problem

If an effect is small but important, such as a fatal drug side effect in a small proportion of patients, it sounds sensible to combine different trials into a big enough sample to see what the size of the effect is. Scientists call this approach meta-analysis. Meta-analyses of health and medical studies regularly appear in major journals, and, again, many journalists assume incorrectly that a peer-reviewed meta-analysis must contain straightforward, unimpeachable results that deserve news coverage.

Meta-analysis is capable of detecting existing effects. However, the mathematics at the heart of this combination procedure require researchers to include all relevant trials that have been conducted and to ensure that those trials have been performed using comparable protocols, definitions of terms, control conditions, participants, and outcome measures.

Few meta-analyses meet all of these criteria. Translating such findings into news stories that dispense alleged clinical implications of combined data to the general public can spread false hope or inappropriate fear about medications and medical procedures.

In 2007, many media outlets reported that a meta-analysis in the *New England Journal of Medicine* had found that Avandia®, a drug for treating diabetes, "significantly" increased the risk of heart attacks. Yet the increased heart attack risk for Avandia® users had barely achieved statistical significance in the meta-analysis. Raw data from the trials showed that 59 people per 10,000 had heart attacks without Avandia®, while 55 people per 10,000 had heart attacks while using Avandia®. A raised heart-attack risk from Avandia® might still have been possible, but the meta-analysis left much unexplained. It included many unpublished studies that had been conducted in diverse ways, with no standard method for defining or validating outcomes. It was impossible to conclude from the study whether Avandia® raised the risk of having a heart attack in a small but statistically significant way or if the finding had been due to chance.

The ambiguities of meta-analysis also surfaced in a recent paper published in the *Journal of the American Medical Association* (Risch et al. 2009). That article generated a negative finding: People who inherit a particular version of the serotonin-transporter gene and who experience child abuse and other early-life stresses do not display an increased risk of developing depression as adults, as had been previously reported in a highly publicized study.

Coauthors of the new meta-analysis combined data from the original study with results from 13 attempted replications that used comparable measures of depression and stressful life experiences. Many studies in the meta-analysis, including some that replicated the original finding, contained small numbers of participants who were interviewed in person about depression and stressful experiences. Two studies that reported no gene–stress link to depression contained large numbers of participants who were interviewed over the phone.

As a result, the meta-analysis may have been unduly skewed toward yielding a negative finding. Phone interviews, such as those used in the two large studies included in the investigation, tend to produce less reliable information about mental illness symptoms and past traumatic events than face-to-face interviews. However, the data-combining technique of the meta-analysis gave greater mathematical weight to the large studies, despite their methodological drawbacks.

This does not mean that meta-analyses should never be reported. Media accounts need to explain the drawbacks as well as the strengths of any particular attempt to wring conclusions from combined data. Meta-analyses provide an opportunity to explain to the public how difficult it actually is for scientists to replicate the investigations of others. Just as with first reports of scientific findings, a clear explanation of statistical and methodological uncertainties tempers the temptation to portray meta-analyses as the source of unimpeachable truth.

Leaving Context Behind

When journalists' statistical illiteracy meets tight publication deadlines and a 24-hour-a-day media cycle, the broader context of new scientific findings usually gets sacrificed in the rush to deliver the news. In the long run, public understanding of medical research suffers and news consumers grow increasingly cynical about science.

It is not uncommon to read or hear separate news stories, one released shortly after the other, portraying the same foods first as dangerous and then as benign. In one case, many news reports on a 2006 randomized, controlled trial of women's diets concluded that a low-fat diet, in which fat accounted for 20% of calories, showed no link to reduced rates of any major diseases. Aside from failing to note lower breast cancer rates among women eating low-fat diets versus those in a comparison group, media stories made no mention of a large 2005 study, which received news coverage when it was first released, in which a low-fat diet reduced the risk of recurrent breast cancer among women already treated for the disease (Dentzer 2009).

Context-free news stories can also fuel public anxiety over mental health issues. A decade ago, the American Association of University Women (AAUW) funded a survey of girls' self-esteem and sent the survey results—which had not been published in any journal—and a press release to a variety of media outlets. News reports soon appeared warning that girls' self-esteem plummeted as they entered adolescence. AAUW officials warned that a national epidemic of girls thinking poorly of themselves, perhaps stimulated by inadequate educational opportunities and negative media portrayals, demanded a fast response. Journalists reinforced that claim.

Media stories largely ignored serious methodological problems with the self-esteem survey (Bower 1991). In particular, the survey had measured self-esteem with a brief self-report questionnaire administered once to girls of various ages, from which the researchers inferred that female self-esteem generally plunges during early adolescence. Only white girls, not black or Hispanic girls, reported low self-esteem in their early teens—a detail left out of most media reports. In addition, the researchers had gathered no evidence from parents and teachers to evaluate whether individual girls were justified in their self-esteem assessments.

Most problematic for the AAUW survey, though, was the fact that several long-term studies of psychological development in children had already found that girls tend to maintain their self-esteem during early adolescence. Researchers conducting those studies dismissed the new survey as inaccurate and methodologically flawed.

After a few months of media palpitations over girls' alleged self-esteem crisis, news reports about the AAUW survey disappeared. No follow-up surveys were conducted to see if the general public had believed the media fanfare or felt alarmed about girls' supposedly dim self-esteem prospects.

Getting the Statistical Story Right

The news about statistical illiteracy in journalism looks bad. Reporters, editors, and other media decision makers usually want to write about scientific findings that are likely to be wrong. Statistical significance is routinely misunderstood and the intricacies of clinical trials and meta-analyses are ignored. Controversial findings are presented without any context or historical background.

But all is not lost. Steps can be taken to increase statistical and scientific savvy among journalists. No quick and easy solutions exist, especially as media organizations scramble to find new business models appropriate for the digital world. The following suggestions provide a general framework at best for fostering statistical literacy in a rapidly changing news environment.

Education, Early and Often

Learning about the mathematics of probability should begin in primary school and continue through the secondary grades. Statistical-thinking classes should focus on solving real-world problems of general interest to students, starting with frequency-based, discrete number formats (Gigerenzer et al. 2007).

A stockpile of basic statistical knowledge would wean journalists from their widespread assumption that scientific controversies simply consist of differing interpretations of data. The relative merits of statistical methods used in medical research and statistical contributions to controversial health findings would attract increasing attention.

Early statistical training would be especially valuable for future journalists because, if taught effectively, it would encourage critical thinking about social problems and scientific studies rather than a reflexive trust in number-wielding researchers. Journalists might even start to question whether new health and medical studies used appropriate statistical models.

A statistical education would also go a long way toward preparing future public affairs officers to write press releases that correctly describe the implications and drawbacks of new medical investigations. Press releases would still, of necessity, put a positive spin on studies. But statistical clarity on issues such as the risks and benefits of a treatment would put the onus on journalists to translate the findings into an accurate story.

Professional Development

With or without a statistical background, journalists would benefit from continuing education about what the numbers in health and medical studies really mean. A few newspapers and scientists have initiated such efforts. In the United States, journalists who take the initiative can attend the Medical Evidence Boot Camp run by the Massachusetts Institute of Technology, the Medicine in the Media program sponsored by the National Institutes of Health, and the Dartmouth Institute for Health Policy and Clinical Practice's Center for Medicine and the Media.

Internet classes on statistical issues related to media coverage of science would reach a large number of journalists, especially if the classes were promoted by editors and publicized through organizations such as the National Association of Science Writers. Publicity for these classes should not portray them as venues to cure journalists of their statistical sins so that they can "see the light" of numerical literacy. Instead, the emphasis should be on the potential for statistical knowledge to give any individual journalist an advantage over his or her competition, both in the workplace and at other media outlets.

In that respect, continuing education in statistics fosters professional advancement, an outcome that all journalists can appreciate. Statistically literate reporters will generate news "scoops" that they otherwise never would have noticed, and publishers and editors will smile approvingly.

Electronic Assistance

Interested organizations, such as those already involved in statistical training for the media, should establish and publicize web sites that provide statistical advice for journalists. These efforts could build on pioneering web sites already devoted to statistical thinking in the media. One-stop web sites for statistical backup on breaking health and medical stories could become an integral part of the news-gathering process.

A step in that direction has been taken by the *Journal of the National Cancer Institute* (JNCI). On its web site, JNCI has posted links to tip sheets with guidance on what to ask study authors, how to interpret common statistical tests, and ways to highlight study limitations (JNCI 2010).

Statistics sites on the web would ideally contain information about a spectrum of statistical methods, use examples from media stories to explain the difference between good and bad coverage of health and medical studies, and allow journalists to email questions about statistical issues for a quick, clear response from a knowledgeable scientist. Web sites could also illustrate how to make statistical findings understandable by using pictorial representations and graphs. Journalists could incorporate these visual displays as needed into their own health and medical stories or blog posts.

Telling Stories with Numbers

Implications of health and medical investigations can be made more compelling and understandable, first to journalists and then to media consumers, through the use of stories about real people, a long-standing tradition in reporting about nonscientific issues. In some cases, such as the controversy over vaccines allegedly causing autism, personal stories have overridden scientific findings. Best-selling books tell stories of parents whose children got vaccinated, stopped interacting with others, and received autism diagnoses. When scientists dismiss these accounts as anecdotes in search of evidence, parents often suspect that the scientists have ulterior motives or do not take them seriously. Science-based explanations of the risks and benefits of childhood vaccines could employ alternative and equally dramatic anecdotes, such as describing an instance of a parent watching a child die of a vaccine-preventable disease (Gross 2009).

Journalists could begin to redress their widespread misunderstanding of the predictive value of medical tests via storytelling. Reading about the trials and agonies of real people who tested positive in routine HIV tests before getting negative results on later HIV tests provides a route to understanding the predictive accuracy of such tests (Gigerenzer 2002).

In the digital age, stories about health and medical issues can instantly reach people across the globe. Organizations involved in statistical literacy could work with journalists to put together brief video interviews and documentaries about individuals with relevant stories to tell about medical issues and the implications of new studies. These videos could be posted on specialized web sites as well broader digital venues, such as YouTube.

Such videos would reach a worldwide audience already generally interested in science and technology information (National Science Board 2008). A large majority of people surveyed in the United States and China say that they have "a lot" or "some" interest in new scientific discoveries. Those figures drop slightly but remain high elsewhere in the world.

Surveys also tap into some public reservations about science. In the United States, a majority of adults feel that scientific research does not pay enough attention to society's moral values. Nearly half believe that science makes life change too fast. Many express skepticism about scientific ideas regarding evolution and the origins of the universe.

Effective statistical communication in the media is not capable of making all areas of science palatable to everyone. Neither will it always win friends for the scientific enterprise or ease public anxiety by illuminating gaping uncertainties in medical research and practice. However, it has accuracy on its side. Over time, accuracy will breed trust in new sources and, with a little luck, a sense of greater personal responsibility for health care among media consumers.

Competing for the Truth

Researchers who want to help people make sense of health statistics have drawn inspiration from the words of Enlightenment philosopher Emmanuel Kant: "Dare to know!" Kant's insightful and succinct statement acknowledges, in its choice of verb, that knowledge can be dangerous. As Jack Nicholson's admittedly less profound character in the movie "A Few Good Men" exclaimed, "You want the truth? You can't handle the truth!"

Journalists will undoubtedly have qualms about reporting statistical truths, especially those that raise embarrassing questions about their previous coverage of health and medical studies. Accurate reporting on the benefits and risks of new drugs and of tests for various medical conditions will also make it difficult to pitch new findings as "hot news" or as revolutionary advances.

But as more and more journalists get a solid grounding in statistical thinking, news gathering and reporting will change—whatever the media environment ends up looking like in the digital age. Embarrassment about past errors in health coverage will give way to concern about avoiding the embarrassment of having new errors exposed by the superior health coverage of media competitors. A new form of investigative journalism focused on statistics and risk will uncover exaggerated claims and erroneous interpretations of scientific data, made by the media as well as scientists.

Among statistically literate journalists, "Dare to know!" will be complemented by a more visceral sentiment: "Don't dare get scooped!"

Acknowledgments

Whatever knowledge I have about statistical illiteracy and scientific misinformation in journalism has benefited greatly from the publications and comments of others:

Gerd Gigerenzer, John Richters, Steven Woloshin, Lisa Schwartz, Geoffrey Loftus, David Funder, and Tom Siegfried. Any errors of fact or interpretation in this paper are mine alone.

11

Improving Health Care Journalism

Holger Wormer

Abstract

To improve health care journalism, criteria and assessment strategies are needed. This has proven difficult due to the various definitions of quality used by science and journalism. Recommendations are made to integrate these varying perspectives into a usable set of quality criteria.

Ranking the quality of health news must be conducted on the basis of consistent criteria. Several strategies are presented to improve evaluation. A two-step model is proposed to increase the quality of investigation and presentation in science journalism. This model is accessible to highly specialized as well as general journalists. An overview is provided of the basic rules in journalistic presentation, and the effects of medical reporting among recipients are discussed. Health reporting in the media and the quality debate concerning direct consumer/patient information (via Internet) is highlighted. Finally, the future role of health care journalism, journalists, and "personal evidence scouts" is discussed in the context of a rapidly changing and fragmented media world.

> Bad science is no excuse for bad journalism. —Victor Cohn
> First get the church full, then start to preach. —Henri Nannen

Introduction

Medical and health care issues rank consistently at the top of all scientific topics covered by the international mass media. In an analysis of three leading German newspapers, research at my institute found that from 2003–2004 medical issues comprised 27.7% of all scientific articles reported; in 2006–2007, this figure rose to 28.9% (Elmer et al. 2008). After medical topics, environmental sciences (15.0%) ranked as the next most popular topic, followed by articles on biology (12.7%). If behavioral sciences are counted as medical topics, coverage climbs to 58% in U.S. papers (Clark and Illman 2006).

The exact reasons for these consistently high rates have yet to be fully understood. However, three factors appear to play a role:

1. "Medicine sells," as shown by the number of copies sold of any news magazine bearing a medical headline on its cover.
2. Output of medical research is greater than in any other scientific field; there are more publications, more conferences, and more press releases.
3. Medical issues meet many criteria of classical news theory (e.g., Galtung and Ruge 1965), such as "relevance," to a very high degree, which raises their chances of being covered (Badenschier and Wormer 2010).

Public opinion on health issues is strongly influenced by the media. According to a national poll taken in the 1990s, the primary source of health news for the average U.S. citizen was television, which ranked ahead of information received from medical doctors (Johnson 1998). In a recent analysis of nine European countries, Gigerenzer et al. (2009) found that the mass media ranked lower as the source of health-related information behind family/friends, practitioner, and pharmacist. However, between one in three and more than one in two participants responded that they use the television as their source of health information "sometimes" or "frequently" (Gigerenzer et al. 2009).

Media reporting has been faulted with "unsettling" patients or "scaremongering." This criticism stems primarily from medical professionals, their professional associations, and pharmaceutical companies, and relates to the following general cases:

1. Past reporting by the media has been very poor and/or inaccurate.
2. Past reporting, though correct, has exposed an "inconvenient truth" for certain stakeholders, who then respond, for example, by discrediting the article or journalist.
3. The meaning of *quality* is defined differently in (medical) science and journalism, and different perceptions exist as to what role journalism should play.

Each of these points affects how we approach "better health care journalism."[1] If we are indeed to improve the state of health care journalism, we must do more than just identify current scientific mistakes in medical reporting; we must also incorporate in our criteria what it means to compose a "quality" article from a journalistic perspective. Some scientists may need to adjust their perception of medical journalism, for the journalist is not merely a translator but also a critic, whose very role may be to "unsettle" patients. With this understanding, we can begin to discuss what it means for scientists and journalists to share in the process of health care reporting. In addition, we must also recognize the dynamic interaction that exists between the media, patients, and health care professionals and be able to evaluate this within the framework of

---

[1] Since the reporting of clinical studies and fundamental medical research can impact patient behavior, a broad definition of "health care journalism" is used. In addition, medical journalism and health care journalism are used here synonymously. For further discussion of the classification of health news, see Brodie et al. (2003).

evolving technologies (in particular, the Internet). With these general cases and issues in mind, let us consider two broad areas:

1. Improving the quality of journalistic *investigation* to lead to "evidence-based journalism," and
2. Improving the quality of journalistic *presentation* in terms of reaching an audience, increasing comprehension, maximizing reception, and addressing the accompanying psychological components.

When we analyze what it means to have "quality" presentation, an interesting conflict arises: in science, quality stands for completeness or differentiation, while in journalism it relates to how well a report is received by the target audience. Thus, in the spirit of Henri Nannen, founder of *Stern*: How useful is a complete and differentiated article that reports on a medical issue if it does not attract the masses? That is, if nobody sees or reads it.

Dimensions of Quality in (Medical) Science and (Health Care) Journalism

To improve health care journalism, the concept of *quality* must be defined. Our starting point is the assumption that the mechanisms and working routines in health care journalism can be regarded as processes that enable the best evidence—from both journalistic and scientific perspectives—to be discovered. I review how medical reporting must combine these two dimensions of quality and discuss assessment models that currently exist.

Quality in Journalism

Do articles from the yellow press or tabloid newspapers exemplify high-quality journalism?[2] According to at least one of three current perspectives in journalism, the answer is yes (Arnold 2008:491). Consider the German tabloid paper *BILD*. From an economic standpoint, *BILD* fulfills one aspect of quality: its daily circulation to nearly nine million daily readers is as high or higher than the next ten major German newspapers (AWA 2009). Even if this "market-oriented, audience-centered" perspective is deemed irrelevant in defining quality, a message's impact factor must be considered. In addition, one must account for a functional, system-oriented perspective (Blöbaum and Görke 2006)

---

[2] "Quality" is a term widely used to distinguish between "quality" and "tabloid" newspapers. Newspapers in a broadsheet format "aim to provide readers with comprehensive coverage and analysis of international and national news of the day together with informed comment on economic, political and social issues" whereas the popular press (e.g., tabloids) is geared primarily toward "entertainment, mostly show-biz gossip, sport and sensational sex scandals" (Entwistle and Hancock-Beaulieu 1992:370). The borders are, however, not clear-cut. Even "quality media" have celebrity sections. In public financed television (e.g., in Germany) "entertainment" is prescribed by law as a necessary mandate along with information dissemination.

as well as a normative-democratic perspective (e.g., Rager 1994; Schatz and Schulz 1992). For our approach, the latter seems to be the most appropriate. There is no generally accepted "theory of quality" in journalism (e.g., Bucher and Altmeppen 2003; Weischenberg et al. 2006). There is, however, a broad consensus that quality in journalism is a standpoint-dependent, multidimensional construct (see also Russ-Mohl 1992:85; Weischenberg et al. 2006:12). Thus, no simple assessment matrix of criteria can be generally applied. Quality in media can be only measured by considering different factors for each individual case: type of media, format, target group (e.g., scientist, laymen), point of reference (e.g., politics, economics, science). Direct comparison seems only possible between similar types of media. Furthermore, the structural context of production must be considered (Weischenberg et al. 2006).

At present, the most widely used criteria for determining quality in journalism are:

- accuracy (correctness), communication (presentation), actuality, relevance (Rager 1994) with ethics added later;
- diversity of sources and frames (Blöbaum and Görke 2006:321);
- diversity, relevance, professionalism, acceptance, and legitimacy (Schatz and Schulz 1992);
- diversity of sources, news factors (concerning the choice of a subject); cross check by a second source, critical assessment of sources (concerning the investigation); actuality, originality, transparency, comprehensibility, objectivity (Russ-Mohl 1992);
- the answering of WH-questions: who, what, when, why, etc. (Weischenberg 2001:79, 110);
- credibility, independence, and provision of context (cited from Arnold 2008).

It is neither possible nor necessary to discuss these in detail (for an overview, see McQuail 1992). However, it is important to know that they exist and that journalism adheres to its own criteria of quality. The question is: To what extent can these be applied in medical journalism, and how should they be measured?

Quality in (Medical) Science

Objectivity, relevance, and originality are often mentioned as criteria for quality in science (e.g., Merton 1985:299). Interestingly, these three criteria are often used to measure quality in journalism as well. Even in science there is no general consensus as to how these criteria should be quantified. Below I discuss different approaches to this and provide a short overview in the context of evidence-based medicine.

Philosophy of Science: Methodological Rules

The philosophy of science has identified several methodological rules to evaluate the quality of scientific work (e.g., the falsification approach by Popper 1963). However, in a review of the different approaches, Neidhardt (2006) admits to capitulation in an attempt to establish universal criteria for quality in science. Hornbostel (1997:166–169) states that there is no standardized scale for quality in a methodological sense because the criteria for an evaluation are variable, due to cognitive and social influences. This does not mean, however, that "anything goes" if there is a methodological argument to explain why a certain claim of knowledge in a certain field is acceptable. As a condition, Hornbostel sees ideals of explanation and strategies of validation and evaluation that are negotiated in the respective field. Evidence-based medicine (discussed below) is an example for such a context-embedded methodological evaluation.

Sociology of Science: Expert Judges

From a sociological perspective, the quality of a scientific work correlates, under ideal circumstances, with recognition from other scientists (Hornbostel 1997:93). Consensus among peers is seen as the best possible solution to replace a methodological evaluation (Neidhardt 2006). However, as Hornbostel points out, this may only be valid within a specialized field, where a certain consensus about methods, relevant questions, and available knowledge has already been established. The "peer-review process" is an example of broadly accepted expert judgment being used to evaluate the quality of a scientific work, with criteria such as pertinence, reception of the literature, originality, methodological correctness, relevance of the results, and clear presentation. Still, the peer-review process is disputed because subjectivity and other influences can affect outcomes (e.g., Fröhlich 2008; Nature 2010). Even when there is consensus from different reviewers, this collective judgment may be wrong. However, most scientific organizations as well as scientific journals see no practicable alternative.[3]

Scientometrics: Objective Indicators?

Throughout science, a necessity or wish exists to quantify the quality of research in different institutions through striking rankings. Such rankings are used often in political decision making as well as in profiling efforts by "winning" institutions. Originally, however, scientometrics was used to quantify

---

[3] In some recent approaches, the classical peer-review system has been combined with "open" or "public" peer review. After initial evaluation, the draft of a scientific paper is posted on the Internet for comment by other experts before it is revised for final publication (Pöschl 2004).

research and, ideally, the structural indicators used should correlate with the acceptance of a certain scientific quality and reputation (Hornbostel 1997:186).

Some of the indicators that have been used include: number of publications (especially in peer-reviewed journals with a high citation index impact factor), number of citations, external funding, and scientific awards. To what extent the various indicators should be used to measure quality remains controversial (e.g., Fröhlich 2008). Many highly cited papers, for example, do not describe a scientific breakthrough but simply report on the nomenclature or lab methods used, which in the meantime have become standard. Surprisingly, the basic idea that the most widely read publications equate to the most important ones brings us back to the argument of market-oriented criteria discussed earlier for tabloid newspapers.

The Criteria for Evidence-based Medicine

Sackett et al. (1996:71) defined evidence-based medicine as "the conscientious, explicit, and judicious use of current best evidence in making decisions about the care of individual patients." Evidence-based medicine contains five steps and includes the defining of a question, a systematic literature research, and a critical evaluation of the available evidence (Sackett and Haynes 1995). Its evaluation is based on strict criteria, as discussed by Guyatt and Rennie (1993) and Greenhalgh (2006). By using these criteria, it is possible to evaluate quality past the reputation of an author. In addition, Guyatt and Rennie (1993) and Greenhalgh (2006) provide ideal study designs to evaluate therapies, diagnosis, or risk factors. Strategies, such as randomizing and double-blind approaches, are introduced to reduce potential bias, and statistical indicators (significance, confidence interval) are used to quantify results. Relevance is measured by considering whether a sample is representative or if there has been a real benefit to the patient. Since 1992, systematic reviews of studies that focus on a specific question have been conducted according to these criteria and have included a statistical summary and weighing of the results (Petticrew 2001).

Although evidence-based medicine is still disputed within the medical profession, its high level of standardization is beneficial for journalists, and some of its criteria (e.g., "relevance") are well known in journalism. Thus, basic checks can be applied schematically without special knowledge in the medical field. This might include, for example, verifying the hierarchy of methods (with a systematic review on the top) used in therapeutic studies (Guyatt et al. 1995). However, the quality of a systematic review is limited by the quality of the original studies available. What happens when no data are available, or only conflicting evidence exists? Topics of this nature are often very important to the media (e.g., vaccination against swine flu, the risks of mobile phones, or correlation between leukemia and living near nuclear power plants). In addition being "correct" in medicine is usually more difficult to define than, say, in mathematics.

Measuring Quality in Science and Medical Reporting: Models and Results

In the broad field of journalism, different, widely varying approaches exist to measure the quality of reporting. In *science* journalism, however, risk communication and accuracy studies have dominated the field (e.g., Peters 1994; Ruhrmann 2003). This has led to an evaluation process based on strict scientific standards—one that unfortunately does not reflect important journalistic principles (for a criticial analysis, see Kohring 2005).[4]

To analyze quality in science journalism, one approach is to assess the extent to which the relationship and interdependency between science and society has been properly reported (Kohring 2005:283). In addition, the role of a science journalist requires careful consideration. A purely educational role—transmitting simple, uncritical descriptions of scientific results to the public without context or comment—is rejected. Journalism entails more than positive public relations for the scientific community. Thus, as we define approaches to empirically measure the quality of the science reporting, we must be mindful to retain established scientific criteria while incorporating important journalist principles (Wormer 2008b:346).

Practical Approaches to Measure Quality in Medical Reporting

The work of Moynihan et al. (2000) has served as a model for several attempts to measure the explicit quality of medical reporting. These attempts focused on the quantification of risks and benefits of medications as well as their costs, and raised the question of sources. Moynihan et al. attempted to "articulate basic principles of high-quality medical reporting, in line with an evidence-based approach to medicine" by adopting the following criteria as:

*   What is the magnitude of the benefit, both absolute and relative?
*   What groups of patients can be helped?
*   What are the associated risks and costs?
*   What possible links exist between the sources of information (studies or experts) and those who promote the therapy (e.g., manufacturers)?

Although their work was limited to a case study of three special medications, it inspired the creation of the Australian "Media Doctor" in 2004 (Schwitzer 2008). This project monitors the health news coverage of 13 Australian news organizations and is "dedicated to improving the accuracy of media reports about new medical treatments" (Media Doctor Australia 2010). Current news

---

4   With his criticism, Kohring follows the conclusion of the newspaper researcher, Otto Groth, who pointed out in the first part of the 20th century that there are different standards and indicators of measuring quality in science and journalism: "Acting under a severe misconception of the character of a newspaper and its resulting working methods and equipment, scholars believe that they can dictate the laws of science to the newspaper" (cited in Kohring 1978:175).

items that report on medical treatments are reviewed by independent and objective sources (approximately 20 clinicians and researchers) according to a standardized rating scale. The results of "good" and "bad" reporting are listed on the project's web site.

The criteria used by Media Doctor follow a classic approach, aided by a peer-review system and rating catalog (Table 11.1). Explicit scientific criteria (e.g., accuracy) are not favored; instead, Media Doctor draws on criteria widely accepted in journalism: novelty, independence, diversity, and contextualization. One important criterion—the quality of the presentation (e.g., Is the story told in an understandable way and interestingly enough to be read by a broad audience?)—is only included in the comment section of a review where, for example, a "sensationalist headline" can be noted (Wilson et al. 2009). In principle, one must ask whether a story that is incorrect and yet presented well could be given a high rating. One could argue that the review system provides a fail-safe in terms of accuracy, because most reviewers are clinicians and researchers, whose judgment should imply a high degree of accuracy. However, some of the criteria (e.g., costs) may be weighted differently in various health systems.

The attempt by Media Doctor to integrate scientific and journalistic criteria is groundbreaking. It allows semi-experts to verify information easily and has since been adopted in Canada and in United States under the project name "healthnewsreview" (Schwitzer 2008).

Others have taken a slightly different approach. Lai and Lane (2009), for example, used a combined form of scientometrics and evidence-based medicine to compare 734 front-page stories from international newspapers. They evaluated how the scientific articles published in these newspapers corresponded to the actual research to derive publication status and evidence level. When they encountered unpublished results, they verified whether the results had been

Table 11.1   Criteria used by the Media Doctor project to evaluate reporting of a journal article (Wilson et al. 2009). Stories are rated "satisfactory," "not satisfactory," or "not applicable." For criteria used to determine scores, see Media Doctor (2010).

Rating criteria: The extent to which a story:
1. Reports on the novelty of an intervention
2. Reports on the availability of the intervention
3. Describes the treatment or diagnostic options available
4. Avoids elements of disease mongering
5. Reports evidence supporting the intervention
6. Quantifies the benefits of the intervention
7. Describes the harms of the intervention
8. Reports on the costs of the intervention
9. Consulted with independent expert sources of information
10. Went beyond any available media release

published in a scientific journal after the story in the mass media appeared. Lai and Lane conclude that journalists should always distinguish between medical research news that is based on mature research and news which is reported based on studies from preliminary findings. This approach relies to a high degree on a functional peer-review system and does not integrate journalistic criteria of quality (e.g., comprehensibility) into its evaluation.

Oxman et al. (1993) have proposed an index of scientific quality for health-related news based on seven key criteria:

1. Applicability: Is it clear to whom the information in the report applies?
2. Opinion versus facts: Are facts clearly distinguished form opinions?
3. Validity: Is the assessment of the credibility (validity) of the evidence clear and well-founded?
4. Magnitude: Is the strength or magnitude of the findings (effects, risks or costs) clearly reported?
5. Precision: Is there a clear and well-founded assessment of the precision of any estimates or of the probability that any of the reported findings might be due to chance?
6. Consistency: Is consistency of the evidence (between studies) considered, and is the assessment well-founded?
7. Consequences: Are all of the important consequences (benefits, risks, and costs) of concern relative to the central topic of the report identified?
8. Based on answers to the above questions, how would you rate the overall scientific quality of the report?

Oxman et al. (1993) tested the reliability and validity of the index among physicians, research assistants, and members from the Canadian Science Writers' Association. Although there was a poor response rate among journalists, the answers given offer insight into the problem of defining quality between the various expert groups. "Judging from their comments, this reflects in part the difficulty some journalists had with the whole notion of separating the scientific quality of an article from its other features (such as the quality of the writing) and of making a numerical rating of this quality" (Oxman et al. 1993:992–993).

Instead of evaluating in detail the quality of medical reporting in the mass media, a different strategy is to alarm the public if an extremely bad, misleading, or even dangerous report appears. This approach is taken, for example, on blog sites such as Plazeboalarm or Bad Science but it must be implemented carefully, otherwise it may have the opposite effect. Fast response time is the primary advantage here. It is much easier to identify an extremely low-quality report than to give a balanced evaluation, and when there is a high potential for bad reporting to harm patients, speed is important. One of the main criticisms, however, is that it indirectly serves to promote the therapy or treatment being reported, at least among those desperately seeking a solution. Thus, this approach needs to be implemented carefully and communicated effectively to avoid deleterious effects.

Preliminary Conclusions

The strategies and criteria employed by Media Doctor and "healthnewsreview" have been implemented but whether these strategies can be universally applied throughout the entire health care system is debatable. Full integration of journalistic criteria (e.g., issue selection, presentation, readability, or vividness of an article) is still outstanding, and it remains questionable whether each criterion should be weighted equally. For example, is it enough for an article to be wonderfully written or must it fulfill other fundamental, important criteria, like being based on accurate facts or figures? To address this issue, let us look at an approach used by the German consumer organization, *Stiftung Warentest*, which weighs criteria independently; when a key criteria (e.g., a security feature in a technical device) fails, the product is rated as defective (mangelhaft) regardless of performance in any other area.

Although there are no final answers, there is initial consensus on some criteria of quality. Preliminary results have yielded recommendations for basic improvements. At the University of Dortmund, a group is currently working to establish a German version of "healthnewsreview" ("medien-doktor") that will be designed to look at reporting via mass media as well as on the Internet (e.g., Google hits).

Status Quo of Health Care Journalism

The mass media report on medicine and health-related topics more than any other scientific issue, and the tone of coverage is mostly positive (see study of German newspaper media by Elmer et al. 2008:886). In the United Kingdom, Entwistle and Hancock-Beaulieu found a proliferation of health-related articles in the 1990s compared to the previous decade; however, they note a clear distinction in quality between the mainstream and popular press (Entwistle and Hancock-Beaulieu 1992:380).

Poor-quality medical reporting has been observed in many countries, although there are signs of improvement. Between March 2004 and June 2008, Wilson et al. (2009) analyzed 1230 news stories in Australia. Comparing these results to similar reports from Canadian and U.S. media they found that despite modest improvements in some areas, "the general media generally fail[ed] to provide the public with complete and accurate information on new medical treatments." Deficits cited ranged from incomplete information, which is often skewed to extremes (underemphasized or exaggerated), to the failure to report complex research data. Coverage by commercial current affairs television programs was especially poor. In an analysis of 500 new stories from U.S. press, Schwitzer (2008) found that 62–77% of these articles failed to address the facts adequately (in particular, costs, benefits, harms, and the quality of the evidence used or methodology).

From 1961 to 2000, Verhoeven conducted a long-term content analysis of medical topics on Dutch television (Verhoeven 2008). Over time, a strong decrease in the speaking time of experts was observed, commensurate with a strong increase in the speaking time allotted to laypeople. To explain this, Verhoeven (2008:470) hypothesized that the "layification of the speaking time might be explained by the transformation in the patient–doctor relationship that occurred between 1961 and 2000, and the rise of patient activist groups and activism around specific diseases like AIDS." Paradoxically, during this same time period, television programs devoted less attention to everyday medical problems and increased coverage of diseases that required "first-class clinical care or new and specialized treatments" (Verhoeven 2008:467).

Long-term studies that analyze the development of medical or health care reporting are rare and are often limited to a single disease. Thus, it is difficult to provide an accurate status report. Nonetheless, based on the existing knowledge base, strategies to improve health care reporting can be entertained.

Strategies to Improve Medical Reporting

Two general areas in journalism could benefit from dedicated strategies to improve reporting: how a story is investigated and how it is subsequently presented. To illustrate the issues involved in journalistic investigation, consider the following anecdote taken from a professional training course entitled, "How to identify a good expert." After imparting some basic knowledge to participants, a journalist working for a well-established online publication remarked: "Why should I know how to identify a good expert when I usually never have the time to contact one?"

Although the argument of "lack of time" may appear to some to be an excuse, it is one of the most serious problems facing a working journalist (Figure 11.1). In his latest survey of 256 members of the Association of Health Care Journalists, Schwitzer (2009) reported that nine out of ten respondents (89%) indicated that ample time constitutes one of the top two ingredients of quality reporting. Over half (53%) stated that the time allotted for investigations had declined in their organization over the past several years. This is verified by Larsson (2003), who cites "lack of time, space, and knowledge" at the top of his list of barriers to the improvement of informative value in medical journalism.[5]

---

[5] Since much of medical reporting is done by an ever-increasing number of freelancers, "lack of time" may translate to "lack of financing" and even an endangered financial existence.

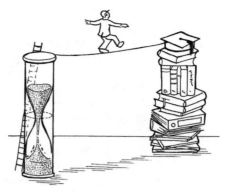

Figure 11.1 Balancing the demands of successful reporting, journalists often work under immense time constraints to get their story out (cartoon by Becker in Wormer 2006).

Despite this general tendency, some journalists still have a certain amount of freedom to decide how much time should be allocated on a particular story. Thus a gradational approach may most likely meet the variable needs of journalists: one flexible enough to account for the timescales involved in different media as well as the diverse levels of scientific expertise.

In terms of journalistic presentation, different issues must be addressed: What kind of information is necessary, and in which hierarchical order should it be presented, for a medical topic to be understood? To what extent is an "ideal information transfer" applicable to the media circus, which has its own rules and is governed by ever-growing competition? From the perspective of current communication theories, one must ask to what extent the media should even be used to communicate complex issues, such as medical or science-based health topics. Neil Postman (1986:7) illustrates the problem as follows:

> Puffs of smoke are insufficiently complex to express ideas on the nature of existence, and even if they were not, a Cherokee philosopher would run short of either wood or blankets long before he reached his second axiom. You cannot use smoke to do philosophy. Its form excludes the content.

Postman postulates that the medium is the metaphor. Transferring this to medical reporting, we must question whether, for example, a one-minute piece of news reported on television is sufficient to qualify as discriminating health advice. Most notably, it is difficult to predict how a certain piece of information will affect listeners and/or readers.

A Two-step Model to Improve the Quality of Investigation

Several authors have proposed checklists for journalists to use when verifying the quality of medical evidence (Levi 2001; Moynihan and Sweet 2000).

However, differences that arise between the various media form a fundamental barrier to the standardization and application of these lists. A science journalist, who is a medical doctor by training and works for a monthly popular magazine, will have to meet different standards than a general news editor, who has to decide within minutes (e.g., on a Sunday) whether an announced medical breakthrough has a high probability of being correct. Based on experience with these two extremes, I have proposed a two-step model for science journalistic evidence (Wormer 2006). Here, again, checklists play a central role but they are more adapted to the needs of different journalists, publications, and timescales (Wormer 2008a, b).

For the first step, the credibility of a scientific source must be verified; that is, reputation of an institution, (peer-reviewed) scientific publications, scientific awards, or external funding by foundations. Here, no special scientific knowledge in a particular field is necessary; instead, an understanding of the overview of general structures and criteria for an evaluation in the scientific system is required. Although this step is intended solely as an initial plausibility check, and contains problems associated with any scientometric-based evaluation, it can potentially weed out bogus announcements of "medical breakthroughs" or dangerous "miracle cures" (Wormer 2008b:351).

The second step involves the scientific (i.e., methodological, statistical) content of a publication, lecture, or announcement. Science journalists should be able to evaluate the presented results in terms of their validity, unambiguousness, and consistency, and to cross check existing scientific literature in the field. Here, an additional checklist may be helpful (e.g., Antes 2008; Greenhalgh 2006). Only in a few cases will journalists have sufficient specialization in the required field to enable a detailed and substantial evaluation of the specific study. However, journalists should be able to identify other scientific experts and turn to them for an evaluation or explanation of the results. If the topic to be reported is based on an existing scientific paper, the peer-review process of the scientific journal will be extended by a second "science journalistic review process" (Wormer 2008a:223). Since the scientific peer-review process itself has been criticized, this additional review process could increase the value of the reporting and even contribute to scientific quality assurance. As Woloshin et al. (2009) criticize, the exaggeration of scientific results often begins in medical journal articles and journal press releases, which researchers believe and read with interest. In such cases, the mass media must "review" and correct such exaggerations. Especially in cases of scientific fraud, the mass media has often played an important role in the past.

The advantage of this two-step model lies in its ability to be applied by nonspecialist journalists and science journalists. It also contributes to a better structuring of each journalistic investigation. Furthermore, training experience with professional (but not specialized) journalists shows that this model has the potential to dismantle the apprehension associated with science issues. Instead of an "I-will-not-understand-it-anyway" attitude, journalists are empowered to conduct an initial, formal check (first step) of the evidence. This can lead to the application of step 2 as well as a deeper application of step 1 (e.g., identifying citation networks by social network analysis).

Improving the Quality of Journalistic Presentation

Even after a thorough investigation is conducted, one must weigh how many details can, and should, be presented to a given audience. How many methodological facts are necessary to present the results and consequences of a certain research?

Usually, articles that report on medical issues contain sparse information about the scientific methods. They also fail to describe the limitations of scientific results, thus creating the impression that the results are more certain than they actually are (e.g., Dunwoody 1999). This has also been observed by the Media Doctor project and "healthnewsreview."

The reasons for this lack in presentation could stem from investigation process itself: A journalist may fail to scrutinize the methods used (Dunwoody and Peters 1992). In addition, he may overestimate the significance of a peer-reviewed article, which still have a high degree of uncertainty, at least until the experiment or study is repeated by other groups. In the worst case, a source may be understood to be proven fact, although its intent was as a genuine "working paper" meant to spur discussion in the scientific community (Wormer 2008a:223; Angell and Kassirer 1994).

Another explanation for the lack of details about scientific methods holds that journalists believe that too much detail will overtax their audience (Dunwoody and Peters 1992). This explanation conforms to a recent survey of the heads of science departments in German media (Wormer and Cavaliere, unpublished). Whereas 51% of 37 respondents regarded knowledge about scientific methods as "very important" for an *investigation*, only 13.5% thought that the *presentation* of the scientific news in articles needed to include this information. The perception is that recipients prefer clear and short messages on how something is—not on how it could be (Angell and Kassirer 1994).

For this reason, controversies may, on the one hand, be intentionally suppressed by journalists who prefer to go with a simple, understandable story over a complete but complex presentation. This conflict between complete versus simple was demonstrated by Weber und Rager (1994:1–15): For journalists, "completeness" is usually not considered to be a central indicator for quality, whereas a simple matter of facts is an important marker for understandability.

In some cases, on the other hand, the uncertainties of results and doubts can be used by the journalist as a kind of rhetorical, dramaturgical means or as the consequence of a political controversy (Zehr 1999). The same phenomena are true not only for uncertainties but also for scientific controversies. Controversies are even considered a trigger for reporting in journalism (Friedman et al. 1999:12; Galtung and Ruge 1965). Furthermore, the usual presentation techniques in journalism can amplify or even construct a controversy. The media tend to present different positions, in some cases even as a kind of surrogate for checking real evidence (Dunwoody and Peters 1992). In addition, the overarching rule that governs good journalistic practice—namely, the presentation of all sides of an issue—can actually get in the way of good scientific reporting because arguments are often presented as if they have equal validity, when in actuality a broad scientific consensus may already exist. Examples of such "balance as bias" phenomena can be found in the reporting on climate change (Boykoff and Boykoff 2004) and the effects of tobacco smoke (Miller 1992). Finally, because of their exotic and special character, self-proclaimed scientists ("mavericks") may be attractive because they promise an interesting, unusual story that sets it apart from the "boring" business-as-usual-scientist.

Lewenstein draws a rather pessimistic conclusion on the ability to improve the presentation of controversial scientific findings (Lewenstein 1995:347):

> Taken together...studies clearly imply that media coverage of controversies cannot be "improved" by better "dissemination" of scientific...information. Rather, media coverage is shaped by structural relationships within communities (including political relationships) as well as by the media's need to present "stories" that have "conflict" embedded in them.

To improve the general perception and understanding of medical and statistical information, many recommendations resulting from educational research, cognition, and psychology (e.g., Gigerenzer et al. 2007) have been made and are applicable to the mass media and its recipients. Their implementation, however, is impacted by the need to attract crowds. This often means that the presentation of every single report, radio, or television piece is subjected to constraints in length, time, or density of information (see Postman 1986). Medical reporting in the mass media must not only attract patients and their concerned relatives, but also anyone who is just a little bit interested in such topics. Given the propensity of switching over to the next interesting topic on another program or page at any given time, attractiveness and comprehensiveness of media pieces (e.g., vividness and narrative style) as well as linguistic aids (e.g., short sentences or use of repetition) play a major role in determining the quality of health news reporting (e.g., Brosius 1995; Kindel 1998).

Possible Effects of Health Care Journalism

Studies about the perception and effects of health care reporting on recipients are usually limited to specific medical subtopics. One exception is a survey by Brodie et al. (2003), where more than 42,000 Americans were asked how closely they follow major health stories and what they understood from the issues covered. Four in ten adults answered that they follow such stories closely. Brodie et al. report that this group of respondents was also more likely to give the correct answer to knowledge questions about these stories. This concurs with the findings of Chew et al. (1995), who observed that participants in the study demonstrated an increased knowledge about nutrition after watching only a one-hour television program, even when tested five and a half months after the broadcast. Although these studies do not allow us to predict a real change in health behavior, Li et al. (2008) report a significant increase of national iodized salt sales in Australia after a brief period of television and newspaper reports about the benefits of using iodized salt. They conclude that even brief news media exposure can influence health-related decisions. A further example is the dramatic decrease of hormone replacement therapy after widespread reporting of its adverse effects or the case of celebrities, such as Kylie Minogue, whose widespread breast cancer diagnosis seems to have contributed to an increase in mammograms among women who had previously never been screened. Finally, Phillips et al. (1991) emphasize the importance of the general press in transmitting medical knowledge to the scientific community itself.

These studies, which look for smaller effects, are at a high risk of only measuring simple correlations. They also are highly uncertain with respect to possible confusing elements imposed by other uncontrolled sources of information or memory effects. Gigerenzer, Mata, and Frank (2009) observe that information sources (including the mass media) appear to have little impact on improving public perception of mammography and PSA, although the poor quality of these sources may be have contributed to this. Furthermore, doubt has been expressed as to how effective simple information in the media can really influence judgment or even change the opinion of people, especially those with strong beliefs (e.g., Brosius 1995). Brosius finds that recipients do not follow a scientific rationality when processing information from the media, but rather adhere to an "everyday rationality," where presentation type and emotions play important roles. Another viewpoint ststes that "newspapers do not exist to be vehicles of health promotion or to further public understanding of medical science, but have the potential to contribute to these" (Entwistle and Hancock-Beaulieu 1992:380).

Whether people can identify good health information and distinguish it from misleading sources remains to be seen. People generally seem to rely on the reputation of a specific journalistic brand name to judge the credibility of information.

In a study involving Internet sources, Eysenbach and Köhler (2002) examined the techniques used by consumers to retrieve and appraise health information. None of the 21 participants checked formal quality indicators, such as "about us" sections of web sites or disclosure statements. This may indicate that a tiered strategy (such as the two-step model for science journalistic evidence or many of the checklists) may be preferable for a broader public as it would avoid overtaxing people (including those without knowledge of the simplest evaluation techniques) with detailed information on how to read the statistics of a clinical study.

Establishing "Evidence as a Topic"

Among journalists, there seems to be little doubt that only a very limited amount of methodological details should be included when reporting on a health care topic. Instead of providing complete methodological information in an article (e.g., addressing the topic of a cancer or the swine flu), background information could be made available separately as a topic of its own. "Evidence as a topic" is attractive for certain types of media (e.g., the popular German magazine, *Stern*). It has also been successful in many recent books, some of which have made various bestseller lists. Focusing on topics such as "popular errors," these books reveal the potential to attract a broad audience, for interest lies not only in medical results but also in good and bad science as well as its methodologies and pitfalls (e.g., Gigerenzer 2002). Another visible, but as yet unquantified, example concerns the interest in special aspects of risk and evidence related to "swine flu" and its vaccination during a period of focused reporting.

In support of evidence as topic, the German Network for Evidence Based Medicine established a new journalism prize, which was recently awarded to Markus Grill (2009) for his article "Alarm und Fehlalarm" [Alarm and False Alarms]. Such efforts to establish evidence as a topic of its own (e.g., by sensitizing journalists to these issues in their formation and permanent training)[6] may be an important complementary component to the formal teaching of risks and evidence in schools (see Bond 2009).

The Future of Health Care Journalism

When discussing the future of health care journalism, we must address the potential of the Internet to communicate medical information directly to the consumer. The general market for medical advice and health reporting can be expected to grow in the future. However, there is also a high probability that this future market will not be controlled by independent reporting.

"Whether directly or indirectly, scientists and the institutions at which they work are having more influence than ever over what the public reads about their work" (Brumfiel 2009:274). At first glance, this statement could be regarded in a positive light, especially for those who lament the poor quality of medical reporting in the mass media. However, a scientist's blog, a medical

---

[6] These aspects have already been integrated into the bachelor degree program for "science journalism" at the University of Dortmund.

doctor's advice page, or the public relation "news" of a pharmaceutical company or scientific institution is rarely void of bias.

If the traditional role of journalism in a democracy as a watchdog—or at least as a moderator of competitive scientific opinions—is undermined, it is uncertain whether the average report from these groups will attain better quality than that from science journalism. It is also unclear whether future recipients will be able to distinguish between journalistic information and public relations (see also Eysenbach and Köhler 2002). Journalists often play a role in blurring this difference by incorporating the content of press releases verbatim in their articles without further investigation, or by using electronic material prepared by outside sources in their TV and radio pieces. Even editors of quality newspapers, such as *The Times* in London, admit: "If there's a good press release and you've got four stories to write in a day, you're going to take that short cut" (Brumfiel 2009:275).

In a fragmented media world that we expect in the future, standards of quality may become even more difficult to install or enforce. It may also become difficult to raise awareness or focus public attention on a specific issue (e.g., an important health campaign).

Need for a "googlehealthnewsreview"

People interested in medical advice on a particular topic often turn to the Internet, instead of the health section of their newspaper, and use a search engine (e.g., Google) to access information. Therefore, it may be useful to track the top results for medical key words from Google and other search engines as well as wikipedia and produce a kind of a new "googlehealthnewsreview" or "wikipediahealthnewsreview." Obviously, the difficulties of defining "quality" would apply here as they do for other media forms.

In a systematic review of 79 studies designed to assess the quality of health-related web sites, Eysenbach found that 70% of these studies regarded "quality" as a problem inherent in the Web (Eysenbach et al. 2002). The most frequently used quality criteria identified by Eysenbach were similar to those widely accepted in journalism: accuracy, readability, design, disclosures, and references provided. In addition, "completeness" was often mentioned.

In a more recent analysis of 343 web sites, which focused on information about breast cancer, Bernstam et al. (2008) came to a more optimistic conclusion: "most breast cancer information that consumers are likely to encounter online is accurate." However, in their opinion, commonly used quality criteria did not identify *in*accurate information.

Several instruments are widely available to judge the quality of consumer health information (DISCERN 2010; Charnock et al. 1999); however, opinions vary as to the potential and limitations of these indicators. Griffiths and Christensen (2005) found that "DISCERN has potential as an indicator of content quality when used either by experts or by consumers." However, Gagliardi and Jadad (2002) criticize that "many incompletely developed rating instruments" appear on web sites providing health information.

Further research is needed to compare and systematically reconcile the proposals that address quality criteria in consumer health information and quality criteria in journalism. This could serve as an external evaluation for both fields and may help direct potential improvements in both.

Future of Journalism in General

The future importance of directly communicating health issues via the Internet is closely connected to the future of journalism in general. Far beyond the acute effects of the recent financial crisis, it is doubtful whether the traditional financing of news media will suffice in an era where information is perceived to be offered for free via the Internet. It is extremely improbable that traditional media will disappear altogether; however, dramatic changes could impact the quality of health reporting. How can high-quality journalism be guaranteed? Weichert and Kramp (2009) raise the following options to support quality journalism in the general media:

1. Foundations could finance investigative quality journalism (e.g., Probublica 2010).[7]
2. A general fee could be imposed not only on public broadcasting (e.g., BBC, ARD) but also on print media.
3. A surcharge could be levied on every Internet account as well as hard- and software, and the resulting funds transferred to the general media.
4. "Rent-a-journalist" or "investigate-on-demand" models, where the user pays for a specific investigation, could provide in-depth information (e.g., Spot.Us 2010).
5. Public institutions, such as universities, academies, and other educational organizations, should cooperate to ensure that quality data gets into the hands of reporters, and newspapers should be given the same tax status as educational institutes.

Although these ideas are relevant to general as well as health care journalism, some may be more applicable to health care journalism with a clear focus on educational issues. All models raise issues that relate to the independence and diversity of reporting, and some emphasize the need to pay for access to the mass media products via the Internet (e.g., Russ-Mohl 2009).

The media competence of the average person can be expected to become more important in the future. To ensure quality reporting on the Internet, it may

---

7 Although this model is less popular in German-speaking countries than in the United States, modest attempts in the field of medical journalism have been made, such as the "Peter Hans Hofschneider Recherchepreis" in Germany, Austria, and Switzerland (Stiftung Experimentelle Biomedizin 2010).

be helpful to examine the strategies presented in this chapter to see whether they can be applied here as well. In addition, the role of journalists in the future may expand to include training the public on how to verify medical information or to work as "evidence scouts" for individuals or interest groups such as NGOs.

Acknowledgments

I would like to thank Eva Prost and Pia Nitz for their preparatory work concerning the question of quality in science and journalism, Gerd Gigerenzer, Christian Weymayr, and two anonymous reviewers for their helpful remarks as well as Paul Klammer for much of the literature research.

Overleaf (left to right, top to bottom):
Richard Smith, Michael Diefenbach, Talya Miron-Shatz
Odette Wegwarth, Opening reception
David Spiegelhalter, Ingrid Mühlhauser, Ben Goldacre
Bruce Bower, Group discussion

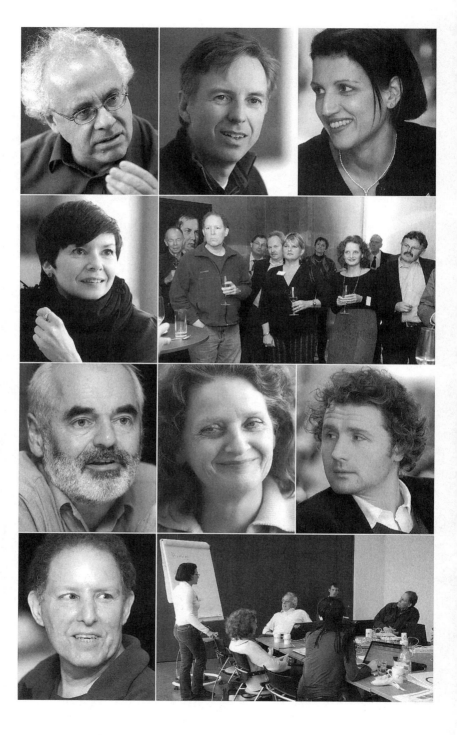

12

Barriers to Health Information and Building Solutions

Talya Miron-Shatz, Ingrid Mühlhauser, Bruce Bower,
Michael Diefenbach, Ben Goldacre, Richard S. W. Smith,
David Spiegelhalter, and Odette Wegwarth

Abstract

Most stakeholders in the health care system—doctors, patients, and policy makers—have not been taught to apply evidence-based information to the many decisions that must be made daily. Little awareness of this problem exists, yet a better use of evidence could improve outcomes for patients, increase patient satisfaction, and lower costs. This chapter considers how the use of information that emerges from evidence-based medicine could be improved.

"Health literacy" constitutes the first step. After a discussion of the barriers that exist to health literacy (e.g., lack of incentive to search for health information, non-standardized reporting of health results, and poor comprehension), possible remedies are presented. Raising health literacy by targeting individual stakeholder groups, such as patients and health care professionals, is debated as is the option of focusing on change in the overall health system. What is required to achieve a change both at the individual and system levels? Solutions are unlikely to generate systemic changes in center-based treatment variations. However, a change at one level may set off change in another. Finally, increasing awareness beyond the immediate professional community is necessary if systemic changes are to be made. The promotion of health literacy requires careful consideration to reach the various stakeholders throughout the health care system.

Introduction

Health literacy is a broad, social concept. The Institute of Medicine (IOM 2004) defines it as "the degree to which individuals can obtain, process, and understand basic health information and services they need to make appropriate health decisions." Statistical literacy can be interpreted as the ability to grasp the meaning of numbers, proportions, and probabilities. However, although statistical competency is important, it is not the essential component in health information. This was recognized by the World Health Organization, which included social competencies and skills into its definition of health literacy (WHO 2010): "Health literacy has been defined as the cognitive and social skills which determine the motivation and ability of individuals to gain access to, understand, and use information in ways which promote and maintain good health."

To appreciate the complexity of health literacy, it is important to realize that it is not a static concept. Experiences in personal health, the health care system, as well as cultural and societal influences all shape a person's ability to obtain, process, and understand basic health information. Zarcadoolas, Pleasant, and Greer (2006:5–6) advocate a broader view of health literacy, which they define as "the wide range of skills, and competencies that people develop over their lifetimes to seek out, comprehend, evaluate, and use health information and concepts to make informed choices, reduce health risks, and increase quality of life." They specify four different domains of health literacy:

1. Fundamental literacy includes the traditional view of literacy according to the IOM definition.
2. Science literacy means that a stakeholder appreciates fundamental scientific concepts and processes, and understands that technological relationships are often complex and can rapidly change. They also understand that there is an inherent element of uncertainty to the scientific process. Zarcadoolas et al. (2006) suggest that only between 5–15% of the general public are scientifically literate.
3. Civic literacy covers the domains of information acquisition and information source. Specifically, civic literate individuals are able to judge the information source as credible, possess media literacy skills, have a basic knowledge of civic and governmental systems, and are also aware that personal behaviors can affect the community at large.
4. Cultural literacy includes the ability to recognize, understand, and use the collective beliefs, customs, world view, and social identity of diverse individuals. Cultural literate individuals are capable of interpreting and acting on cultural information and context, and are aware that certain information can only be interpreted through a cultural lens.

This expanded concept has profound implications when constructing appropriate messages intended to be understood easily by health literate individuals. Clearly, the use of plain language and simple numbers is not enough; the broader civic and cultural context must also be considered.

Steckelberg et al. (2007, 2009) suggest that teaching competencies that enhance consumers' autonomy in health care issues requires combining the concepts of evidence-based medicine, evidence-based health care, and health literacy. Competencies originating from this new concept are referred to as *critical health literacy*. Some aspects are absent from existing definitions (e.g., the information that patients are not receiving and their ability to request such information). Patients need to know how to pose questions and to be suspicious when, for example, a brochure specifies the benefits of a drug or treatment but neglects to list possible harms or the merits of alternative routes of action. Indeed, everyone exposed to health information should be able to pose questions as to the knowledge source and its bias.

We suggest that definitions of health literacy apply to all stakeholders. The levels at which any one particular stakeholder needs to obtain, process, and understand information will obviously vary, as will the specific area of focus. However, all stakeholders can be included in a definition if the extent of the knowledge to be obtained, processed, and comprehended depends on whoever is pursuing it. Notably, differences will exist not only between but also within stakeholder categories; information should be available so that individuals can choose how much or how little of it they need.

For the clinician, information must be obtained from the patient: What are the patient's preferences, life circumstances, and history? Once elicited, this information should be used to establish the alternatives which the professional presents and recommends. It is the clinician's responsibility to communicate health information to a patient and to ensure its comprehension. Improving skills to obtain, process, and understand patient-specific information remains a challenge.

For journalists, policy makers, and public communicators, health information must be conveyed so that the patient, reader, consumer, or citizen understands it. However, this must be done without compromising the evidence base. When communicating to the general public, journalists, policy makers, or public communicators must consider the potential hurdles that their stories or accounts will invoke and help the public overcome these. Reports need to be intelligible, though not at the cost of accuracy.

Existing definitions of health literacy have focused on the individual person—primarily the patient. They take into account the individual's ability and skills, yet ignore elements that could influence and help the individual understand and interpret medical information. Some of these factors are internal, such as the patient's beliefs and their impact on comprehension. Others are broader in context: cultural and social aspects, or even the extent to which health literacy is pursued. The way systems are structured affects a patient's ability to obtain, process, and understand health information. If such information exists only in specialized journals, if it is presented in an incomplete manner, if media reports sensationalize it or omit "boring" details (e.g., sample size or numbers needed to treat), then obtaining, processing, and understanding health information is greatly impaired. Focusing on any stakeholder at the individual level may not be the most beneficial way of promoting health literacy.

We suggest a dual approach: top down and bottom up. We discuss remedies at the individual level, but also at the level of the information as conveyed throughout the health system and beyond, including industry and government.

Obtaining, Processing, and Understanding Health Information

In an ideal world, society would be made up of health literate citizens, yet this is not the case. Here we discuss potential barriers that exist to hinder the process of accessing health information. Not every obstacle will be easy to overcome. Still, there is value in drawing attention to them so that their impact can be addressed in the future.

Social Construction of Roles

The chain of events whereby a person sets out to obtain information requires motivation. A person who is content with the information they have is unlikely to contemplate obtaining further knowledge. People need to feel unsettled and be urged into actively seeking information. While acquiring new knowledge requires action on the part of an individual, the motivation to do so does not solely stem from the individual. Motivation can involve a shift in the way society constructs the "sick" role; that is, whether a patient is a mere recipient of information or someone who assumes an active role in health-related decision making, including the decision of whether to engage with the medical establishment. Such construction of prevailing narratives has been shown to be influential in selecting treatment options (Wong and King 2008). Likewise, for health care professionals, it would be conducive to health literacy if greater emphasis were put on reflective practice. The active pursuit of information by a patient does not necessarily equate to an inherent mistrust of health care professionals, but is often perceived as such. This needs to be addressed in the role construction of both the patient and health care professional.

Perceiving Information Seeking as Mistrust in Health Care Professionals

If patients and other stakeholders perceive information seeking as a sign of mistrust, they might be reluctant to engage in this behavior or to encourage others to do so. The misinterpretation of trust as blind acceptance is most often imposed on patients, though it may apply to other stakeholders as well. Those who provide information often struggle with numbers or may have conflict of interest. Thus, blind trust in the health care professional who presents information can be a barrier to health literacy.

Onora O'Neill argues that trust has fallen dramatically in many institutions: "Mistrust and suspicion have spread across all areas of life" (O'Neill 2002:8). The usual answer to the growth in mistrust is to insist on transparency and greater accountability in everything. Further, O'Neill argues that "if we want to restore trust we need to reduce deceptions and lies....well placed trust grows out of active inquiry, not blind acceptance" (O'Neill 2002:70, 76).

One would hope that health care professionals and other stakeholders, who are sometimes mistrusted, would view the opportunity to refer patients to information they can check and assess themselves as advantageous rather than threatening. For example, Nannenga et al. (2009) demonstrated that a decision aid designed to help patients decide about statin use was associated with both increased knowledge and enhanced trust on the part of patients. Trust increased with patient participation.

David Mechanic (2004) reminds us that patients cannot always assess their health care professionals' skills, which then leads to trust or mistrust accordingly. He mentions other bases for trust, however, which coincides with the notion of professionals both conveying information and eliciting patient-specific input: "Patients' trust is how doctors communicate and whether they listen and are caring. Patients do not expect intimacy but they do seek respect and responsiveness…patients want to know that their doctors are committed to protecting their interests" (Mechanic 2004:1419).

Paternalism

When health care professionals, policy makers, insurers, or other stakeholders avoid presenting evidence to patients, decline to share uncertainty, and/or make decisions on their behalf, they erect barriers to health literacy. Paternalism supports the notion of a patient as a passive, non-inquisitive recipient of whatever information the professional wishes to impart. Health professionals may do this with the best of intentions, believing that it actually protects patients, as has been the traditional style of doctors for centuries. Yet increasingly, doctors do share evidence and uncertainty with patients. Unfortunately, many health care professionals continue to insist that patients do not want to share in the decision-making process. It is undoubtedly true that some will choose, under some circumstances, to allow health care professionals to make decisions on their behalf, but strong evidence indicates that doctors assume all too often a paternalistic attitude (Stevenson et al. 2004; Coulter and Jenkinson 2005). Professionals should adopt a default position that patients want to be informed and, at the very least, should ask patients how much information they would like and whether they would like to share in the decision-making process.

Paternalism is not confined, however, to the doctor–patient encounter. It is evident between the media and the public, the government and the public, and health care professionals and policy makers.

Perceived Inadequacy in Handling Medical Information

A de-motivating factor for seeking health information is the feeling that even if accessible, it will not be understood. In a study on prostate cancer patients (van Tol-Geerdink et al. 2006), about half of the patients (69 of 148) indicated an initial low preference to participate in medical decisions. However, after receiving information about treatment options from a decision aid, 75% of these patients wanted to be involved in choosing their radiation dosage. Contrast this with the group of patients who expressed an initial high participation preference, where 85% wanted to be involved in choosing their radiation dose.

This suggests that although patients may have initially refrained from seeking information or making health decisions, preferring to defer to professional opinion instead, once information is available in a clear and understandable way, these same patients now feel equipped to participate in decision making.

Barriers to Obtaining Health Information

Lack of Evidence-based Information

Although there is an abundance of communication on health issues targeting patients and the general public, it rarely adheres to criteria deemed by researchers as necessary for making decisions on health issues (Bunge et al. 2010; Steckelberg et al. 2005; Trevena et al. 2006). Information must be relevant to the individual patient, its content must be based on the best available evidence, and its presentation must follow specific criteria to allow understanding of the information. Elements that are often missing include quantitative estimates of the benefits and harms of treatment options, diagnostic or screening procedures using numbers, and verbal and graphical presentations. All options should be presented, including the option not to intervene or to postpone the intervention. Outcomes relevant for patients should be reported rather than surrogates. At present, such information is provided only for a few areas of interest; structures are missing to ensure that updated, comprehensive, and understandable information can be used by all stakeholders.

Non-standardized Reporting

It is difficult to develop the skills to seek out health information if such information is not reported in a consistent form. Clear, transparent templates need to be developed and consistently utilized: in textbooks, drug information, patient brochures, newspaper reports, and white papers. Standardized reporting is also a key component in the development of a scheme to address existing and missing knowledge.

Existing and Missing Knowledge

To pursue information, one needs a scheme involving the kind of information that is needed within a particular decision situation. If such a scheme is absent, one does not know what is missing, or even that the information they are receiving is incomplete. An overview of questions to ask, to know what information must be sought, has been provided by Gigerenzer et al. (2007). These questions can serve as informal guidelines for designing risk information.

Listed below are some of the most important questions and concepts that need to be clarified when examining health information.

- Risk of what? Does the outcome refer to dying from the disease, not getting the disease, or developing a symptom?
- What is the time frame? Time frames such as the "next ten years" are easier to imagine than the widely used "lifetime" risks. They are also more informative because risks can change over time but ten years may be long enough to enable action to be taken. For example, for every thousand female nonsmokers (age 50), 37 will die within the next ten years; however, for every thousand smokers (age 50), 69 will die (Woloshin et al. 2008).
- How big? Since there are few zero risks, size matters. Size should be expressed as absolute rather than relative risks.
- Benefits and harms: Screening tests, as well as treatments, have benefits and harms. Thus information on both is needed. Always ask for absolute risks of outcomes with and without treatment.
- Screening tests can make two errors: false positives as well as false negatives. Understand how to translate specificities, sensitivities, and other conditional probabilities into natural frequencies. Ask how common the condition is in the population: Out of 1,000 sick people, how many will the test correctly identify (sensitivity) and how many will it miss (false negative rate)? Out of 1,000 healthy people, how many will the test correctly identify (specificity), and how many will it mistake as ill (false positive rate)?

Conflicts of Interest

A conflict of interest occurs when an individual or organization is involved in multiple interests, one of which could possibly influence the other. A conflict of interest can only exist if a person or testimony is entrusted with some impartiality. Thus, a modicum of trust is necessary to create it.

An Institute of Medicine report on the topic states that "conflicts of interest threaten the integrity of scientific investigations" (Lo and Field 2009:2), and "evidence suggests that...relationships [between industry and researchers] have risks, including decreased openness in the sharing of data and findings and the withholding of negative results" (Lo and Field 2009:9). However, the authors are also explicit in saying that empirical evidence is limited and that "data are suggestive rather than definitive" (Lo and Field 2009:4).

In 2001, American-based pharmaceutical companies sent out some 88,000 sales representatives to doctors' offices to hand out nearly US$11 billion worth of "free samples" as well as personal gifts (Angell 2004; Chin 2002). The expectation is that when the free samples run out, doctors and patients will continue to prescribe or take them. An editorial in *USA Today* (2002) painted a vivid picture: "Christmas trees; free tickets to a Washington Redskin game, with a champagne reception thrown in; a family vacation in Hawaii; and wads of cash. Such gifts would trigger a big red "bribery" alert in the mind of just about any public official or government contractor."

Even though the Office of the Inspector General of the U.S. Department of Health and Human Services issued a warning in 2003 that excessive gift-giving to doctors could be prosecuted under the Anti-Kickback Law, critics stress that the laws are still full of loopholes (Angell 2004). In recognition of these pervasive influences, some major hospitals in the United States have denied pharmaceutical representatives entry onto their premises and have forbidden the sponsoring of meals where products are advocated. In addition, existing conflict of interest regulations have been tightened to enforce strict reporting of any incomes or stock holdings of health care-related companies, of hospital employees, as well as their family members. It is too soon to tell whether these efforts have been effective in curbing the influence of the pharmaceutical industry on health care delivery.

Alongside health care professionals, patient advocacy groups also meet the criteria for assumed impartiality. Such groups have become a target of the industry's marketing efforts (Grill 2007) and have been found to be strongly entangled with pharmaceutical companies, who often design their web sites and pay their public relations agencies (Angell 2004). Company representatives sometimes even take leading positions on their boards (Schubert and Glaeske 2006). Such entanglement may cloud any objective view of a pharmaceutical product portfolio and prevent doctors' and patients' advocacy groups from either requesting or reporting transparent numbers on the real benefits and harms of a drug or medical intervention. In general, little is known about the exact extent of influence that pharmaceutical promotions have on the behavior of patient advocacy groups.

Barriers to Processing Health Information

During elementary, middle, and high school education, children are seldom taught risk, probability, and the concept of uncertainty. This lack of education is at the root of the prevailing levels of low statistical literacy. Teaching schoolchildren how to approach frequencies and probabilities helps prepare them for the complexities and uncertainties of the modern world; it also equips them to make sound decisions throughout their lives (Bond 2009; Gigerenzer et al. 2007). Yet the attainment of these necessary skills is not part of the curricula in every school and in every country.

Health statistics and randomized trials are an indispensable part of clinical practice. In 1937, an editorial in *The Lancet* stressed the importance of statistics for both laboratory and clinical medicine, and criticized the "educational blind spot" of physicians. In 1948, the British Medical Association Curriculum

Committee recommended that statistics be included in medical education. Ten lectures were proposed with additional time for exercises, ranging from teaching core concepts such as chance and probability to interpreting correlations (Altman and Bland 1991). Despite this, it took until 1975 before statistics became a mandatory subject in medical schools within the University of London, and it took an additional ten years before adoption in Austria, Hungary, and Italy (Altman and Bland 1991). Although statistics has received a mandatory status, statistics and risk communication are far from being an essential part of medical education: Only 3% of the questions asked in the exam for certification by the American Board of Internal Medicine cover the understanding of medical statistics (clinical epidemiology), and risk communication is not addressed at all. Similarly, biostatistics and clinical epidemiology do not seem to exceed the benchmark of 3% in curricula of medical schools, and transparent risk communication is completely lacking (cf. Wegwarth and Gigerenzer, this volume). Another important aspect in improving literacy is an understanding of what information is missing. For example, in the case of screening, does the report include numbers needed to treat, does it include health outcomes of control groups that have not received screening, and does it include information on potential harms? If society wishes to have literate doctors, medical schools need to devote time in their curricula to teach the concepts of transparent and nontransparent statistics, as well as which information is necessary and which is not. Teaching medical students transparent representations fosters understanding (Hoffrage et al. 2000) and so does teaching doctors (Gigerenzer et al. 2007). Every medical school should require graduates to exhibit at least minimal statistical literacy, with a longer-term goal of requiring more advanced understanding.

Barriers to Understanding Health Information

There are transparent and nontransparent formats for statistical information. Much of the mental confusion that defines nontransparency seems to be caused by the reference class to which a health statistic applies (Gigerenzer and Edwards 2003). Single-event probabilities, by definition, specify no classes of events, and relative risks often refer to a reference class that is different from the one of which a patient is a member. Sensitivities and specificities are conditional on two different reference classes (patients with disease and patients without disease), whereas natural frequencies all refer to the same reference class (all patients). Survival and mortality rates differ crucially in their denominator; that is, the class of events to which they refer. Clarity about the reference class to which a health statistic refers is one of the central tools in attaining health literacy.

Understanding could also be improved by providing numbers as well as words. Patients have the right to know the extent of the benefits and harms of a treatment, and qualitative risk terms are notoriously unclear. Contrary to popular belief, studies report that a majority of patients do prefer numerical information to care alone (Hallowell et al. 1997; Wallsten et al. 1993). Providing patients with accurate, balanced, and accessible data on disease risk and treatment benefits could, however, influence their choices in ways that doctors may consider undesirable. Patients may be very surprised at how negligible many of the risks or benefits are. Consequently, they may dismiss interventions that physicians might deem extremely valuable.

In one example, participants in a study were very optimistic about the effectiveness of three different drugs; in each case, these perceptions dropped substantially after seeing the actual data (Woloshin et al. 2004). This was a cause for concern, since one of the drugs—a statin used to treat men with high cholesterol but no prior myocardial infarction—showed a reduction of overall mortality over five years from 4 in 100 patients to 3 in 100 patients. It seemed that many respondents did not appreciate the real magnitude of this effect. Few drugs now being manufactured can match this reduction in all-cause mortality among relatively healthy outpatients.

To judge how well a drug (or other intervention) works, people need a context; that is, some sense of the magnitude of the benefit of other interventions. Reactions to benefit data will change as people have more exposure to them. Consumers will be better able to discriminate among drugs and interventions as they become better calibrated to effect sizes. This context is necessary so that people do not discount small but important effects.

How Can Stakeholders Be Motivated to Obtain Good Quality Evidence?

We live in an era where knowledge abounds and time is pressing. Assuming that a general practitioner needs only five minutes to skim an academic article, it has been estimated that 600 hours per month are required to read all of the published academic items pertinent to primary care alone (Alper et al. 2004). Work on cognitive limitations and information overload leads us to question whether simply providing more information will result in a higher comprehension levels (Shaughnessy et al. 1994). Clearly, the existence of information is not enough. For information to be utilized, it needs to be deemed useful, a concept Shaughnessy et al. defined as:

$$\text{usefulness} = \frac{\text{relevance} \times \text{validity}}{\text{time required to obtain}}.$$

While clinicians often claim that they consult medical journals or the library when they are unsure how to proceed, research suggests they may actually consult with their colleagues instead (Shaughnessy et al. 1994). This clearly fulfills the requirements of efficiency and relevance (a sense of local practice norms may also be a source of reassurance to the anxious practitioner), but the information may not be of the highest quality.

It has proved challenging to develop systems capable of ensuring that information is relevant at the point of delivery. Even when there are attempts to make clinical advice context dependent (e.g., notifications on evidence in practitioners' computer systems, like EMIS), these may be deactivated by practitioners, who regard them as intrusive or unhelpful. A system that sets red flags, when several medications prescribed to the same patient are determined algorithmically to be incompatible, may be disenabled if it raises alerts so as to be overwhelming. Thus too much information, given in an automated and unsolicited way, may not be the ideal structure.

Humans are good at judging relevance. "Information prescriptions," given explicitly by health care practitioners to patients, provide an example and could be improved by considering when the information is most relevant. For example, it may be most useful for people to have access to information contextualizing a discussion with a clinician before an appointment, requiring that information prescriptions are routinely sent out in anticipation of an appointment, and ensuring that such information exists. The concept of alerting patients to a range of treatment options prior to meeting with clinicians is the subject of research in shared decision making. At the Decision Laboratory (2010) in Cardiff University, parents of children referred for possible tonsillectomy are sent a checklist, based on a national guideline, which stipulates the criteria for surgery. Parents are asked to assess whether their child meets these criteria. The impact of this checklist is being evaluated.

Guessing what consumers of information will find relevant, however, is not enough: the information needs to be evidence based. Most decision support systems assume that patients would like to know, for example, the probability of suffering a heart attack with different treatments over a one- and five-year period. Thus, decision support systems are designed to answer these questions, even though they may not be the ones that a patient asks. Some support systems do present patients with alternatives in vivid terms. The Prostate Interactive Education System (PIES 2010), for example, displays the harms and benefits of prostate cancer treatments in film format, using real doctors.

An individual's own search activities provide a valuable source of information and may prove the most valuable resource. Similarly, just as we must identify areas of clinical uncertainty to drive the generation of primary and secondary research (trials and systematic reviews), we may need to consider systems to identify where there is the most need for the evidence-based information.

Good quality evidence-based information should be available online. Ideally, such information needs to be organized rationally, preferably in a standardized format, and accessible with consistent search tools. The Finnish Medical Society, Duodecim, has been producing national evidence-based current care guidelines since 1995. This web-based tool is administered by expert groups, who select core clinical questions to be answered; systematic literature searches are conducted, articles critically appraised and summarized, and detailed evidence reviews linked to the text as background documents. Guidelines also include a patient version and an English summary. Ninety-eight guidelines are available from a single web site (Current Care 2010) free of charge. In 2004, physicians accessed 3.2 million articles from this database; this corresponds to each Finnish physician reading one guideline per working day (Kunnamo and Jousimaa 2004). In 2009, the number of annual readings had reached 12 million, which means that health professionals consult the guidelines four times per day on average (Jousimaa, pers. comm.). This statistic is encouraging; it indicates that when up to date, standardized information is accessed by people who need it, when they need it.

Standardized Reports and Common Health Literacy Vocabulary

Non-standardized reporting impairs comprehension as well as health literacy by increasing the risk that flawed or misleading reporting can become accepted as the truth. If we could develop a prototype of a transparent and comprehensive report, information transfer might be optimized and health literacy might be more easily attained. Due to the nature of reporting, meeting this goal will not be easy. However, unless we impose a structure in this complex and rapidly changing field, the framing and transfer of information will continue to be unnecessarily difficult.

We deliberately interpret the term *reports* loosely. We envisage standardized reporting in (a) professional medical journals and subsequent press releases; (b) newspaper stories, feature articles, commercials, or advertisements; (c) patient communications (e.g., brochures, support-group web sites, or mammogram screening invitations); and (d) official documents intended for policy makers, commissioners, insurers, and other major players. In terms of medical content, our suggestions relate to individual decisions, whether concerning treatment, prevention, or diagnostics, as well as to population decisions regarding public health interventions.

Are There Precedents?

Whether discussing an intervention, screening or diagnostic test, or even a recommended behavior change, information needs to be presented and clearly delineated so that any stakeholder can weigh the possible benefits and harms. At a minimum, these can be listed and informally weighted. Often there is sufficient evidence to quantify the likelihood of specific benefits and harms. In our discussion of how these "probabilities" might be displayed, we reviewed several suggestions for conveying information in a stratified, standardized fashion (for a review, see Politi et al. 2007).

The Cochrane Collaboration utilizes a layered structure in its reports and has developed a plain-language summary, which includes the use of numbers. The inclusion of a "summary of findings" table for the main comparison in the review is gradually becoming the standard (Schünemann et al. 2008). Cochrane appears to believe that this does not compromise the quality of their reports and has positively evaluated the format. Cochrane has standardized as many elements of the reports as possible (Higgins and Green 2009); for example, although the effect of the intervention may be reported as an odds ratio, the absolute risks with and without the intervention are reported as frequencies (with the same denominator used throughout the report). Both "high" and "low" baseline risks are considered, and "GRADE" assessments (GRADE Working Group 2004) of the quality of evidence are provided for each benefit and harm.

Review users often become overwhelmed when more than seven outcomes are presented; more than this is confusing and cannot be integrated. Thus, in line with memory constraints, Cochrane Tables list no more than seven benefits and harms (or, more commonly, outcomes) (Higgins and Green 2009). These are ordered by degree of benefit, followed by potential harms. Cochrane also includes a "plain language summary" intended for patients, but accessible to all (Higgins and Green 2009, Chapter 11).

In Germany, guidelines are presented at three levels: a short version (no numbers) for doctors, a longer version (with numbers) for doctors, and a version for patients that includes practical suggestions (e.g., what to do if you are at particular coronary risk and feeling unwell: should you rush to the hospital or wait until the morning). The German Disease Management Guidelines (NVL 2010) also includes an evaluation of the quality of the evidence; this transparency allows clients to be critical users of the information.

The "drug facts box" is another clear example of a successful precedent. Developed by Schwartz and Woloshin (this volume), its goal is to provide accurate information on prescription drugs to the public. By utilizing a standardized 1-page table format, it summarizes the benefits and side-effect data on prescription drugs in a concise manner. Descriptive information about the drug is provided: its indication, who might consider taking it, who should not take it, recommended testing or monitoring, and other things to consider doing to achieve the same goals as the drug.

How Can Statistical Information Best Be Presented?

We suggest that this can best be achieved by combining the strengths of the "drugs facts box" (Schwartz and Woloshin, this volume) and the "summary of findings table" (Schünemann et al. 2008) using a layered format and a vocabulary accessible to all stakeholders. Principles for "basic" representation are as follows:

1. Represent probabilities as whole numbers using a constant denominator (e.g., 1000). Probabilities could also be shown as miniature icons representing people.
2. Provide a list of probabilities with and without intervention (as two columns) to allow comparison between options. The difference between interventions could then be presented in a third column.
3. Include harms and benefits.
4. Reproduce tables for different baseline risks (but do not include relative risks).
5. Include an indicator of quality of evidence (but do not include confidence intervals in the basic presentation).
6. Provide a common format for patients, health care professionals, policy makers, and the media.
7. Encourage an electronic version, with links to supplemental information for those sufficiently motivated. This would allow multiple graphical formats, animations, resources, references, etc., depending on the desires and sophistication of the user.

These principles will not apply in all circumstances, but are intended to spur further development. The challenge and goal for the future will be to develop standardized reporting formats for qualitative as well as for diagnostic research.

Who Can Help Make Standardized Reporting Happen?

Multiple strategies—both bottom up and top down—are necessary to implement standardized reporting. It will never be enough to embed it within guidelines alone, since guidelines are often not adhered to or enforced.

The U.K. Academy of Medical Sciences is proposing uniform requirements for reporting benefits and harms in medical journals. There is already an expanded CONSORT statement to include harms (Ioannidis et al. 2004), but no evidence on compliance. Editors and referees of peer-reviewed and other journals are best positioned to ensure adherence to guidelines. We note, however, that editors in the mass media may lose influence if publishing continues along its present trajectory. Continuing medical education (CME), or an equivalent professional organization for journalists, could help disseminate the prescribed reporting formats, should editors become obsolete.

In line with the mandate to provide patients with helpful, agenda-free information, patient advocacy groups could help enforce implementation. Some major charitable organizations (e.g., the U.S. National Breast Cancer Coalition) already present information in this way.

The pharmaceutical industry provides another avenue, since it is in their interest to make clear the balance of harms and benefits. Hormone replacement therapy information leaflets provide current examples of risk reporting. Paradoxically, this is one place where legislators can mandate the ways information needs to be presented. Even if a company cannot list all alternatives to their proposed product, they could be required to note the efficacy of their treatment compared with a placebo or no treatment, as is the case in the drug facts box.

A model by which good practice can be enforced may be found in Finland. There, a consumer organization reviews every type of patient-oriented communication according to pre-determined and well-publicized criteria, and either grants or withholds its stamp of approval.

Standardized reporting could also be enforced through a bottom-up approach. If consumers are trained in reading statistics (when these are provided in natural frequency format) and become familiar with a standard format, we can expect that they will, in turn, demand that information is presented in this way—be it from the media, industry or other source. Trained citizens would not be susceptible, for example, newspaper stories consisting solely of relative risk information and, likewise, would be wary of advertisements devoid of information on numbers-needed-to-treat. Equipped with the necessary tools and skills, informed consumers will be able to demand better, clearer, more transparent information from their physicians, media, and others.

What Could Stop Standardized Reporting from Happening?

We should expect the call for standardizing report formats to be met by objections. One possible source could come from health care professionals, who might perceive that standardized information (and patient aids) would interfere with their professional judgment—making them obsolete or turning them into automatons. Yet there is a big difference between presenting numbers clearly and implementation. Accessible information to the patient makes the doctor's role all the more crucial: doctors will be able to discuss implications and patient-specific recommendations, rather than regurgitate information already available. Rather than debilitating, doctors should view this change as emancipating and enabling. Standardized reporting does not eliminate health care professionals; it simplifies and streamlines the processing and understanding of information, thus leaving room for more substantial discussions to take place.

Another objection concerns the modification to original data, which involves judgment. Take the Cochrane list of harms and benefits for example: Who determines the importance of each of these? A reasonable way to address such objections is to make the judgment process transparent. In addition, the multi-layered presentation used allows anyone to go back to the original paper or raw data to generate their own impressions and ratings.

Inevitably, various groups and stakeholders have agendas and would prefer to select information to coincide with their interests. Thus, it is imperative for the public to become trained in reading standardized reports to detect information gaps and distortions.

Improving Health Literacy Skills

In this section, we discuss different ways to improve public comprehension of health information. Our ideas are not comprehensive, but serve to highlight areas which should be further explored.

Targeting Young People

The need to change existing educational school curricula to promote statistical literacy throughout the population has been discussed elsewhere (e.g., Gaissmaier and Gigerenzer; Smith, this volume). Early statistical teaching must overcome the assumptions that the mathematics of certainty (e.g., algebra and geometry) is more important than the mathematics of uncertainty. Martignon and Kurz-Milcke (2006) provide an encouraging study that shows the effectiveness of early training: fourth graders were able to master combined probabilities after participating in structured games using colorful cubes.

While structured education offers one method, another avenue might be through computer and board games. Games appeal to young people and could be an appropriate platform to turn something that appears difficult to understand into something that is assimilated naturally. For example, in the United Kingdom, computer games designed to teach probabilities have utilized aspects of gambling and have proven to be very appealing to young people (Spiegelhalter 2010). At a later age, visualization software such as Fathom (Finzer and Erickson 2006) and TinkerPlots (Konold and Miller 2005) help young people explore and manipulate data sets (Garfield and Ben-Zvi 2007). By starting with concrete representations of risks, children can accumulate confidence in basic concepts and will less likely develop a math phobia when more complex concepts are introduced at a later stage.

Although computer probability games for children exist already on several Internet sites, the extent to which young people take advantage of these games is unknown. Use of those designed explicitly for children, such as Club Penguin (2010) or Webkinz (2010) provides a starting point to incorporate modules to teach probability. These popular resources often have modules geared toward spelling, have attractive designs, and award children points for successful performance. Providing incentives to commercial companies to integrate relevant modules into resources widely used may be a feasible means of reaching and capturing the attention of children.

Another example can be drawn from a curriculum of critical health literacy for secondary school students, age 17 years, successfully piloted by Steckelberg et al. (2009). The curriculum's objectives were to develop and enhance statistical knowledge and competencies, to appraise medical information critically, and to gain understanding of how medical information is developed.

From Patients to Doctors

Simple decision aids for interpreting the meaning of medical test results provide a possible means of educating patients. Human mediators (e.g., health coaches who inform patients on how to pose questions about the benefits and risks of tests administered by their physicians) might also facilitate access to health information.

Increasingly, patients' interests are being represented on health care boards, agencies, and institutions. Training courses for patient and consumer representatives to cope with these roles have been successfully piloted (Berger et al. 2010).

Computer games that involve probability might help health care consumers, medical students, and clinicians explain the benefits and risks of various tests and screening instruments to their patients. In addition, handheld devices (e.g., touch phones) could be equipped with probability guides so that medical students and clinicians can calculate key measures (e.g., base rates of diseases, frequencies of medical conditions, and the absolute risk of having a disease after testing positive) or access information to key questions.

A more direct route to medical students would be through the Medical College Admission Test (MCAT), which is administered by the American Association of Medical Colleges (AAMC). Since every prospective medical student is required to take the MCATs, there is high motivation to perform well. Thus, if probability, uncertainty, and other core concepts of statistical literacy were integrated into the exam, students would be motivated to acquire this competency. As with children's computer games, the trick is getting people to want to know.

Journalists

Journalists exert a powerful influence on how the public perceives health and health care. Much of what people—including many physicians—know and believe about medicine comes from the print and broadcast media. Yet journalism schools tend to teach everything except the understanding of numbers. Journalists generally receive no training in how to interpret or present medical research (Kees 2002). Medical journals communicate with the media through press releases; ideally, they provide journalists with an opportunity to get their facts right. Unfortunately, press releases suffer from many of the same problems noted above (Woloshin and Schwartz 2002). Some newspapers have begun to promote correct and transparent reporting, and efforts are underway to teach journalists how to understand what the numbers mean. As in Finland, statistical training courses for journalists exist at several universities and are conducted by some government agencies. Opportunities for statistical learning remain rare in the media, however.

Editors play a central and powerful role in the presentation of new stories, at least in traditional media outlets. Even a minimal amount of training for editors (e.g., knowing which questions to ask about statistical procedures in health and medical studies written by reporters) could improve general news coverage.

Another push to make journalists report more carefully about medical facts could come from statistically literate observers. Internet sites in the United States and Australia, for instance, rate the quality of medical reporters and medical news in major news publications. One such site (Health News Review 2010) evaluates the quality of health reporting in major U.S. newspapers and magazines. Although this form of watchdog effort has not yet been evaluated, it seems plausible to assume that by intensifying the monitoring of press coverage of medical statistics, improved reporting will result.

Change from Within

It is difficult to define the level at which change should be pursued. It is people who understand information, but the problem neither starts nor ends at the individual level. Should the focus be on the patient and his/her maladies, history, and choices? Or should the emphasis be on the policy maker who determines funding, resource allocations, treatments, screenings, and bed numbers for millions?

The best way to change a system is from within. Those who set health policy and fund health care are in the strongest position to ensure that more health promotion and care is based firmly on evidence, that formats are standardized, and that people are helped and encouraged to obtain, process, and understand evidence.

There is strong evidence to indicate that the amount of health care that people receive is largely determined by the supply of health care institutions (i.e., "supplier-induced demand") (Fisher et al. 2004). For example, people in Los Angeles receive twice as much health care as people in Minneapolis simply because there are twice as many health care providers in Los Angeles. Far from producing benefit this leads to increased adverse outcomes Los Angeles: people are more likely to suffer from errors that are common in the health system because they come into contact with it more often. Wennberg (pers. comm.) argues that improving health literacy among the people of Los Angeles is unlikely to reduce the amount of care they receive. Yet providing his compelling data to those who organize and fund health care could potentially reduce the health care supply in Los Angeles and encourage care based on evidence.

Do We Need to Demonstrate the Benefits of Health Literacy?

In a room full of psychologists and physicians who have been practicing shared decision making for decades, the benefits of health literacy appear obvious. Yet, this skill is neither prevalent nor actively fostered by most major players in the health and education arena. To promote health literacy, especially if this endeavor entails a major change in the way risks, benefits, and probabilities are conveyed in every report, we need to transmit the merits of health literacy beyond the scope of its current advocates. Presently, two main justifications exist for promoting health literacy, representing two different viewpoints that are not necessarily contradictory. We discuss these benefits (ethical and economic) in turn. The widespread exploitation of this lack of literacy through biased report of evidence can also be seen as a moral issue (see Gigerenzer and Gray, this volume).

Improving Health Literacy: An Ethical Imperative

Since the Age of Enlightenment, efforts have focused on educating citizens for their personal and the greater societal good. It has become an ethical obligation to educate young members of society. Over time, general educational efforts have been applied to health issues: individuals' knowledge about diseases, risks to health, and ways to maintain a healthy lifestyle. Yet, health literacy levels, as defined previously, have generally been found to be insufficient among large segments of the population. A recent report by the American Medical Association (AMA) estimates that over 89 million American adults have limited health literacy skills (Weiss 2007). This estimate is based on the AMA's interpretation of the results of a National Assessment of Adult Literacy survey conducted in 2003, wherein AMA reclassified anyone "below basic" or "basic" (Weiss 2007:10) health literacy as being "limited" and multiplied this percentage by the number of adults in the population.

To address this remarkably low level of literacy, efforts to increase health literacy have been advocated as a necessary condition for a better educated population—one capable of making appropriate and informed health decisions and engaging in recommended health behaviors. Increasing health literacy has even been called an ethical imperative for health care professionals, who are tasked with ensuring that individuals process and comprehend relevant public health messages, treatment options, and recommended regimens (Gazmararian et al. 2005; Woloshin and Schwartz 2002).

Improving Health Literacy: A Means of Reducing Costs and Improving Care

In the present era of cost containment, it is questionable whether the ethical imperative is sufficient to remedy the dismal situation of low literacy levels and to develop and sustain the resources for an effective health literacy campaign. One argument put forth by the AMA is that individuals with limited health literacy incur up to four times greater cost in unnecessary doctor visits and hospital care, compared to individuals with average health literacy.

Increasing health literacy has been associated with a number of positive outcomes: improved decision making, better understanding of disease and treatment regimens, and adherence to prescribed treatment options. It is thus possible that increased health literacy could translate to lower costs associated with increased adherence and fewer unnecessary doctor visits and hospitalizations. Indeed, studies on the health outcomes of low-income individuals (controlling for education, insurance, race/ethnicity, sex, language, insurance, depressive symptoms, social support, diabetes education, treatment regimen, and diabetes duration) have found that those with higher health literacy had better health outcomes than those in the low literacy group (Schillinger et al. 2002).

However, the assessments of detailed costs are hampered by the fact that multiple outcomes could be considered and standards for assessments do not exist. The question therefore arises as to how outcomes can best be measured.

What Are the Most Appropriate Outcome Measures?

A number of outcomes have been associated with improved health literacy. For example, adherence to diabetes treatment regimens (Mühlhauser and Berger 2002) increased after patients received an intervention designed to improve understanding of the disease and self-management of its treatment. Other outcomes frequently mentioned are the reduction of unnecessary care and its associated monetary savings. Another measure, which resides between the ethical imperative and economic benefit, is that of quality of life. If health literacy is associated with reducing the severity of chronic diseases (e.g., diabetes or hypertension), patients' lives may become more bearable and acute outcomes can be avoided.

Marketing Implications: Promoting Systemic Change

There is a strong sense that psychologists and health care professionals have valuable health literacy tools and information which are underused. If we assume that a need exists among stakeholders in the health domain for obtaining, processing and understanding information, we can state that our products, as it were, address a pressing need. That this need is seldom met, or even identified, by stakeholders is a problem that could be solved through improved coordination and marketing.

Marketing is a word rarely used in the world of health literacy. However, drug companies, diagnostic tool manufacturers, and other commercial players use appealing strategies to promote their information. Often, their products do not represent the totality of the evidence in the most readily comprehensible fashion, and yet they are widely and efficiently disseminated. Evidence-based patient information and evidence-based information sources targeted at health care professionals compete in the ideas market alongside these materials.

In marketing our insights, knowledge, and tools, we have several resources at our deposal. The public and clinicians have considerable trust in academics and other health care professionals. Several strategies are available to us to exploit this receptiveness. Just as individual case studies of patients may be appealing, case studies of clinicians who had a positive experience around improved health literacy may be helpful in marketing (e.g., positive experiences in shared decision making, improved statistical literacy). As the media is often drawn to stories of personal interest, we could attempt to create such stories demonstrating, for example, how a city, a school, or a retirement home achieved better health outcomes due to a literacy intervention. There are publication venues for these positive stories in "personal view" sections of professional journals, and these could be written or solicited by anyone in the field.

For resources to be obtained, they need to be easily accessed. To date, however, there is no single information resource linking all the many available decision aids and risk calculators. At the most basic level, a Wikipedia page could be created, producing background references and a table of available tools. It would be trivial—yet surprisingly novel—to install a piece of wiki software on a server such as "decisionscommons.com" where trusted and registered academics in the field could update a central structured list of resources. The same could readily be done for structured and updatable lists of educational resources, probability games for children, and other resources.

A top-down approach also needs to be applied, as change cannot only come from below. Lobbying politicians to improve the quality and transparency of patient information provided by industry may bear fruit. Sites funded by the state (e.g., NHS Choices 2010) also represent good examples of state-funded, patient-facing, evidence-based information. Another strategy would be to offer assistance in developing statistical features to add into existing online communities and games. This will require funding and infrastructure but would be extremely helpful in reaching audiences far beyond what conventional interventions can accomplish.

"Translational medicine" or the concept of knowledge translation (Davis et al. 2003) is a relatively new principle which is also relevant here. Generally characterized as taking research work "from the laboratory to the bedside," it improves the application of basic science research to clinical research and practice (Lean et al. 2008). At its simplest level, it may be beneficial for all who work in the field to keep in mind that their work could be applied when communicated in professional and lay media.

In all of these actions, there is a strong argument to have a single professional organization for those engaged in improving health literacy: one that will reflect the interests of the community; act as a central contact point for clinicians, academics, journalists, politicians, civil servants, and patients seeking further information and expertise; coordinate lobbying; fund outreach activities and share information. Such an organization would also serve as a valuable resource for generating and sharing ideas on promoting the field of health literacy, in addition to this early and speculative list.

Acknowledgments

Our discussions benefited from the input of Angela Coulter, Glyn Elwyn, Ralph Hertwig, Marjukka Mäkelä, France Légaré, Albert G. Mulley, Jr., and Holger Schünemann.

Health Care 2020

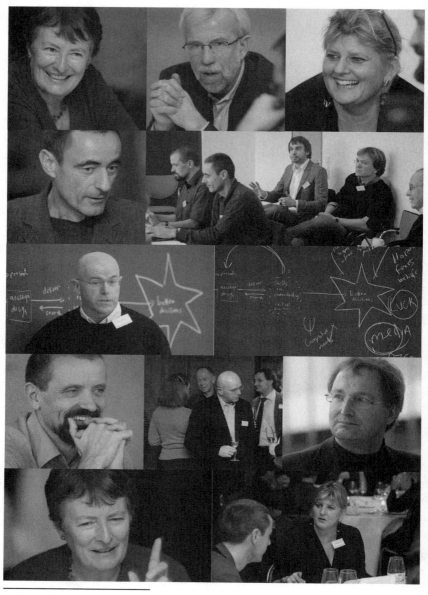

Left to right, top to bottom:
Angela Coulter, Wolf-Dieter Ludwig, Hilda Bastian
David Klemperer, Group discussion
Glyn Elwyn, Group work
Norbert Donner-Banzhoff, Evening disucssion, Günther Jonitz
Angela Coulter, Dinner discussion

13

How Can Better Evidence Be Delivered?

Norbert Donner-Banzhoff, Hilda Bastian,
Angela Coulter, Glyn Elwyn, Günther Jonitz,
David Klemperer, and Wolf-Dieter Ludwig

Abstract

Bias impacts all aspects of research: from the questions formulated in the study design to the dissemination of results and perceptions by different target groups. The implementation of evidence is not a simple, unidirectional pipeline, nor do target groups operate in a vacuum, eagerly waiting for any information. The information landscape can be likened to a crowded marketplace, with multiple vendors shouting at potential customers. People must be able to process information overload from multiple sources that strive to promote their interests actively in this pluralistic environment.

Recommendations are made to improve the evidence base and message design through (a) public funding of clinical trials, (b) development and reinforcement of information standards, (c) improvements in the delivery of information in continuing medical education, (d) support and development of information sources independent of commercial interests, (e) helping clinicians communicate uncertainty to their patients.

Information from many sources is exchanged between multiple audiences within a pluralistic environment. Messages from valid clinical trials addressing relevant questions must compete with ideas of obscure origin, often with the intent to manipulate clinicians, patients, and the general public. Recommendations are made to correct and/ or avoid imbalances.

Powerful players can influence the production of evidence (research) as well as its dissemination. In most countries this poses a greater threat to pluralism than the suppression of individual opinions. The interplay between private sources (industry), voluntary and academic organizations, and a broad range of media and government regulation is necessary for a balanced expression and promotion of information. To ensure this, public regulation and intervention may be needed.

Introduction

In evidence-based medicine, the term "bias" is usually used to refer to a systematic error in the design, conduct, or the analysis of a study. We will use the term in a broader sense to include manipulation of information, intentional or not. Bias can result during the production and dissemination of information as well as when it is received and interpreted.

We realize that the delivery of "unbiased" evidence, in the strict sense, is not possible, for this notion implies an objective truth, deviations from which can be defined unequivocally. This assumption can neither be justified from a philosophical point of view nor does experience with published clinical studies and reviews support the view that a single truth exists. Still, the concept of "biased" and "unbiased" evidence is useful as we attempt to understand and improve the dissemination of information to health professionals and patients/ citizens at a pragmatic level.

In our discussions, emphasis was given to results derived from clinical studies as the paradigmatic content for the delivery of information. Given the amount of resources invested in formal research, as well as its potential to relieve human suffering, there is ample justification for this emphasis. However, this emphasis was not made to exclude ethical deliberations, personal insights and observations, qualitative studies, guidelines, etc.

Many actors are involved in the delivery of evidence: researchers (e.g., clinical, health services research, psychology, education, social science), professional societies, patient organizations, industry (pharmaceutical, devices), those who pay (e.g., insurance companies, patients), government institutions, and regulatory agencies (e.g., NICE, IQWiG, and Unabhängige Patientenberatung [independent patient advice]). All actors have their particular perspective which is likely to influence how they produce and disseminate information.

Information is disseminated through various forms of media. Over the past few decades, profound changes have impacted the media, as evidenced by the Internet which has revolutionized the information management of professionals and citizens alike. However, issues of access (technical as well as literacy) and provision (funding) remain as important today with electronic media as it was twenty years ago with print media.

The dissemination processes discussed here take place in the global capitalist environment. New drugs and devices are constantly being developed and marketed, and interconnected industrial, governmental, scientific, and media groups exist to promote their interests. Still, we wish to emphasize that "villains" and "heroes" are not always distinguishable. Plenty of examples exist of manufacturers who provide important and useful information, as well as nonprofit organizations that distort evidence to promote their interests. In the case of individualized medicine, the research community often drives the premature adoption of new practices before effectiveness can be adequately evaluated.

In this chapter, we suggest measures to reduce the amount of bias in information for professionals and citizens. Where possible, we mention countries or organizations where they have already been adopted. More often than not, these measures have not yet been formally evaluated. Their impact, therefore, is difficult to quantify. Whereas for some measures, scientific evidence on effectiveness is unlikely or even impossible to emerge in the future, for others, scientists are called to study the effects and unintended consequences.

Origins of Bias

In Setting Research Questions, Study Design, and Reporting

Conflict of interest can distort professional judgment. Defined as "circumstances that create a risk that professional judgments or actions regarding a primary interest will be unduly influenced by a secondary interest" (Lo and Field 2009), conflict of interest can be found in the setting of research, the design of its study, as well as in how it is eventually reported.

A large proportion of research relevant for clinical decisions is sponsored by the pharmaceutical industry. For instance, more than 75% of randomized controlled trials which are published in major medical journals are funded by manufacturers of drugs or medical devices (Smith 2005). Thus, research topics often reflect commercial interests or those related to requirements of regulating authorities. Issues of high importance to clinicians (Tunis et al. 2003) or patients (Gandhi et al. 2008) are all too often not addressed. Moreover, "seeding trials" (i.e., clinical trials or research studies where the primary objective is to introduce the concept of a particular medical intervention to physicians, rather than to test a scientific hypothesis) do not address relevant research issues but rather serve to promote particular treatments or strengthen networks of local opinion leaders (Hill et al. 2008).

A slightly different source for bias can be the tendency on the part of the investigator to reach a desired result. This phenomenon has been referred to by Wynder et al. (1990) as "wish bias." They state that "from the initial hypothesis, through the design of the study, the collection and analysis of the data, and the submission and publication of the results, the possibility that the study may reflect the wishes of the investigator must be recognized if bias is to be adequately eliminated." Wish bias appears to be a ubiquitous phenomenon. In the 17th century, Sir Francis Bacon described it (Bacon 1620) and it has also been referred to as "confirmation bias" (Nickerson 1998).

Separate to the formulation of the research question, study results can be limited or biased by design and/or analysis in many ways:

- selection of patients,
- selection of too low dose of the control drug (efficacy) or too high dose of the control drug (safety),
- measuring multiple end points and selecting those for which favorable results are obtained,
- analyzing subgroups and publishing results selectively,
- ending a study when the results are favorable,

- interpreting results overoptimistically,
- withholding studies with "negative" results,
- multiple publication of positive results (Lexchin et al. 2003; Turner et al. 2008; Melander et al. 2003),
- overt fraud (Fanelli 2009; Lenzer 2009; Smith 2008).

Several of these points concern publication practices and lack of critical review. The integrity and usability of a medical journal is threatened when powerful interests (e.g., commercial, health service organizations, governments) are able to disseminate their bias, or when there is failure to correct for this bias.

In 2003, Bekelman et al. (2003) conducted a systematic review of quantitative analyses to see if financial conflicts of interest impacted clinical trial results. Assessing the relation between industry sponsorship and outcome in original research, a meta-analysis of eight publications showed a statistically significant association between industry sponsorship and pro-industry conclusions. Bekelman et al. also found that industrial funding is associated with certain methodological features of clinical studies (e.g., the use of inappropriately dosed controls) as well as with restrictions on publication and data sharing.

Lexchin et al. (2003) carried out a similar systematic review of quantitative analyses on the relation between source of funding and publication status, methodological quality, or outcome of research. They found that studies sponsored by pharmaceutical companies were more likely to have outcomes favoring the sponsor than were studies funded by other agencies. In a survey of commercially funded comparative trials of nonsteroidal anti-inflammatory drugs, the sponsor's drug was shown, without exception, to be superior (Rochon et al. 1994). This result, although extremely unlikely, suggests bias in the design and/or analysis of comparison. Different analyses have shown that clinical studies financed by pharmaceutical companies frequently report favorable results for products of these companies when compared to independent studies (Bekelman et al. 2003; Lexchin et al. 2003; Bero and Rennie 1996; Schott et al. 2010b).

Pharmaceutical companies routinely withhold data of adverse drug reactions (Psaty et al. 2004; Psaty and Kronmal 2008). Despite efforts to improve public access to study results through study registration (e.g., by medical journal editors; DeAngelis et al. 2004), clinical trials still remain inadequately registered (Mathieu et al. 2009). The use of ghost writers and guest authors is an additional problem associated with industry-initiated randomized trials (Gøtzsche et al. 2007; Ross et al. 2008).

It must be noted, however, that this research only demonstrates an association; causation is open to interpretation. Given the high quality of most trials funded by the pharmaceutical industry, there are alternative explanations, such as the careful selection of experimental treatments before phase III trial is conducted.

In the Dissemination of Information

The process of disseminating information causes bias in many ways. The financial power of manufacturers often creates an imbalance in the information landscape. The industry is in a position to provide excellent information, but often this is not done. Search engines can be manipulated so that search results emphasize certain products and approaches at the expense of others. Financial dependency creates self-censorship situations in the media. For example, glossy journals produced for continuing medical education (throwaway journals), which are read by most physicians, depend on advertisements for their production; this, in turn, can and does impact, or bias, the journals' content (Becker et al., submitted).

Industry, researchers, and medical professional societies are often criticized for transforming life or lifestyle difficulties into diseases to create markets for drugs or devices ("disease-mongering"). They are also criticized for lowering the thresholds for conditions to be treated medically, such as hypertension (Hopkins Tanne 2003) and hyperlipidemia (Moynihan and Cassels 2005). Although in some cases, this may be justified by improving the quality of life through the use of a particular drug, it creates a bias toward drug treatments. Non-pharmacological interventions are no longer an option, and the choices presented to the public diminish. This situation leads to what we term the "disempowerment of citizens."

Coverage in the general media can influence the acceptance of treatments. A particular form of this is found in disease awareness campaigns in countries where direct-to-consumer advertising is not permitted (see Ludwig and Schott, this volume). Examples are campaigns by different manufacturers for fungal toenail infections in the Netherlands ('t Jong et al. 2004) or erectile dysfunction.

Delivery of Evidence: Pipeline versus Crowded Marketplace

When the implementation of evidence is being discussed, the process is often understood as a simple, unidirectional pipeline (Figure 13.1): Results from clinical studies are fed into a linear process eventually producing easy to understand messages aimed at changing provider behavior. The target group is often assumed to be waiting eagerly for the message so that successful implementation is simply a matter of money and effort. Proponents of this model often assume that some clearly definable clinical policy does emerge from clinical studies so that deviations from this can easily be defined as irrational or aberrant.

The model has several limitations. First, insight that emerges from clinical studies is often cloudy, conflicting, and/or patchy. Apart from the biological, psychosocial, and system complexity, bias arises from the research process

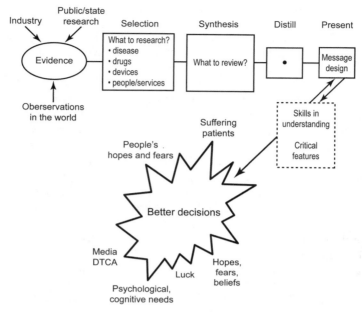

Figure 13.1   Schematic depiction of how evidence is delivered.

itself and thus limits the usability of the evidence. Health providers, educators, and scientists further down the line are well aware of these limitations. As a result, they are selective in receiving information from this continuum.

Second, health professionals and patients do not operate within a vacuum or based on a tabula rasa. They receive a range of messages, all aimed at changing their behavior. In addition, professional traditions and individual experience play influential roles. We suggest that research evidence, like any other information, enters a crowded marketplace where multiple vendors hawk their wares. This metaphor helps us understand how individuals, as well as collectives, must process multiple pieces of information as well as interact with players ("vendors") who promote their interests in a pluralistic environment.

Although most industrialized countries can be regarded as pluralistic, this does not mean that each person has the same chance to make their message heard and heeded. Consider a small town market, where there are rich and powerful vendors with large stands (big manufacturers, pharmaceuticals and manufacturers of medical devices). Such vendors may not only be more successful at selling their goods than their smaller competitors, they may be able to shape the perception of their products and to manipulate related values and attitudes. As in a municipality which sets conditions, governments influence markets through regulations. For information dissemination, the type of media is as important as the government regulation in terms of technical level, ownership, and the degree to which it is dependent on commercial interests.

Individual customers (clinicians, patients) wield much less influence than groups or institutions (health service organizations). The message received, and eventually adopted, depends only to a small degree on the scientific quality of the evidence base. Patients' and professionals' emotions and related expectations, payment systems, commercial interests, and cultural influences can be much more influential than the scientific validity of the message.

In this complex environment, critical awareness is required of patients, health professionals, and also those who process and disseminate information. Our recommendations in this chapter focus on improving the evidence base and message design.

Reducing Bias

Public Funding of Clinical Trials

The pharmaceutical industry invests up to 20% of its annual income in research and development (the sum invested worldwide in 2008 exceeded 65 billion US$). These funds are invested in the projects designed to elucidate the etiology and pathophysiology of disease, both within industry and in the research and clinical communities, as well as in clinical evaluations of the safety and efficacy of its products.

The quality of trials funded by industry is high. However, as discussed above, favorable outcomes may arise through the biased choice of a research question or selective publication of positive results. A more extensive mandatory registration of trials may resolve selective publication, but it will not address problems that arise from the other types of bias mentioned above.

Patients and doctors want head-to-head trials that compare all possible treatments of a condition, including nondrug treatments. Understandably, drug companies are not willing to fund such trials and, even if they were, there would be anxieties among competitors, patients, and doctors about bias in the results. Thus a strong case can be made for public funding of clinical trials.

Research funding bodies have been reluctant to fund drug trials because of multiple demands placed on their budgets. In addition, there is an unspoken belief that drug trial funding can be left to the wealthy pharmaceutical industry. An increasing recognition of the substantial scale of bias in industry-funded studies, the absence of head-to-head trials, and the bias toward drug rather than nondrug treatments has caused a shift toward greater public funding of clinical trials (Lewis et al. 2007; 't Jong et al. 2004).

The main benefit from publicly funded trials would be an evidence base, accessible by doctors and patients, containing research evidence unrelated to immediate commercial interest (e.g., head-to-head comparisons of established treatments). However, there might also be economic benefit. For example, the publicly funded ALLHAT trial showed that off-patent anti-hypertensives were just as effective as newer, more expensive drugs (ALLHAT Collaborative Research Group 2002). Given that hundreds of millions of patients are treated globally every day for hypertension, the financial savings could be substantial. Similarly, a study of acne treatments revealed that most treatments were not very effective and that cheaper treatments were just as effective as more expensive ones (Ozolins et al. 2004). The CATIE study showed similar results for recently marketed antipsychotic drugs (Lieberman et al. 2005). These examples demonstrate the potential to inform clinical and policy decisions.

The cost of conducting such studies will, of course, be high. However, Italy provides an example of how they can be funded: To finance independent drug research, a 5% tax was levied on the marketing costs of drugs (Agenzia Italiana del Farmaco 2003). Proposals were required to cover three areas: (a) orphan drugs for rare diseases and drugs for non-responders, (b) comparison among drugs and therapeutic strategies, and (b) strategies to improve the appropriateness of drug use and pharmacoepidemiology studies (Garattini 2007).

One can expect resistance to such a tax and perhaps any move to increase the number of publicly funded trials, based on the argument that the results would be slowed innovation and reduced profitability to an industry that is important to the economy of many developed nations. Governments cannot always be expected to be on the side of an improved evidence base. Recent debates about drug regulation (e.g., direct-to-consumer advertising) reveal the presence of a competing objective in support of the pharmaceutical and medical device industry. Similarly, the evidence gap is unlikely to be filled by regulatory authorities demanding comparative studies.

Message Design

From an industry point of view, imbalance in the information landscape is normal; from a public point of view, this constitutes a problem. Just as regulatory authorities require manufacturers to submit studies on the efficacy and safety of commercial products, public institutions can help establish balance in the "crowded marketplace." Publicly funded institutions and voluntary groups could process evidence from clinical trials and present them to the public. Examples of the former include NICE and NHS Choices (United Kingdom) and IQWiG and Unabhängige Patientenberatung (Germany), and independent drug bulletins for the latter.

One approach developed in a number of countries has been to encourage the evaluation of health information materials against a standardized set of criteria. Large numbers of rating instruments have been developed. One study found 98 examples of Internet rating tools (Gagliardi and Jadad 2002); however, many of these have not had sufficient institutional support to encourage and sustain their adoption and continued use.

Health on the Net (HoN 2010) is an exception to this rule. Established in 1995 to promote quality standards in web-based health information and to help users find reliable information, its voluntary certification scheme has been used by nearly 7,000 web sites worldwide. It has been effective in sensitizing users to the factors affecting information quality.

Despite the plethora of different rating instruments, there is a broad, general consensus on the key factors to look for in assessing health information. Gute Praxis Gesundheitsinformation [good practice health information] is a recent example that describes a standard for the content and presentation of health information (Klemperer et al. 2010). This standard (see Table 13.1) was developed by the Fachbereich Patienteninformation und Patientenbeteiligung [division of patient information and patient involvement] of the German Network for Evidence Based Medicine in cooperation with a group of scientists,

Table 13.1 Quality criteria for health information, based on *Gute Praxis Gesundheitsinformation* (Klemperer et al. 2010).

Criteria	Description
Clear purpose	The information product clearly explains its aims and purpose.
Relevance	The material meets a clearly defined need and has been tested with representatives of the target audience; where possible, links to sources of further information and support are provided.
Evidence-based	The information is consistent with up-to-date clinical evidence, medical and social research; personal opinion is clearly distinguished from evidence-based information.
Authoritative	Sources of evidence are clearly indicated; names and credentials of authors, funders and sponsors are clearly stated; any conflict of interest is disclosed; any advertising is clearly identified.
Complete	Where relevant, all alternative treatment, management or care options are clearly stated and all possible outcomes are clearly presented.
Secure	Where users' personal details are requested, there is a clear policy for safeguarding privacy and confidentiality.
Accurate	The product has been checked for accuracy; in the case of user-generated content there is a clear procedure for moderation.
Well-designed	The layout is clear and easy to read; if necessary, the product contains specific navigation aids such as content lists, indexing and search facilities.
Readable	The language is clear, where possible conforming to plain language standards.
Accessible	There is a clear dissemination plan for the product; the material conforms to accepted standards for accessibility, where possible including versions for use by people with sensory and learning difficulties.
Up-to-date	The date of issue or latest update is clearly indicated along with the planned review date.

representatives of patient organizations, and service providers. Already it has garnered the support of many influential groups.

The Information Standard

The Information Standard (2010) is an initiative of the U.K. Department of Health to develop a certification scheme for producers of health and social care information for the public. Launched in November 2009, the scheme covers multiple types of information, including print as well as electronic materials. Any information producer (e.g., NHS organizations, local authorities, voluntary organizations, patient groups, commercial publishers, or industries) can apply for certification. The Information Standard evaluates development processes rather than individual pieces of information and, in that respect, is similar to other producer accreditation schemes, such as Fairtrade. Organizations that apply for certification must produce clear documentation of the procedures that were used to develop the health information, together with a sample of their information materials. These are independently assessed by an accredited certification agency. Certification entitles the organization to include the scheme logo on all materials that meet the criteria.

Patient Decision Aid Standards

Not being properly told about their illness and potential treatment options is the most common cause of patient dissatisfaction (Coulter and Cleary 2001; Grol et al. 2000). The desire for more information and participation in treatment decisions (i.e., shared decision making) has been expressed by many patients. In shared decision making, patients work together with the clinician to identify acceptable medical options and choose a preferred course of clinical care (Sheridan et al. 2004). The availability of reliable evidence-based information is an essential component in the shared decision-making process.

Patient decision aids have been developed to support shared decision making. These aids take a variety of forms including web applications, videos or DVDs, computer programs, leaflets or brochures, and structured counseling. Most share the following characteristics (O'Connor, Wennberg et al. 2007):

1. They provide facts about the condition, options, outcomes, and probabilities.
2. They clarify patients' evaluations of the outcomes that matter most to them.
3. They guide patients through a process of deliberation so that a choice can be made that matches their informed preferences.

A large number of decision aids are now available, the majority of which were developed in North America. The Cochrane Register (OHRI 2010) lists decision aids that meet certain criteria. Table 13.2 lists the principal developers of these decision aids and the number of tools they have developed.

Table 13.2   Decision aids, developers, and number of tools.

Developer	Country	Decision aids	No.
Health wise	U.S.A.	Decision points	137
www.healthwise.org			
FIMDM/Health Dialog	U.S.A.	Shared decision-making programs	26
www.informedmedicaldecisions.org			
www.healthdialog.com			
Mayo Clinic	U.S.A.	Treatment decisions	16
www.mayoclinic.com			
Midwives Information and Resource Service	U.K.	Informed choice	7
www.infochoice.org			
University of Sydney	Australia	Decision aids	6
www.health.usyd.edu.au/shdg/resources/decision_aids.php			
National Cancer Institute	U.S.A.		5
www.cancercontrol.cancer.gov			
Ottawa Health Decision Center	Canada	Patient decision aids	3
www.ohri.ca/decisionaid			
Agency for Healthcare Research and Quality	U.S.A.	Consumer summary guide	2
www.ahrq.gov			
Centers for Disease Control and Prevention	U.S.A.	Decision guide	2
www.cdc.gov			
Cardiff University	U.K.	Decision explorer	1
http://www.informedhealthchoice.com			

The International Patient Decision Aids Standard (IPDAS) was established to help ensure that aids conform to high-quality standards. A Delphi process involving a group of researchers, practitioners, policy makers, and patients from 14 countries was used to develop the standards and assessment criteria (Elwyn, O'Connor et al. 2006, 2009). IPDAS is still being tested and further refinements are likely. In the meantime, however, discussion is underway about the possibility of developing a certification scheme for decision aids, potentially under the auspices of an organization with experience of running such schemes.

Continuing Medical Education

Although difficult to prove, it is reasonable to assume that at least a portion of the overuse of commercially marketed drugs and devices can be traced to continuing medical education (CME). Used for credit, and generally formatted as lectures or workshops, the CME enterprise in the developed world has been largely supported by commercial interests. For example, in the multibillion dollar industry of CME in the United States, over half is paid for by industry, particularly the pharmaceutical industry. Health systems, medical schools, governments—and physicians themselves—contribute much less. Furthermore, most physicians are directly affected by CME: the majority must attend hours (generally on the order of 50 hours) of lectures or workshops on an annual basis, as required by state and other regulatory bodies. The support of this large enterprise by interests not always aligned with quality of care or patient-centered care, leads to questions of bias and decision making based on less-than-ideal evidence.

In recognition of the potential bias, authorities responsible for the delivery and accreditation of CME increasingly require conflict-of-interest disclosures for faculty within the CME setting. This disclosure, regulated in the North American setting to occur at the beginning of a lecture or educational activity, includes a listing of grants, monetary rewards, speakers' fees and other sources of income which might produce bias in presentations on the part of the faculty member.

Despite its wide adoption and enforcement, problems still occur. For example, new information on side effects, risks and benefits, numbers-needed-to-treat (NNT), and other aspects is often not presented or fully explored. This stands in sharp contrast to a wider movement of transparency falling under the rubric of patient-centered, evidence-based decision making.

Two proposals are suggested to remedy this situation on a programmatic or institutional level: The first concerns the presentation or activity itself: by using a standardized form, which would include absolute risk, NNT, and other factors, clinical options could be made clearer. A structured abstract format is recommended for use whenever a clinical intervention, screening procedure, medication, or other therapeutic option is presented. This should be accompanied by a checklist for use by program planners, teachers, and participants in the CME setting. The checklist could be based on the IPDAS framework or other instruments designed to measure qualities related to active patient participation in decision making.

The second proposal includes the establishment of a CME review board. This board would be made up of educators, clinical teachers, bioethicists, and perhaps patients and charged to oversee the institutional or programmatic acceptance of commercial expenditures in support of educational activities. The board would review the general content of CME, the flow of funding, and its impact on educational programming. In addition, it would oversee the micro process involved in the first suggestion. Again, an evaluative tool is needed and should be in line with the above checklist. Apart from intervening in cases where bias from funding is shown, a preventive effect can be expected as well as raised consciousness within the professions.

We believe these two approaches would broaden the ethical approach to conflict-of-interest bias and CME—doing no harm, doing good, providing balance, equity and full disclosure. In addition, we believe that, regardless of commercial support, a structured risk assessment format is useful at the level of the participating physicians, the faculty member, and perhaps the health care system itself. In both proposals, a deeper commitment is advocated to the Kirkpatrick model of assessment (Kirkpatrick 1979)—one that stresses evaluation of CME activities beyond the perception of an activity and includes competency, performance, and health care outcomes. This advocacy would ensure, in our opinion, a concurrent commitment to shared, evidence-based decision making.

A similar process has been established in France, where any promotional material, including advertisements in professional journals, must be presented to the Haute Autorité de la Santé for approval.

Continuing Medical Education: A Dissenting Opinion

This proposal highlights a number of situations where bias and conflict of interest are inherent or have been allowed to develop. Prime reasons for this can easily be found in the profit orientation of industry, as information provider and sponsor, and the reliance of the CME system on such sponsorship.

Our group discussion did not yield consensus. A few wanted to stress the positive roles that industrial sponsorship has played in providing information on the latest scientific developments and/or novel principles for disease treatment, diagnosis, or control. In addition, industry contributes substantial financial support to the CME system—annually US$1.1 billion alone in the United States—which offsets the costs of many programs; costs that would otherwise fall onto institutions and/or health care providers themselves.

As to the criticism that industry uses CME unduly as an advertising platform, one must also weigh the role that others bear. Take, for example, the expectations of many health care professionals, who have come to view the luxury aspects of CME offerings as their right. There may also be a certain reliance on the current level, if not mode, of funding.

To address the first example, conflict of interest can be minimized by requiring full disclosure from all who participate: key opinion leaders, contributors, lecturers, instructors, participants, etc. An effective remedy, and perhaps deterrent, may be to make this mandatory disclosure the subject of review, with the results publicly available.

To address the issue of funding (i.e., its flow and impact on educational programming) the establishment of a CME review board has been suggested. In the interest of achieving balance among the various players as well as to optimize the responsible usage of funds and secure access to the large amount of useful data generated by the pharmaceutical industry, particularly in the science of disease, it seems counterproductive, if not naïve, to exclude industry from this board. Of course, efforts can be made to minimize reliance on industrial funding through the procurement of alternate funding sources. For example, funds could be raised by levying a tax on the sales of drugs, through voluntary contributions, as well as by charging higher fees for participation from health professionals who receive CME credits. It seems unlikely, however, that a cost-neutral solution will be possible, and that one could expect for these costs to be passed on to the health care system in one form or another.

A final note to the harmonization of curricula and presentation formats: It appears that there is a working framework upon which this can be achieved. However, any form of harmonized curriculum should most certainly contain the teaching of critical awareness.

Drug Bulletins

Drug bulletins are periodicals that report on issues related to drug therapy, but they are produced independently of the pharmaceutical industry. They aim to provide balance to the large number of journals that depend more or less on advertising by manufacturers.

Their circulation and their impact on prescribing vary widely from country to country. Their influence not only depends on their quality and the willingness of the profession to subscribe, but also on financial incentives. Where clinicians are made responsible for their prescribing cost there is an increased demand for independent information.

This is illustrated by the ambulatory care sector in Germany. Here, physicians are required to prescribe economically. There are strict rules in place to reduce their income if prescribing targets are not met. The demoralizing effect of this is frequently expressed. However, this requirement has fostered a culture of quality and provides practitioners with critical feedback on their prescribing practices. A number of independent periodicals help counterbalance the hundreds of CME journals dependent on advertising.

Learning to Express Uncertainty: Creating a Safe Space

At the level of the individual clinician as well as at a system level, uncertainty is rarely discussed. Despite the presence of evidence-based medicine and statistics in medical curricula, physicians are "determinists by training" (Tanenbaum 1994). When asked to provide a prognosis (e.g., after cancer has been discovered), physicians are prepared to express uncertainty. However, this happens much less frequently when diagnosis or treatments are discussed.

Patients, citizens, and often even decision makers are not usually aware of the uncertainties inherent in the clinical process. One of the most basic misconceptions holds that anything expressed in numbers must be certain. Clinicians often feel that admitting uncertainty will undermine patients' trust.

How can a space be created that will enable both clinicians and patients to recognize the role that uncertainty plays in most medical decisions? The measures we suggest relate to the structure of health care and information systems, with education playing a key role.

In terms of a physician's training, proficiency in the concept of uncertainty should be a prerequisite for entry into medical school. During basic science training, "facts" (e.g., the Krebs cycle) are presented as givens, although they are only theoretical approximations for very complex realities (Fleck 1980). Later, as residents/registrars or clinicians, "decision points" must be able to be identified. As new clinicians, trust and uncertainty are not contradictions, and the communication of uncertainty is complex: Excellent communication and people skills are necessary, as is the cultivation of a good doctor–patient relationship.

Viewed from a different perspective, patients must be capable and prepared to acknowledge and live with uncertainty. Equipping patients with this knowledge can be best achieved through educational efforts, either in a formal setting or through other means (Spiegelhalter 2010). In addition, preparing patients to discuss relevant questions before a consultation is important.

Decision support tools exist to aid the understanding of uncertainty (Spiegelhalter 2010; Arriba 2010). As discussed by Schwartz and Woloshin and Ludwig and Schott (this volume) drug labeling should express information to clinicians and patients in a transparent and understandable manner (see also Schwartz and Woloshin 2009). This information could also be collected and made available by independent bodies (e.g., UK Database of Uncertainties about the Effects of Treatments) to help the public learn about knowledge limitation (NHS 2010).

Clinicians could be more aware of stochastic and collective professional uncertainty if guidelines relied less on algorithmic prescriptions and more on honest presentations of effectiveness measures and study quality. This is a difficult issue because, in general, clinicians need a certain level of confidence in order to function properly. However, they also need to reflect on professional uncertainty in an honest way.

Likewise, the willingness of the patient to confront uncertainty is shaped by the general public's understanding of science. Numerous examples can be found where scientists emphasize "certainty," when addressing the public, rather than that which has not been fully resolved.

The primary care sector is a privileged place in which to address the uncertainty of treatments, since hospital structures often do not allow for discussion and reflection of options and their respective benefits and harms. However, primary care can assume this role for only common conditions. Primary and secondary care need to clarify their respective roles and flow of information at the regional level so that the information needs of patients are adequately addressed.

In the early 19th century, it was not clear which way medicine would develop. The scientific determinist, the artist, and the statistician were the options available at the time (Gigerenzer et al. 1989, Chap. 4). While the deterministic scientist has prevailed, at least in the academic field, the statistician–clinician has gained ground over the last twenty years and will hopefully continue to do so.

Patient Feedback for Monitoring Information Delivery

The systematic measurement of patients' experience is a good way to monitor performance in terms of information provision and shared decision making. In the United Kingdom, the NHS survey program has been implemented in all NHS trusts and primary care units since 2002. It includes surveys of inpatient, outpatient, and local health services as well as mental health, maternity, and long-term conditions (NHS Surveys 2010).

These surveys measure most aspects of patient-centered care, including access and waiting time, communications with staff, privacy and dignity, information provision, involvement in treatment decisions, physical comfort and pain relief, support for self-care, coordination and continuity, environment and facilities, involvement of family and friends, and an overall evaluation of care. Relevant questions could be adapted for use in other health systems to monitor performance of evidence-based information (see Table 13.3). In addition, in the United States, the Consumer Assessment of Healthcare Providers and Systems (CAHPS surveys) includes questions about receipt of information to inform treatment decisions (CAHPS 2010).

Media Literacy

Inappropriate use of statistics is sometimes part of a deliberate, albeit often well-meaning attempt to influence beliefs and actions. However, it is far from being the only way societal knowledge and emotions are biased. If we want the least biased evidence to compete effectively in the battle for people's hearts and minds on health-related matters, then society needs to become more statistically literate.

The mass media is a major source of bias in society's perceptions of disease (M. E. Young et al. 2008), and more. Whether it is the impact of disease-mongering (Doran and Henry 2008) or other forms of awareness creation, we, as citizens, need to ensure that we are resilient to manipulation in this era of sophisticated media and advertising.

One key area that has emerged to increase media literacy is intervention programs in schools (Bergsma and Carney 2008), including the call to action of a group convened by the World Health Organization (Tang et al. 2009). A small body of evidence is growing that even brief encounters with media literacy interventions can have a positive effect, for example, on adolescents' body image and may be able to contribute to the prevention of eating disorders (Pratt and Woolfenden 2002; Ridolfi and Vander Wal 2008; Wilksch and Wade 2009). These initial experiences show that the study and development of effective interventions to increase media literacy warrants increased attention and investment.

Media literacy is an essential skill for a healthy citizenry in an information age. However, media literacy is also an important issue for health professionals.

Table 13.3   Questions used to monitor the delivery of evidence-based information.

Question	Response options
Operations and procedures:	
Beforehand, did a member of staff explain the risks and benefits of the operation or procedure in a way you could understand?	☐ Yes, completely ☐ Yes, to some extent ☐ No ☐ I did not want an explanation
Were you involved as much as you wanted to be in decisions about your care and treatment?	☐ Yes, definitely ☐ Yes, to some extent ☐ No ☐ I did not want an explanation
Medicines:	
Were you involved as much as you wanted to be in decisions about the best medicine for you?	☐ Yes, definitely ☐ Yes, to some extent ☐ No
Were you given enough information about the purpose of the medicine?	☐ Yes, enough information ☐ Some, but I would have liked more ☐ I got no information, but I wanted some ☐ I did not want/need any information ☐ Don't know/can't say
Were you given enough information about any side-effects the medicine might have?	☐ Yes, enough information ☐ Some, but I would have liked more ☐ I got no information, but I wanted some ☐ I did not want/need any information ☐ Don't know/can't say

The appraisal skills typically described in textbooks of evidence-based medicine are not always suitable for finding quick answers to clinical questions. Since evidence-based medicine has been suggested as the preferred approach to professional decision making in health care, learning and reflection, the media and related customer behaviors have changed considerably. In response, a simple three-step heuristic has been suggested to help primary care practitioners judge the validity of a claim regarding treatment, diagnosis, and screening (Donner-Banzhoff et al. 2003; Eberbach et al., submitted). This heuristic makes explicit use of the bias of a particular source and is therefore adapted to our information landscape.

Conclusion

The dissemination of evidence is not a single process that can be carefully planned and implemented. No single actor exists whom everyone would trust as being objective or competent. Instead, we must accept that ours is a pluralistic environment where information from many sources is transferred between multiple audiences. The message from valid clinical trials addressing relevant questions must compete with numerous ideas of obscure origin as well as with manipulation on many levels.

An all-knowing information demon that disseminates comprehensive and unbiased information to all is not a realistic response. The recommendations we have made aim at correcting and/or avoiding imbalances. Powerful players, above all commercial interests, can influence the production of evidence (research) as well as its dissemination. In most countries, this poses a greater threat to pluralism than government suppression or the threat to free thought. The solution will be found in a balanced interplay between private sources (industry), voluntary and academic organizations, a broad range of media, as well as government regulation; under this, a balanced expression and promotion of information will be more likely.

As in other areas of society, public regulation as well as public intervention may be needed for this to happen. For initiatives that are neither linked to commercial interests nor government initiated, lessons should be drawn from industry, for they have to create trusted brands, use persuasion methods, and support tools (Hastings 2007).

14

The Drug Facts Box

Making Informed Decisions about Prescription Drugs Possible

Lisa M. Schwartz and Steven Woloshin

Abstract

The idea that people should be able to participate meaningfully in personal medical decisions is so widely accepted that it is hard to believe that things were ever otherwise. The idea that doctors should routinely withhold important information from patients, order treatments without informed consent, or should not consider patient preferences—once routine practice—would be as acceptable now as blood-letting to purge bad humors.

The modern shared decision-making model has two basic inputs. First, people need the facts: What are their options and the likely outcomes of these options? Second, they need some clarity about their values: How much do they care about the various outcomes and what do they have to go through to get them? Good decisions require a combination of facts and values. Without the facts, good decision making cannot happen.

Ironically, the daily barrage of medical news, advertisements, and public service announcements do not actually deliver a lot of useful facts. Direct-to-consumer prescription drug advertising offers perhaps the best illustration of this problem. Pharmaceutical companies spend nearly US$5 billion a year (DTC Perspectives 2008)—more than twice the total budget of the U.S. Food and Drug Administration—advertising directly to consumers. These ads sorely lack useful facts and, instead, magnify the benefits and minimize the harms of prescription drugs.

This chapter reviews how drug information generally gets to the U.S. public and recommends how this can be better accomplished through the use of "drug facts boxes."

Direct-to-Consumer Prescription Drug Advertising: Lots of Ad, Few Good Facts

Direct-to-consumer prescription drug advertising exists only in the United States and New Zealand. In the United States, the first direct-to-consumer advertisement (an ad for the pneumonia vaccine) appeared in *Reader's Digest* in 1981. Today it is hard to find any American magazine or television show without finding drug ads.

In theory, drug ads could raise consumer awareness about important diseases and educate the public about treatment choices. In practice, however, ads usually omit the most fundamental information that people need: how well the drug works (Bell et al. 2000; Frosch et al. 2007; Woloshin et al. 2001; Kallen et al. 2007). Instead, ads simply assert that the drugs work very well. For example, in a Claritin® (loratadine) ad (Figure 14.1), Joan Lunden (a celebrity) tells consumers that the drug "works for me." However, the ad says nothing about how well, thus leaving consumers only to guess, and often they guess incorrectly. In one survey, more than 20% of the public falsely believed that the U.S. Food and Drug Administration (FDA) only permitted the advertisements of very effective drugs (Bell et al. 1999). In fact, any drug can be advertised as soon as it is approved by the FDA, and FDA approval can (and often does) mean simply that the drug had a statistically significant benefit over a placebo, and that benefit appeared to outweigh harm.

A minority of ads do quantify benefit, but often in a misleading way, typically focusing on numerically large relative changes rather than smaller corresponding absolute differences (Woloshin et al. 2001). This technique, known to magnify perceptions of benefit, is illustrated in the ad for Lipitor® (atorvastatin, a cholesterol lowering drug) reproduced in Figure 14.1. The ad states that "Lipitor® cuts the risk of stroke in half" (a large relative risk

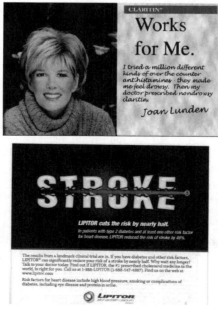

Figure 14.1   Examples of drug advertisements which focus on perceptions of benefit.

reduction), but does not provide the base rate; that is, "half of what," which would give the relative reduction statistic its meaning. The actual figures (not reported in the ad) are as follows: for people with diabetes and other risk factors, Lipitor® reduced the chance of a stroke over the next four years from 2.8% to 1.5% (Colhoun et al. 2004).

Do these ads violate FDA regulations? Unfortunately, the current answer is no. The FDA regulation for drug advertisements which mention the drug by name requires that the ad must promote the drug for approved uses only, must be true and not misleading, and must present a fair balance of information about effectiveness and harms (FDA 2010a). Ads that appear in print media must also include a "brief summary" of side effects and warnings; broadcast ads need only to mention major drug side effects and contraindications and refer consumers to a print ad or other reference with a brief summary. There are no specific FDA regulations about if or how drug efficacy data should be presented in ads. To comply with "effectiveness" criteria, an ad must merely mention the drug's indication (e.g., it treats allergies).

Historically, enforcement of regulations has generally been passive: consumers or others complain about an ad, and the FDA reviews the materials and can request changes, fine companies for noncompliance with regulations, and request that ad campaigns stop, although these actions are unusual. Since 2007, FDA regulations require more active surveillance: FDA is supposed to review broadcast ads prior to dissemination and can request—but cannot require—changes to ads (FDAAA 2007). There is still no pre-dissemination review of print ads.

Public Drug Information: Lost Facts?

In contrast to the highly visible but highly limited drug ads, FDA review documents are a difficult to access but extraordinarily rich source of drug information for doctors and patients alike.

When companies apply for FDA drug approval, they submit the results of (usually) two or more randomized controlled trials ("phase 3 trials") that test the drug in patients with the condition of interest. FDA staff reviewers with medical, statistical, epidemiological, and pharmacological expertise evaluate the evidence and if benefits are felt to outweigh harm, they approve the drug. FDA review documents record the data and reasoning behind approval decisions (FDA 2010b). Unfortunately, the review documents are lengthy, inconsistently organized, and weakly summarized.

The package insert (called the "professional drug label"), which is written by drug companies and approved by the FDA, is supposed to summarize the essential information from the review documents. Sometimes, however, important information about drug benefit and harm gets lost between the review documents and the label (Schwartz and Woloshin 2009). For example, the label for Lunesta® (eszopiclone), a popular sleep drug, states only that the drug is "superior to placebo." In the 403-page review document, the findings from the phase 3 study are clearly reported: patients with insomnia randomized to Lunesta® fell asleep an average of 15 minutes faster and slept 37 minutes longer than patients given placebo (yet Lunesta patients still met the study's criteria for insomnia).

The brief summary—the small-print second page that accompanies an ad— is an excerpt of the label that the FDA requires in drug ads. While the brief summary may contain data on side effects, it never contains any data on how well drugs work.

In its current forms, public drug information does not adequately inform doctors or patients about drugs. FDA review documents are comprehensive but overwhelming, and key information often gets omitted from labels and the brief summary.

The Drug Facts Box

To get accurate information to the public, we created the "drug facts box." The box is designed to highlight the key facts from the FDA review documents, which are missing in drug ads. A drug facts box is a standardized 1-page table that summarizes prescription drug benefit and side-effect data. The top of the box provides descriptive information about the drug: its indication, who might consider taking it, who should not take it, recommended testing or monitoring, and other things to consider doing to achieve the same goals as the drug. Table 14.1 shows a drug facts box for Lunesta®, a drug for chronic insomnia.

The heart of the drug facts box is a table summarizing data drawn from randomized trials used in the FDA's drug approval process. The table includes two columns of numbers providing the chance of various outcomes for people who do or do not take the drug (i,e., those who take a placebo or an active comparator drug). The first half of the table summarizes the benefit of the drug; the second half summarizes side effects. The last element of the box reports how long the drug has been in use (i.e., when it was approved by FDA) and reminds consumers that unanticipated safety issues sometimes emerge after approval—generally within the first five years after a drug comes on the market.

While drug facts boxes are intuitively appealing, there has been concern that numeric data may be too difficult to understand, even for highly educated members of the general public. Our research suggests that this is not the case. Indeed, our work demonstrates that people—even those with limited formal education—can understand absolute risks in tables and that drug facts boxes can improve consumer decision making.

Table 14.1   Drug facts box for Lunesta® (eszopiclone).

Drug Facts Box: LUNESTA (eszopiclone) for insomnia in adults	
What is this drug for?	To make it easier to fall or to stay asleep
Who might consider taking it?	Adults age 18 and older with insomnia for at least 1 month
Who should *not* take it?	No blood tests, watch out for personality changes (like uncharacteristic aggressiveness) and abnormal behavior (like sleep driving)
Other things to consider doing	Reducing caffeine intake (especially at night), increase exercise, establish regular bedtime, avoid daytime naps

LUNESTA Study Findings		
788 healthy adults with insomnia for at least 1 month—sleeping less than 6.5 hr per night and/or taking more than 30 min to fall asleep—were given LUNESTA or a sugar pill nightly for 6 months. Here's what happened:		
What difference did LUNESTA make?	People given a sugar pill	People given LUNESTA (3 mg each night)
Did LUNESTA help?		
LUNESTA users fell asleep faster (15 min faster)	45 min to fall asleep	30 min to fall asleep
LUNESTA users slept longer (37 min longer)	5 hr 45 min	6 hr 22 min
Did LUNESTA have side effects?		
Life-threatening side effects:		
No difference between LUNESTA and a sugar pill	None observed	None observed
Symptom side effects:		
LUNESTA users had more unpleasant taste in their mouth (additional 20% due to drug)	6% (6 in 100)	26% (26 in 100)
LUNESTA users had more dizziness (additional 7% due to drug)	3% (3 in 100)	10% (10 in 100)
LUNESTA users had more drowsiness (additional 6% due to drug)	3% (3 in 100)	9% (9 in 100)
LUNESTA users had more dry mouth (additonal 5% due to drug)	2% (2 in 100)	7% (7 in 100)
LUNESTA users had more nausea (additional 5% due to drug)	6% (6 in 100)	11% (11 in 100)

How long has the drug been in use?

LUNESTA was approved by the FDA in 2005 based on studies that involved about 1200 people. As with all new drugs, rare but serious side effects may emerge when the drug is on the market after larger numbers of people have used the drug.

Table 14.2   Simple table, or benefit box, used to present the benefits of the theoretical drug Avastat which is similar to pravastin.

Benefit of Avastat

In a study, people with high cholesterol took either Avastat or a sugar pill. Here are the percents of people who experienced the following over 5 years:

	Sugar pill	Avastat	Effect of Avastat
Have a heart attack	8%	6%	Fewer
Die from heart attack	2%	1%	Fewer
Die (from anything)	4%	3%	Fewer

Consumers Understand Simple Tables

In 2003, we conducted a study to test how well consumers understood simple tables (i.e., three rows and two columns of data), each summarizing the benefit of a drug (Woloshin et al. 2004). Trained interviewers showed 203 individuals in the greater Boston area actual direct-to-consumer advertisements (only the name of the drug and the drug company had been changed) and then showed them the same ads with the drug facts tables. Table 14.2 shows one of the simple tables, also called "benefit boxes," that was used in the study.

Most (91%) participants rated the information in the benefit box as "very important" or "important." Almost all said the data was easy to understand: median rank of 9 on a scale from 0 (extremely hard) to 10 (extremely easy). Most were able to navigate the table above: 97% correctly identified the percentage of people given Avastat who had a heart attack. In a similar example, as shown in Figure 14.2, consumer perception of the drug's effectiveness was diminished—appropriately, given the data—after seeing the benefit data.

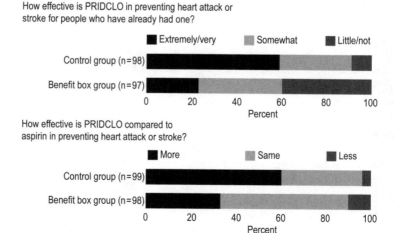

Figure 14.2   Perceived effectiveness of Pridclo® (clopidogrel) by people randomized to see an advertisement with ("benefit box group") or without ("control group") a benefit box.

Consumers Can Understand Complex Tables

We conducted another study to test how well consumers understood a complex table (i.e., nine rows and two columns of data) that summarized the benefit and side effects of drug information that is included in a complete drug facts box (Schwartz et al. 2007). This study included a convenience sample of 274 people with a wide range of socioeconomic status; they were mailed a drug facts box (without any training on how to read it) and asked to complete a survey. In this way, we could test how people used the table in a realistic setting. Table 14.3 shows the complex table which summarized the data on tamoxifen (Nolvadex®) for the primary prevention of breast cancer.

Participants were asked five comprehension questions which tested their ability to (a) find specific data in the table, (b) use data to calculate an absolute risk difference (i.e., subtractions), and (c) compare the effect of tamoxifen to hypothetical drugs with different benefits. Comprehension was high. For example, 89% of participants correctly wrote in "0.8%" as the answer to what percentage of people given tamoxifen got a blood clot in their leg or lung; 71%

Table 14.3 Summary of data on tamoxifen (Nolvadex®) for the primary prevention of breast cancer.

Tamoxifen Study Findings		
13,000 women at high risk of getting breast cancer were given Tamoxifen or a sugar pill for 6 years. Here's what happened:		
What difference did Tamoxifen make?	Women given a sugar pill	Women given Tamoxifen (20 mg/day)
Did Tamoxifen help?		
Fewer women got invasive breast cancer	2.7%	1.4%
Fewer women died from breast cancer	0.09%	0.05%
Did Tamoxifen have side effects?		
Life-threatening side effects:		
More women had a blood clot in their leg or lungs	0.4%	0.8%
More women had a stroke	0.4%	0.6%
More women got invasive uterine cancer	0.2%	0.5%
Symptom side effects:		
More women had hot flashes	69%	81%
More women had vaginal discharge	35%	55%
More women had cataracts needing surgery	1.1%	1.7%
Other things to know:		
Dying for any reason	1.1%	0.9%

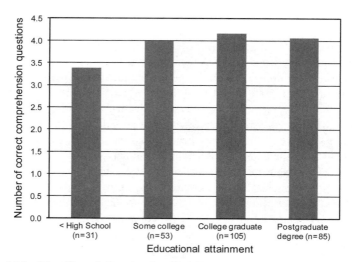

Figure 14.3   The effect of educational attainment on comprehension of a complex table.

correctly answered that tamoxifen "lowers the chance of getting breast cancer by 1.3%." On average, participants correctly answered four of the five comprehension questions. As shown in Figure 14.3, comprehension was good even among participants with the lowest levels of educational attainment.

Consumers Can Choose the "Better" Drug

We tested the effect of complete drug facts boxes in a national randomized controlled trial using direct-to-consumer ads for a histamine-2 blocker and a proton-pump inhibitor to treat heartburn (Schwartz et al. 2009). These drugs were chosen because one had substantially greater benefit, but both had similar side effect profiles; that is, one drug was objectively "better."

To test the box, we invited a nationally representative sample of adults, aged 35–70 years, identified by random digit dialing to complete a mail survey. Surveys in the symptom drug box trial were returned by 231 participants (49% response rate). The control group received two actual drug ads. The drug box group received the same ads, except that the "brief summary" (the fine print second page of ads with detailed information about side effects) was replaced by a drug facts box.

The study results (see Figure 14.4) showed that the drug facts box improved consumers' knowledge of prescription drug benefits and side effects. It also improved decision making, a very high-level task since it entailed integrating data about benefit and harm from two separate boxes: when asked what they would do if they could have either drug for free, 68% of the drug box group, but only 31% of the control group, chose the objectively better drug.

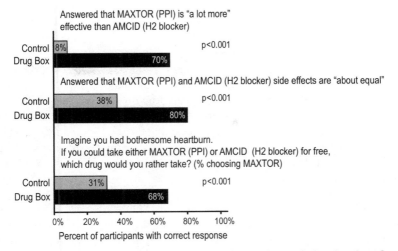

Figure 14.4 Improvement of consumers' knowledge of prescription drug benefits and side effects as a result of using the drug facts box. The black bar gives the percent with the correct answer.

Changing Policy

We presented the results of the national randomized trial to the FDA's Risk Communication Advisory Committee, which had been reviewing FDA's methods for communicating drug information to consumers. The committee voted unanimously that the FDA "should adopt the drug facts box format as its standard." Although the recommendation is non-binding, the FDA often adopts advisory committee suggestions.

The *New York Times* covered the advisory committee meeting and the drug box presentation (Singer 2009). Senators Reed (Rhode Island) and Mikulski (Maryland) saw the article, liked the idea, and eventually submitted a bill to Congress calling on the FDA to adopt drug boxes. The bill was eventually incorporated into the health care reform bill, which was signed into law in March, 2010 (U.S. Congress 2010). Unfortunately the bill is not clear about two fundamental issues: who writes the boxes, and where the boxes will appear. We think that FDA reviewers should write the boxes because the reviewers are independent of industry, have the requisite medical, statistical and epidemiologic expertise, access to (at least theoretically) the totality of the published and unpublished drug performance data, and the time (reviewers spend up to a year analyzing data). We think that drug facts boxes should be used in a variety of ways: as an executive summary of the FDA approval documents, in drug labels, and in place of the brief summary in direct-to-consumer drug ads.

Conclusion

The U.S. public currently lacks accessible and accurate information about prescription drug efficacy and side effects. Instead, people are exposed to billions of dollars in marketing, designed to generate enthusiasm for new products, leaving them vulnerable to persuasive marketing techniques and selective presentations of information. Good, independent drug information does exist, but it can take substantial work (and patience) to find. We developed the drug facts box to make it easy for doctors and patients to find the information they need to make good decisions about drugs. These boxes use tables to summarize what the FDA knows about the benefits and harms of prescription drugs. We have shown in a series of studies that people value the information provided in the boxes and use it sensibly.

The challenge now is one of implementation. Policy makers can show that they are serious about empowering patients and promoting informed decision making by requiring FDA reviewers to create drug facts boxes as a routine part of the FDA approval process.

15

Reengineering Medical Education

David A. Davis

Abstract

This chapter outlines the needs and goals of physicians and expectations relative to their training, and the roles of the medical schools central to that training, with a focus on North American health care and medical education. In the United States, health care reform calls for a realignment of physician roles, to include (a) teamwork and interdisciplinary collaborative care, (b) continuing education and lifelong learning, and (c) workplace learning. Embedded in these constructs are the principles of shared decision making and patient-centered care.

A sizable shift in the concept of the "medical school" is described to enable greater attention to lifelong and workplace learning, and in support of interprofessional care. To accomplish this broad goal, faculty development is needed—that is, a (re)training of "faculty," teachers, and course planners—to address the changes required in a patient-centered health environment. Such shifts will require institutional reorganization and integration, increasing the use of human, technological, and clinical resources from clinical, educational, and research entities within an integrated and functional, effective academic medical center. In addition, the shifts will require thinking along an integrated educational continuum, not only from the standpoint of admissions to a health professional career to retirement, but also across health professional divisions. Finally, a shift to patient-centered care will require reform in educational methodology: an increased use of a wide variety of educational tools and methods as well as more focus on measurable and meaningful uptake of content and less on the process of the simple dissemination of information.

Introduction and Background

Long before calls in the United States were made for health care reform, it was clear that a reengineering of health care and subsequent training of health professionals to match such was urgent. Among many reports that articulated the need for change in health care systems, the U.S. Institute of Medicine (IOM) identified the need to reengineer the way in which all health professionals were educated in its 2003 report: "Health Professions Education: A Bridge to Quality." In summary, IOM called for training to deliver patient-centered care as members of an interdisciplinary team, a commitment to evidence-based practice, quality improvement approaches, and informatics (Greiner and Knebel 2003). The Association of American Medical Colleges (AAMC), the primary organization in the United States devoted to medical education and support of academic medicine, issued several papers related to educational reform under the rubric of its Medical School Objectives Project. Among many are those focused on the quality of care (AAMC 2001), rational prescribing (AAMC 2008), and informatics and information management (AAMC 1998). A major, recent example of work in this area, "Lifelong Learning and Continuing Education" (the final report of a jointly sponsored conference between the American Association of Colleges of Nursing and the AAMC), formed much of the thinking behind this chapter (AACN 2009).

Although compelling, meaningful health care reform and its educational implications pose many challenges for health professionals and the health care system, perhaps especially in the American context. Geographic variations in care, workforce shortages, funding of the health care system, academic inertia, and other factors pose additional challenges. No realization of these goals can occur without a sizable educational reinvestment in individually focused and team- and organizationally-based lifelong learning, beginning with admission to health professional schools and ending with retirement. In particular, patient-centered care, a concept with growing attractiveness in an age of health care maldistribution, comprises an important element in health care and educational reform.

In many ways reports such as those put out by the AAMC appear to begin at the end, describing needs, rather than raising questions: What are the appropriate roles of health professionals? How might we derive them? How might they be described?

Here, I attempt to outline the needs and goals of physicians, relevant training expectations, and the roles of the medical schools central to that training question. The description of the more specific needs of allied health professionals (e.g., nursing, pharmacy, and the other health professions) will not be addressed. In addition, focus is primarily on a North American view of physician education and health care systems, recognizing, of course, that these form only a small part of the global medical education and health system field.

In examining the roles of physicians, several major areas are targeted as the result of health care reform and current needs of the health care system: (a) teamwork and interdisciplinary collaborative care; (b) continuing education (CE) and lifelong learning; and (c) workplace learning. Embedded in these constructs are the principles of shared decision making. Much of these constructs are embedded in and exemplified by the principles of patient-centered care.

In undertaking this exercise, the following assumptions were made:

1. While the present focus is on medical schools and medical training, the importance of the health care team and all its members is explicitly acknowledged.
2. The traditional construct of the "medical school" as an institutional entity and training platform of four years' duration is abandoned. The "medical school" of the future may be an interprofessional experience. Furthermore, "medical education" ends at retirement; thus, emphasis is placed on the skills of lifelong learning and the role of CE.
3. It is suggested that medical school education occurs in a vacuum. A more holistic view of the academic health center is advocated, one that comprises hospitals, community-based clinics, primary, secondary and tertiary care intermingled closely with educational activities and efforts.

Roles of the Health Professional, with Emphasis on the Physician

If one had the time, remit, and energy to do so, how would one begin to craft a curriculum to meet the needs of today's patients, populations, and health care systems?

One project undertook this challenge: "Educating Future Physicians for Ontario," funded by the Associated Medical Services of Ontario and the Ministry of Health in the 1980s (Maudsley et al. 2000). Based on an extensive series of interviews with patients and other policy-level and health care manager stakeholders, the project developed several key physician roles and helped reshape the curriculum of Ontario's medical schools, at least to some extent. It is interesting to observe the (slight) migration of these key roles into the CanMEDS project of the Royal College of Physicians and Surgeons of Canada in the late 1980s, and subsequently into the competencies of the Accreditation Council for Graduate Medical Education (ACGME 2010) in the United States in the 1990s. Given its currency and scope, I refer to the ACGME competencies throughout this chapter.

While the roles overlap sizably, for purposes of simplicity, they may be divided into these major areas:

- clinical/patient care,
- medical knowledge,
- communication and interpersonal skills,
- systems-based practice,
- practice based learning and improvement, and
- professionalism.

These six domains have occupied residency program directors and others, and have been modified and explored for almost a decade in the United States; similar activity has occurred elsewhere in response to other calls for educational reform. In many ways, the ACGME roles have transformed residency education in the United States much as the CanMEDS roles have done in Canada. In the United States, they have led to the development of an extensive set of competencies and assessment methods within each role (ACGME 2010).

Several of these competencies share a common basis on which to build curricular change in medical education, including those directed at incorporating shared decision making into education and health care. They comprise suggestions for the goals of education (to create lifelong learners able to work in team-based, collaborative settings), its methods, and its settings (in the workplace and at the point of care) and are briefly described below.

Lifelong Learning

Lifelong learning comprises the voluntary, self-motivated pursuit of knowledge for either personal or professional reasons. It incorporates an ability to reflect on one's practice and determine learning needs; efficiently and accurately search for and critically appraise learning resources; apply these resources to clinical and other questions; manage large and changing bodies of evidence; and evaluate one's competencies and practice based on subjective and objective feedback. In many ways, this construct may be differentiated from current models of undergraduate medical education, which stress knowledge acquisition and retention. Further, there is a notion of an iterative loop in this model: learning is based on patients, team, and performance feedback.

Interprofessional, Team-based Learning

Interprofessional education refers to the teaching and learning—together— of individuals from different professions during professional training and in practice; it is designed to promote collaborative care practices (CAIPE 1997). While this construct has been evident for over thirty years, much of a health professional's education and practice is carried out in isolation, and this limits integrated collaborative care and shared knowledge and experience (Reeves et al. 2008; Royeen et al. 2008).

Educational Methods

The methods of education (e.g., lectures, rounds, printed materials, Internet-based education) have come under close scrutiny, perhaps most importantly in CE. While some emphasis is given to the full educational continuum, it is also important to focus on CE, given the length and scope of practice and the urgent need for reform in this area. Continuing education is defined as the provision of educational materials, resources, and teaching methods to practicing clinicians after their formal training is complete; attention is given here to the effect of CE on the competence and performance of health professionals and on the health care outcomes of their patients. Several shifts in thinking have led to this construct.

First, studies have shown the nature and size of the clinical care gap (McGlynn et al. 2003), a portion of which is due to the failure of a comprehensive, effective, and systematic approach to CE, as well as a content potentially, seriously biased by support by commercial interests. Second, CE providers—in response to systematic reviews of the literature (Davis et al. 1999; Forsetlund et al. 2009) —have begun to augment didactic teaching methods with interactive and other adult-learning techniques. Third, recent systematic literature reviews of the effect of CE (at least for physicians) have confirmed that educational activities—when undertaken using interactive, multiple methods, and sequencing techniques—can change provider behavior and health care outcomes while maintaining competence, knowledge, and skills (Marinopoulous et al. 2007). It is interesting and possibly informative to imagine that the transition of didactic continuing medical education (CME) to more adult-learner focused learning methods may in some ways parallel notions of shared decision making in the clinical encounter. Taken together, some have called for the use of the phrase continuing professional development (CPD) to encompass this broader construct of CE. For the sake of simplicity the common term, continuing education or CE, is used here.

Workplace Learning

Workplace learning is defined as "the way in which individuals or groups acquire, interpret, reorganize, change or assimilate a related cluster of information, skills and feelings, and a means by which individuals construct meaning in their personal and shared organizational lives" (Marsick 1987:187). This construct is an important element in quality improvement (reflected in the competencies of practice-based learning and improvement and systems-based practice) and allows for a better means of studying behaviors related to professionalism and communication. Point-of-care learning, a subset of workplace learning, is defined as learning that occurs at the time and place (whether virtual or actual) of a health professional/patient encounter. It comprises activities occurring at the time and "place" of a clinician–patient visit and is therefore most often distinguished by its context—the active encounter between the clinician and the patient in the health care site, home, or elsewhere. It, too, is closely aligned with shared decision making and provides a tool for such discussions in the clinical encounter.

Lifelong Learning and Continuing Education

As biomedical knowledge expands to better serve the public, so has the need to "keep up to date." Thus most physicians value the idea of lifelong learning and the need for CE. Although clearly a means to enhancing professional identity

and preventing burnout, an abundance of externally imposed credit requirements limit the view of lifelong learning, reducing it to a mandatory obligation,
frequently unrelated to patient care in many physicians' minds. In a developmental sense, pre-professional education, training and life experiences may
lead to an individual's adoption of lifelong learning as a value and the development of skills needed to translate the value into behaviors articulated by health
professional organizations and adopted by individual health professionals.

Competencies of Lifelong Learning

The "competencies" that lead to appropriate learning and optimal care provision are termed lifelong learning. They comprise the ability to reflect on one's
practice and thereby determine learning needs; the skill to search efficiently
and accurately for learning resources and to appraise them critically (Sackett et
al. 2000); the skill of applying these resources to clinical and other questions;
the management of large and changing bodies of evidence; and the ability to
evaluate one's skills and performance and practice based on external feedback.
Professional education programs hold a key role in providing students with
multiple opportunities to develop these and other skills as the means of continuously acquiring evidence and translating it into professional behaviors. At
least in theory, the process of completing professional training would appear
to ensure that lifelong learning competencies are important components of the
accountable, self-directed professional. However, medical school curricula
frequently fall short and, while focusing on knowledge retention, may fail to
promote and test for the competencies of lifelong learning, given their heavy
dependence on factual learning.

While studies provide evidence of a strong interest in CE among nurses and
other health professionals at the individual level (Griscti and Jacono 2006),
they also suggest that lifelong learning and concomitant self-assessment should
extend beyond individual wants or desires and be supported, if not directed,
by health professions' schools, health care organizations, and regulatory bodies. Lifelong learning needs to be aligned with health systems' need for safe
practices, better patient outcomes (Galbraith et al. 2008), and better, up-to-date
evidence.

The Process of Working and Learning Together:
Interprofessional Education

Interprofessional education (IPE) is defined as "any type of education, training, teaching or learning session, in which two or more health and social care
professions are learning interactively (CAIPE 1997)." The definition embraces
learning across the professional education continuum, but remains relatively
undeveloped and unvalued in traditional curricula. This lack of development
is in the face of recognition by many health and social care disciplines as a

primary vehicle to improve health professional collaboration and health care delivery, their endorsement by academic institutions and others, and research demonstrating that IPE and interprofessional (or interdisciplinary) collaborative care improves efficiency and efficacy of patient-centered care (Greiner and Knebel 2003).

According to this view, IPE appears to maximize the strengths of individual disciplines within the integrated delivery of relevant and optimum care. It is not new. Over three decades ago, Halstead et al (1976) reviewed the outcomes of interprofessional team approaches in the area of chronic illness and rehabilitation. Outcome studies of interprofessional care delivery in many other areas of care (e.g., primary care and mental health) have appeared in the literature subsequently. Implicit in these interprofessional approaches has been their response to critical issues in health care delivery such as geriatrics and, more recently, in chronic illness care. In primary care, workforce shortages, access to care for underserved populations, as well as family-oriented and preventive care needs have driven the development of interprofessional care models, including the creation and growth of the nurse practitioner role in the 1960s and beyond (Charney and Kitzman 1971). Each role demonstrates potential or promise for increased, shared decision making.

Educational Methods

The foot soldiers of "education" remain the traditional, formal teacher-centered approach: lectures, conferences, rounds, courses, lectures, printed materials, and their computer-mediated counterparts. Most health professionals and educators think of education in terms of such methods—a formal transmission of a predetermined body of knowledge. In CE, these activities are frequently provided with designated accreditation and generate "credits" for practitioners, necessary for most credentialing processes, and they reflect undergraduate experiences.

A large literature in CE describes educational effects on knowledge and other competencies. Given its proximity to the workplace and interactions with practicing clinicians, the literature highlights its generally positive role in acquiring knowledge, skills, and attitudes—and an important, but lesser effect on physician performance and patient health outcomes In terms of more distal outcomes, concern has been raised about the impact of formal, classroom-style CE on practice performance or health care outcomes (O'Brien et al. 2001), especially when delivered in didactic, noninteractive modes in CE. More recent systematic reviews (Marinopoulous et al. 2007) confirm this evidence but suggest that well-designed educational activities employing a variety of educational methods, as well as better needs assessments and more interactive designs, can alter clinicians' behavior and even health care outcomes.

Today, "classroom" education—while often still didactic in nature—may encompass a number of such interactive formats, enabling their uptake and positive effect. These formats vary from passive, didactic, large-group presentations to highly interactive learning methods, such as workshops, small groups, and individualized training sessions. Studies highlight several areas of importance to formal educational methods, based on adult education and learning principles.

1. Establishing learning objectives based on learners' and system needs and individual readiness to change: Clinician-learners frequently progress at their own rates, depending on their experience, motivation, knowledge, or the perception of a gap between current knowledge and skills and those needed (Fox et al. 1989). In this respect, then, it is important to determine learning and system needs from both subjective and objective perspectives, recognizing that activities based on more objective assessments appear to have more positive effect given the lack of ability to self-assess one's own performance without external feedback (Davis et al. 2006).

2. Envisaging the "lecture" as only one element in learning: Evidence exists to suggest that among the educational techniques and media outlined above, some methods can be distributed at the time of the educational activity, enabling the practice changes desired by course planners. These include patient education materials, flow-sheets and other checklists to serve as reminders, and links to web sites and other learning resources. Some CE providers have used email and other post-course methods to deliver to participants, materials, or resources such as printed educational materials or reminders. This is considered a passive dissemination strategy to improve knowledge and awareness (Farmer et al. 2008).

3. The modification of classroom education to include interactive techniques to improve its effect in achieving goals such as performance change (Moore 2008). Nowlen (1988) describes one method that uses peer discussion and interaction, stressing the role of the group in adopting new information. Bandura's (1986) Social Learning Theory stresses the importance of personal, environmental/situational, and behavioral factors. Such methods include (a) increasing and improving question and answer periods (e.g., by using electronic audience response methods), (b) using case discussion methods, (c) encouraging small groups to form within the context of large group sessions, (d) role playing, and (e) brainstorming, quizzes, or inviting patients to participate, among others (Steinert and Snell 1999). In addition, the use of multiple media techniques (e.g., simulations, videotapes or role-playing) may provide advantages over the use of a single technique, and multiple exposure to a topic appears more effective than a single exposure (Marinopoulous et al. 2007).

4. Educational interventions beyond the course or conference model have arisen as the product of earlier evidence about the relative weakness of more "formal" didactic education. Generally considered to be more effective than didactic methods in CE, these interventions employ proactive techniques and strategies to effect learning and change in health professionals. Among other methods, they include: community or practice-based efforts (e.g., academic detailing, opinion leaders); computer-generated reminders, protocols and decision-support systems; clinical database-driven audit and feedback methods; and multifaceted educational programs/activities (Grol 2001).

It is interesting to suggest (but difficult to prove) that several of these adult-learning principles operating in the CE of clinicians, also operate at some levels in the doctor–patient relationship especially as it relates to shared decision making, which treats the patient (much as the learner) as a fully capable adult. Might it be true that physicians trained in a paternalistic and didactic fashion, are thus more likely to operationalize it when interacting with patients?

Settings for Lifelong Learning and the New Continuing Education: Learning in the Workplace and at the Point of Care

While formal education using a predetermined curriculum may have prepared students to enter the world of work in the early 20th century, concerns have been expressed in the vocational and professional education literature unrelated to health that this type of education may not prepare learners for their roles in contemporary society, described by some as "complex adaptive systems" (Christensen et al. 2000). The contingent nature of the health care setting requires professionals to go beyond previously learned "scripted" approaches to resolve novel, frequently ambiguous work challenges. In this environment, skilled performance reflects the expertise distributed among the members of a group or team. Further, since successful performance is dependent on factors not yet known or predictable, workers are confronted on a regular basis with problems and challenges not fully addressed by their formal education program. Thus they add, replace, enhance, and mold their practices as changes in work processes (the Internet, for example, or discovery of new clinical technologies) gradually eliminate the need for skills previously learned and necessitating the development of new ones.

Point-of-care learning is seen as a component of workplace learning, occurring generally at the time and place of a health professional/patient encounter. Such learning can deliver information based on needs identified during the clinical encounter, uses primarily evidence-based biomedical and other health-related literature and information resources, and carries the potential to provide an answer either at the time of the patient encounter or soon after. Methods such as reminders offer a "push" effect by being able to promote more actively the dissemination and possible implementation of best evidence at the point of care (Kahn et al. 2007; McGowan et al. 2008). Point-of-care learning is most often characterized by its context (i.e., the active clinical encounter in the health care site, home, or elsewhere). It is during this process that information needs are identified and the opportunity for clinician and patient education, clinical decisions, and patient management all intersect. However, in an era of growing information and communication technologies and new approaches to health care delivery, patient encounters may also include clinician–patient interactions such as telephone calls, email communications, and video conferencing.

Several key elements, similar to those considered as lifelong learning skills, operate within the framework of point-of-care learning. The most basic of these skills is knowledge management, which includes the abilities to identify learning needs, know and understand what resources to use, how to access and critically appraise the information, and how to apply it. A second basic skill is the ability to self-assess (i.e., the appropriate assessment of one's own learning needs, outcomes, and performance change). These elements apply to the question of shared decision making— process that values and uses those resources available at the point of care, enabling patient understanding of complex medical problems and treatment options.

Medical Schools: What Changes Do We Need?

If physicians are to acquire new competencies in the 21st century, curricular reform in medical education is imperative. Figure 15.1 outlines the key elements of this reform, which will need to occur in the workplace, in the individual and team, as well as in the methods used to bring about better learning and outcomes. Infrastructure needs for this to occur include faculty development, institutional reorganization/integration, educational integration (across the educational and health professional continuum), and educational methodology reform.

Workplace and Point-of-Care Learning

Effective workplace learning shows promise in preventing errors, supporting health professional interaction, allowing for reflection on practice and performance, sustaining ongoing professional development, and enhancing individual and organization performance outcomes (Stolovitch et al. 2000). It can also address the incorporation of shared decision making into practice by providing feedback and support. Learning strategies employed in the workplace setting have the potential to address the rapid increase in biomedical and other health information. Because of such information overload, health professionals can no longer be educated with the expectation they will be able, or should try during each patient encounter, to recall information necessary for making

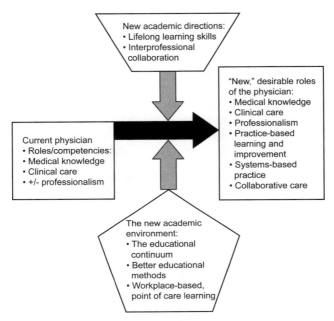

Figure 15.1 Achieving new competencies: the 21st-century academic imperative.

decisions that impact the patient's health status. Current approaches to point-of-care or "just-in-time" information can be modified and fully integrated into the workplace and work routine across the entire health system. The goal of "just-in-time" learning is to match educational resources with a clinician's immediate needs. Just-in-time or point-of-care methods allow learning and self-assessment to be embedded into health professionals' daily workflow, using links to information and clinical systems; thus it promises to be an effective approach to CE delivery (Kahn et al. 2007; McGowan et al. 2008).

This vision for lifelong learning embedded in the workplace includes formative assessment of performance and continuous learning. Learning while one works can be incidental and informal; however, greater impact may be gained if the learning is organized and supported by an integrated and coordinated education and workplace information system (Evans et al. 2006). In such a learning system, performance and outcomes are assessed continuously, supported by the presence of virtual or real workplace coaches and the use of methods like cognitive apprenticeship or scaffolding (Oliver and Herrington 2003). In the United States, this notion is also supported by the constructs of focused and ongoing professional education, recently articulated by the Joint Commission (Greiner and Knebel 2003). Further, in the course of normal work activities, learning resources (e.g., reminders and "just-in-time" information) may be provided to clinicians. Integrated into the normal work patterns, and ideally through an electronic health record, "just-in-time" information can provide health care professionals immediate answers to questions generated by patient encounters. The vision possesses measurable characteristics including:

- a clear focus on patient outcomes and extensive use of data in the form of performance measures,
- a common, shared electronic health record linked to evidence-based content resources,
- the use of the educational resource as a tool to enable shared decision making wherever possible, and
- a team-based, interactive learning culture and processes.

From the standpoint of increasing patient-centered care, such point-of-care resources can prompt and optimize shared decision making.

Formal, current educational approaches may not provide adequately for clinicians as they manage the highly contingent nature of the work and distributed expertise in the work place. Attending traditional CE activities may meet the clinician's perceived learning requirements or provide updated information in specific areas but may not reflect practical, day-to-day learning needs related to practice performance or patient's needs with regards to informed decision making. In response to the growing complexity of the health care system and its knowledge base, as well as the pervasive need for evidence-based knowledge at the point of care, I suggest that a data-driven, participatory, and patient-centered approach to health professional education be established and embedded within the workplace (Billett 1996).

This process would engage a full spectrum of health care professionals and practice settings and would account for business models to support workplace learning systems. These business models would link learning strategies to patient and population outcomes and consider appropriate reorganization of the clinical learning environments to accommodate and support point-of-care learning. In addition, to ensure success, we need to incorporate considerations of the practice culture, context, and structure to enable effective point-of-care learning strategies and provide a better understanding of the impact of point-of-care learning on the identification and application of appropriate resources. Finally, faculty development in this area would not replace the need for information specialists but would allow for more meaningful and effective collaboration between content experts and continuing education providers. Experts in point-of-care learning (i.e., informaticians, information specialists, and health sciences' librarians) are necessary agents to (a) collaborate in the translation of content, especially at the patient level; (b) validate point-of-care learning tools; (c) provide support to improve content and tools; and (d) assist in the integration of best evidence into educational and point-of care learning processes as well as in the development of a research agenda.

Lifelong Learning

Given the "high velocity environment" or "information overload" in medical science, lifelong learning skills need to be integrated into professional schools' curricula to ensure that health professionals are better equipped in knowledge acquisition, appraisal, and application (Kell 2007). An additional reason, given the focus of this paper, is also to assist patients with their decision making. Yet how is this to be achieved?

Academic institutions, curriculum designers, and planners should (a) develop, test, and refine curricula that emphasize and reflect the value of lifelong learning and (b) incorporate and test lifelong learning skills. The latter process should include promoting educational curricula that focus on individual and group responsibility for self-directed learning while building a foundation of responsibility for internally and externally directed continuous learning throughout the professional's working life. This could include the following:

- Creation of a sustainable educational infrastructure to enable lifelong learning throughout health professionals' working lives. Such an infrastructure would emphasize information and communication technology usage to prepare clinicians to learn throughout their careers and to aid in the process of shared decision making. Technologies useful in this regard are informatics, telehealth, computer-based instruction, and virtual simulation.
- Creation and/or adaption of current academic curricula and experiences to generate and assess skills in knowledge acquisition, appraisal, and application.
- Development and testing of tools to assess lifelong learning skills, self-assessment abilities, and knowledge management competencies.

Interprofessional Education: Team Learning

Educators, curriculum planners, and others must begin to incorporate meaningful, formal, and experiential, interprofessional education in entry-level and advanced training of all health professionals. This should include elements of curricular redesign, developing experiential learning opportunities, evaluating IPE activities, and designing IPE CE programs specific to workplace settings.

This process would incorporate an identification of core IPE competencies for all health professionals, a determination of the types of interprofessional experiences appropriate for different learning levels, and the search for ways in which these experiences can best be integrated into health professions' curricula and IPE experiences. Further, CE providers and teachers need to support and create strategies for meaningful, outcomes-oriented IPE. Such methods could include better aligned programming and the development of certification processes to encourage IPE to complement individual professional accreditation components and systems.

Partnerships among health professional schools can enable the exchange of resources and best practices to promote IPE innovation and curricular development, and to support the construct and reality of IPE. The integration of IPE curricula and skills into health professions' education requires:

- faculty and staff development focused on the development and implementation of interprofessional content and learning strategies;
- the identification by health professional education accrediting bodies of clear and meaningful standards for IPE that establish objectives, facilitate curricular change, and require performance measurement and translation into practice;
- collective actions by education, research, and clinical practice leaders to enable the testing of innovations and subsequent curricula modification to foster IPE.

Educational Methods

Academic institutions are responsible for the development of faculty (including teaching and providers of undergraduate, residency training) and continuing education to achieve the goals of a newly envisioned, cost-effective educational system. These goals are twofold:

1. Educational methods must fit the context of learning and change in practice and the learning styles of modern students.
2. The focus of education must shift from disseminating information to assessing its uptake (i.e., "competency-based education"). This process may include attention to shared decision making as one of its many endpoints.

As in other areas, such a shift requires that extensive effort be given in the professional development of faculty members to ensure a broad understanding of the health care system and effectiveness of educational methods. Professional development activities would enhance skills in data use to foster performance improvement—critical skills which influence system administrators and organizational culture.

Such a process would also emphasize the exploration of multiple media methods; allow for creativity, innovation, and personalization of education accessible to clinicians in various settings and integrated into clinical practice; close participants' performance gaps; and address the needs of individuals, teams, and practice groups. In addition, educational strategies would also include the use of interactive techniques, online methods, and follow-up to support the way health professionals learn and change (Davis et al. 2003). Information and communication technology training would include the use of audio/videoconferencing, the Internet (which provides a single point of access to an array of resources computer-based simulations and other methods), and a computer-based instructional program directed to a specific skill or knowledge area (Anderson and Jay 1997).

In addition to educating faculty in the use of such techniques, increasing understanding of potential funding sources and modes of integration into local or regional health care systems is also necessary. This might involve closer collaboration between educators and colleagues in quality improvement, informatics, shared decision making, population health and/or health services research, among other disciplines.

Better Teachers, Better Education: A Focus on Shared Decision Making

Taking the imperative of shared decision making as an example, faculty development could assume several forms: workshops, online learning techniques, and more didactic sessions. Such professional development would also include content in the areas of evidence-based health care and comparative effectiveness research, the detection and mitigation of commercial bias, and a broader understanding of ethics, independence, cost-effectiveness and cost-benefit analysis, and related topics. Educational efforts should also be considered from the perspective of a broad organizing framework that addresses learning needs related to not just clinical but cognitive, interpersonal, moral/ethical, and skill development needs at the individual and system level. One could easily imagine some practical teaching examples such as:

- targeting learning using social networking principles,
- balancing the use of simulation and technology with human interaction and mentorship,
- incorporating real-time technology, increasing accessibility for users and allowing for evaluation,
- improving self-assessment through the use of metrics related to health professional knowledge, skills, behaviors, and health care outcomes across the educational continuum,
- developing mechanisms for external validation and feedback from colleagues in similar clinical practices, and
- assessing and documenting changes in care processes and patient outcomes attributable to such activities.

Summary: New Directions, New Infrastructure Needs

A sizable shift in the current concepts of "the medical school" is needed if a greater emphasis on lifelong learning is to be achieved and teaching methods are to be altered to facilitate interprofessional care and workplace learning. In particular, movement toward the uptake, application, and sharing of best evidence resources is advocated. To enable these shifts, whether in an evolutionary or revolutionary manner, specific infrastructure needs are evident:

1. "Faculty" (teachers and course planners) development or (re)training is needed to address the changes required in a patient-centered health environment.
2. The institution itself needs to be reorganized so that the increasing use of human, technological, and clinical resources from clinical, educational, and research entities can be integrated into a functional, effective academic medical center.

All of this requires a rethinking our concept of medical education, not only from the standpoint of admissions to a health professional career to retirement, but also across health professional divisions. Finally, a shift to patient-centered care will require reform in educational methodology: a wide variety of educational tools and methods need to be employed and more focus given to measurable and meaningful uptake of content, less on the process of the simple dissemination of information

Changing Medical Schools

Barriers to Implementation

The current system contains barriers that inhibit the full evolution of a system supportive of patient-centered care and shared decision making. Such barriers exist in the several of the domains explored above (e.g., health professionals' lifelong learning, interprofessional learning and teamwork, and better educational methods and setting anchored in health care). In this section, using a "force field analysis," I will attempt to outline those forces which align against change, and those which argue for it.

In Lifelong Learning and Continuing Education

The stages of undergraduate and residency training allow for testing of new educational models within current educational standards. The inclusion of patient-centered care, as well as professional and communication skills as a requirement for residency training serves as an encouragement to change in the U.S. context. Continuing education, however, presents its own challenges:

1. Inadequate funding for CE development and programs are reflected in the competing priorities of corporate educational systems, affected by regulatory bodies, higher education institutions, and health care organizations.
2. Differing roles and priorities of health care authorities and professional bodies operate to support lifelong learning, and are molded by their culture, history, political, public, and institutional views of their roles.

3. Inadequate knowledge about the uptake of appropriate and effective curricula and traditional educational methodologies restricts the creation of learning situations conducive to the lifelong learning needs of health professionals.

4. Rapid changes in professional knowledge and technology—and the need to share information with patients in a meaningful way—affect both the learner and the systems in which the learner works—including educational, accreditation, certification, and care delivery aspects.

5. The need to develop an integrated lifelong learning system—one that is closely tied to patients' health outcomes, health system needs, and health professionals' competencies.

Despite evidence of a potential positive effect, the use of interactive and learner-centered activities in planned conferences and other more interventionist approaches pose additional challenges. Frequently developed and tested in research settings, such innovations are less often employed due to cost and other factors (Harrison Survey 2008). Faculty members responsible for the delivery of CE often lack the skills required to develop and use these learning methodologies.

Challenges related to the business aspects of CE slow the uptake of alternative, outreach interventions. Commercial interests and even physicians have, in the past, valued traditional, more passive formal CE; funding sources appear to be limited when the funding for alternative interventions is considered. In addition, alternative learning interventions are often not considered "educational," and thus "credit" is not able to secured. Finally, while such methods may be more proactive, they can fail to engage or to interact with the clinician in a meaningful fashion, thus failing to accomplish their objectives.

In Interprofessional Education

Many issues impede the planning, implementation, and evaluation of IPE models in practice and education. These include interprofessional differences from a long list of subject areas:

- history, language, culture, scheduling, accountability, payment and rewards,
- professional and interprofessional professional identity and clinical responsibility,
- levels of preparation, qualifications, and status, and
- requirements (Ho et al. 2008), regulations, and norms of professional education (Headrick 2000).

More specific barriers exist in academic health centers (Steinert et al. 2005), where there may be weak administrative support, financial and human resources for faculty development. This may be especially the case in IPE; that is, in the time required to plan and implement IPE faculty development for interprofessional learning (Steinert et al. 2005).

In Workplace and Point-of-Care Learning

Multiple barriers exist to the implementation and use of workplace learning as a key educational strategy. The culture and perception of CE as a classroom—not a work-based enterprise—limits the uptake of the concept, as does the previous experience of most faculty members and other teachers of formal education as the primary dissemination vehicle. Further limitations to the construct occur because faculty members are not able to use informatics effectively and other components of point-of-care learning in workplace learning and patient-centered care. A large barrier exists in the awarding of educational credit primarily for classroom participation in formal CE activities. This has been offset somewhat in the United States through new requirements by the Joint Commission, enabling a focus on ongoing and focused education. This barrier may be the most significant impediment to progress in this area.

Forces for and against Change

Change as a Disruptive Process

It is possible to view reform in medical education that would lead to better patient-centered care as a "disruptive" concept. Coined by Christensen (2000), disruptive technology describes innovations that unexpectedly displace an established technology. Use of the term "disruptive" indicates that the learning needs of health professionals working in today's complex health care environment cannot be met by merely fixing pieces or small components of the current approach to health professionals' education. Reflecting this "disruptive" approach, I wish to stress that sizable efforts must be undertaken by health care organizations, health care systems, CE providers, and other stakeholders to ensure the adequate incorporation and testing of workplace learning strategies in health care settings designed to lead to better patient-centered care and shared decision making.

A Force Field Analysis

Kurt Lewin's force field analysis is a useful means by which to assess the degree of readiness of academic medicine to change—both at the level of educational reform, in a general sense, and at the more specific level of improved patient-centeredness in care. Table 15.1 outlines forces arguing for and against change at the more global level of educational reform. They include academic culture, the educational–clinical interface, business issues, accreditation and regulatory concerns, team learning, political realities, individual learning

Table 15.1   Forces for and against change at the global level of educational reform.

Element	Forces for change	Forces against change
Academic culture	New faculty; increased use of IT and other methods	Traditional methods of "teaching," promoting and tenure
Linkages between health care delivery and education	Identification of clinical care gap; recognition that education is at least a part of this gap	Unperceived linkage
"Business models"	Studies outlining effectiveness of alternative models, especially in CE	Relative ease of traditional models of dissemination
Accreditation and regulatory issues	Increased attention to preparation of learners for complex medical practice	Standard accreditation process, focus on educational delivery, hours of content,
Team/interprofessional learning	IOM and other health care delivery reports; physician shortages	Medical "culture"; physician accountability, liability
Individual learning styles	The new millennial learning patterns: multi-tasking, IT-dependent	More traditional teaching styles, acculturation in formal educational settings
Infrastructure	Advent of new IT learning systems	Old concepts of "schools" and learning

styles, and infrastructure. They are useful headings by which we might explore and analyze the question of patient-centered care. Patient-centered care is also affected by many factors, parallel to those impacting educational reform more globally.

Many argue against change. Academic and clinical culture play a major role here: physicians, view themselves as knowledgeable, as many trained decision makers, not considering that patients need or want to share in the decision-making process. This somewhat paternalistic perspective in care is also reflected in education—the expert teaching the novice, the specialist teaching the generalist—echoing issues of power differential and the teacher (much as the physician) as the one-way disseminator of knowledge. Further, arguing against the incorporation of patient-centered care is the primary business model of care and its physical infrastructure, at least in a fee-for-service environment. Here, little time is available—or is made available—to the primary care clinician or the specialist to engage in information-sharing and joint decision making. Further, limitations may be placed on the clinician–patient interaction by the lack of availability of point-of-care resources—computer, human, or other— which might enable the shared decision-making process. Similarly, there is little pressure to change communication styles when there is no, or only vague reference to patient-centered care in regulatory or accreditation standards, apart from the need to employ informed consent processes when surgery or other interventions are used. Shared decision making, however, encompasses a much broader construct, well beyond the notion of informed consent. There are also many educational or "learning" issues involved: physicians and others may not know or be comfortable with the full risk/benefit profile of clinical interventions, either because they have not had time to absorb and consolidate these, or such information is lacking for other, proprietary reasons.

Nevertheless, while many issues and forces argue against change in this area, an equal—perhaps greater—number argue for it. Cultural and business issues, embodied in interprofessional, collaborative care, new and expanding patient-centered models of care, and the success of highly integrated systems, are slowly shifting toward more patient involvement. The political reality of health care reform in the United States, as well as health care demands internationally, may compel significant change in the system—most likely of an incremental nature. Further, new accreditation requirements in U.S. residency training have increased attention to communication and related skills—a feature of patient-centered competencies. Adding to this has been a growing focus on evidence-based medicine, aided by new funding for technology assessment or comparative effectiveness.

Next Steps in Reforming the System

Given that change may be a slow and patchy process, several strategies may assist in overcoming these barriers and in developing a more inclusive, patient-centered health care professional role. These include, but are not limited to, the following three steps.

First, a prime mover in this area is the concerted, systematic implementation of faculty development efforts, across the health professional educational continuum, so that new educational methods, team-based and workplace-centered learning are embraced and incorporated into teaching, role modeling, and mentoring activities. Such faculty development will ensure the preparation of teachers to train learners to practice in modern, rapidly evolving health care environments. Further, faculty training must incorporate a patient-centered model of care approach—modeling and paralleling efforts in educational reform. Not without its cost in monetary and human resource terms, a strong case can be made for its necessity and clear role in health care and educational reform.

Second, the development of highly flexible, competency-based curricula in a patient-centered culture can permit and even encourage the transfer of knowledge and shared roles between and among health professional streams, learning integrated with health care (workplace settings)—an approach to education that takes the learner from admissions to retirement. Inherent in this step is the creation of assessment mechanisms to document learner progress toward goals outlined here by developing new competency assessment methods, performance measures, interprofessional collaborative tools, and other means to document progress. As such measurement tools are developed, curricular planners will need to embrace the concept of mastery learning in which less emphasis is placed on time measurements and more on the demonstration of competency in a variety of skills, including patient-centered care, communication, evidence based medicine, and related topics.

Third, progress toward achieving a patient-centered agenda requires the active engagement of systems of care, including health care delivery systems along with relevant health care and education accreditation bodies to increase the uptake and support of these processes. The former may require increased collaboration between health care settings (hospitals and community-based clinics) to provide meaningful educational experiences. In the context of linking the health care and educational setting, the increased use of innovative IT and other educational methods are needed to assess learners' needs, identify the best resources to address these needs, provide timely and appropriate answers based on evidence-based principles, document learning, and capture the impact of learning on patient management and care outcomes.

Summary and Conclusions

Many limitations are inherent in this chapter. First, it was not based on a systematic literature search, and thus studies supporting—or not supporting—the educational directions or its corollaries in patient-centered care may have been missed. Second, arguments in this chapter were based on work from a Macy Foundation-supported conference on lifelong learning (Moore 2008), and although its major focus supports educational reform, this reform was not validated in the context of patient-centered care. Third, it has focused on physicians providing a heavily North American, especially U.S.-based perspective.

Nonetheless, clear directions have emerged for the future of medical education. These incorporate elements of interprofessional, team-based learning centered in the workplace and use more effective adult-learner and proactive educational methods. Embedded and clearly made more easily attainable within this context is the notion of patient-centered care, which emphasizes shared decision making in addition to other attributes of a patient- and population-centered health care system.

16

The Chasm between Evidence and Practice

Extent, Causes, and Remedies

Richard S. W. Smith

Abstract

Many patients do not receive optimal care, and there is huge variation in all aspects of health care. "Statistical illiteracy" and "health illiteracy" among patients and providers of care contribute to this, but it may be most useful to think of statistical and health literacy as a function not simply of individuals but of the health and education systems.

Studies consistently show that health care practitioners are poor at processing statistical information on risk. Indeed, almost everybody in health care, apart from a few people with advanced training, is poor at processing statistical information. The inability to process statistical information among health care practitioners is one cause of patients failing to receive optimal care. But there are many others, including a flawed and biased information base, unawareness of evidence, unwillingness to accept the evidence, lack of applicability of the evidence, inability to implement treatments, failures to act, unwillingness of patients to accept evidence, and failure to adhere to treatments.

Commissioners of health care and those who set policy may be in a much stronger position than practitioners to follow evidence, as they have access to expert advice and are not under the same time pressures as practitioners. The reductionist ideas of evidence-based medicine, however, are not simply applied in commissioning and the making of policy. Commissioners and policy makers must consider many sorts of research evidence and evidence not derived from research, and it might be that a new type of professionals, "evidologists," are needed to help build evidence more effectively into commissioning and policy making.

Many information tools have been developed to help practitioners apply evidence more effectively, but they have probably had limited impact. Improvement is most likely to come with a systems approach, making it easy for practitioners to use interventions based on evidence and more difficult to use those not based on evidence.

Defining Statistical and Health Literacy
and Evidence-based Practice

We have huge amounts of evidence that many patients do not receive optimal care and that many people do not receive preventive interventions that could benefit them (IOM 2001). This has been the case for a very long time, and it is not clear whether this situation is better now than it was 25 years ago. We also have substantial evidence of dramatic variations in every aspect of health care (Wennberg and Cooper 1999). For example, fivefold variations in one year survival from cancer have been observed from different institutions in New York (Quam and Smith 2005) and a 50-fold variation in people receiving drug treatment for dementia has been reported (Prescribing Observatory for Mental Health 2007).

Why are there these large gaps in optimal care? What causes them, and what accounts for such large variations?

Statistical illiteracy in health can be defined as the inability to understand, describe, and implement the statistical information that is fundamental to health care. Gigerenzer at al. (2007) have listed the insights that constitute "minimal statistical literacy in health":

1. Understand that there is no certainty and no zero-risk, but only risks that are more or less acceptable.
2. Understand what the risk is, the time frame and size of the risk, and whether it applies to the patient.
3. Understand that screening tests may have benefits and harms.
4. Understand that screening tests can make two errors: false positives and false negatives.
5. Understand how to translate specificities, sensitivities, and other conditional probabilities into natural frequencies.
6. Understand that the goal of screening is not simply the early detection of disease; it is mortality reduction or improvement of quality of life.
7. Understand that treatments typically have benefits and harms.
8. Understand the size of those benefits and harms.
9. Be able to assess the quality of the evidence behind the numbers.
10. Recognize any conflicts of interest.

This fascinating and useful list comprises very different sorts of competencies. Intelligent patients might lack every competency, including the fundamental concepts that there is no such thing as zero-risk and that all screening tests and treatments have both benefits and harms. Physicians are probably familiar with these concepts, but they tend to be poor at manipulating numbers and most are not competent in translating specificities, sensitivities, and other conditional probabilities into natural frequencies. Being able to "assess the quality of the evidence behind the numbers" is a broad and complex competency, and perfection in such a competency is probably impossible—but incredibly limited skills are very common among physicians, most of whom have never received any training in assessing the quality of evidence.

Statistical illiteracy is thus very widespread among doctors, patients, politicians, journalists, and, indeed, almost everybody apart from a small trained minority (Gigerenzer et al. 2007).

Health literacy is a broader concept than statistical literacy in health in that it also requires the competency to process nonstatistical information, but statistical literacy might be regarded as an essential requirement for full health literacy. In its report on health literacy, the Institute of Medicine (IOM 2004) defines health literacy as "the degree to which individuals have the capacity to obtain, process, and understand basic health information and services needed to make appropriate health decisions." This definition is broader than simply statistical illiteracy in health, but the report immediately recognizes that its definition is too narrow. Health literacy is not simply a property of individuals but "a shared function of cultural, social, and individual factors." It is, in other words, a property of the system.

A Nordic workshop defined evidence-based health care as "the conscientious use of current best evidence in making decisions about the care of individual patients or the delivery of health services. Current best evidence is up-to-date information from relevant, valid research about the effects of different forms of health care, the potential for harm from exposure to particular agents, the accuracy of diagnostic tests, and the predictive power of prognostic factors" (NIPH 1996).

Evidence-based health care concerns the totality of health care, not simply medicine. It involves all health disciplines, including nursing, health management, and health policy. For the Nordic workshop, it was about the use of research evidence, which contrasts with the widely quoted definition of evidence-based medicine that puts a strong emphasis on clinical expertise (Sackett et al. 1996).

I think that the Nordic definition is too narrow, and thus will use as my working definition the following: *Evidence-based health care* is the careful use of evidence, not simply research evidence, in the making of all decisions in health care and the promotion of health.

I define *providers* as everybody involved in the delivery, organization, and planning of health care and health promotion. The definition includes not simply doctors, nurses, and other health professionals delivering care but also public health practitioners, health commissioners, health managers, and those who make health policy. The use of the word provider is potentially confusing as a distinction is often drawn between "providers" and "commissioners, payers, or purchasers," but I'm using the word broadly.

"Commissioner" is word that is unfamiliar to many in the context of health but is widely used in the English National Health Service. I use it to mean those who employ the resources available for health care and health promotion to achieve maximum value from those resources in treating sickness and promoting health. It implies more than "purchasing" and includes reshaping health care and the environment to promote health.

Extent of Illiteracy in Evidence-based
Health Care among Providers

The extent of illiteracy in evidence-based practice might be measured as the gap between optimal health care, health promotion, and health policy and what actually happens. The Institute of Medicine has reviewed the gap within health care and called it a chasm (IOM 2001). The gap for health prevention is probably bigger than that for treatment because many health systems lack methods for identifying and contacting those who might benefit from prevention and because far fewer resources are devoted to prevention than to treatment. The gaps between optimal and actual health policy are probably impossible to measure but huge because the creation of health policy is a complex, contested, and political process.

Before considering the full range of factors that stand in the way of optimal care, I want to consider briefly the narrower issue of statistical illiteracy among health care providers. This subject is addressed in far greater depth by Gigerenzer at al. (2007) and Wegwarth and Gigerenzer (this volume). In a study from 1998, a group of 48 doctors with an average of 14 years of professional experience were asked the probability that somebody who had a positive fecal occult blood test had colorectal cancer (Gigerenzer and Edwards 2003; Hoffrage and Gigerenzer 1998). They were told that the prevalence of cancer was 0.3%, the sensitivity of the test 50%, and the false positive rate was 3%. The correct answer is about 5%, but the doctors' answers ranged from 1% to 99%, with about half of them estimating the probability as 50% (the sensitivity) or 47% (sensitivity minus false positive rate).

In a more recent study, 1502 randomly selected licensed pediatricians in the United States were sent a case vignette of a five-month-old girl with perioral cyanosis and a hacking cough and told that the pre-test likelihood she had pertussis was 30% (Sox et al. 2009). They were told that she was admitted to hospital, given a direct fluorescent antibody test of her sputum for pertussis and started on erythromycin. Three days later she was somewhat better, and the test proved negative. The pediatricians were asked to calculate the post-test probability that the patient had pertussis. They were given either no further information, told that the test had a sensitivity of 50% and a specificity of 95%, or were given more information on the meaning of sensitivity and specificity. The pediatricians were asked to estimate the probability that the patient had pertussis. The probablilty estimates of the pediatricians ranged from 0 (patient does not have pertussis) to 1 (patient definitely has pertussis). The correct answer was 0.18 but, as Figure 16.1 shows, many people gave an answer of 0.5. Out of the 1502 pediatricians, only 80 gave the correct answer.

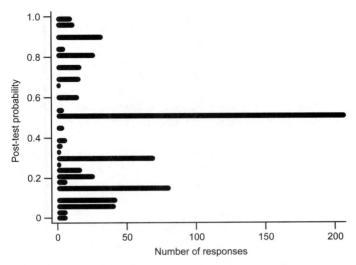

Figure 16.1 Results of pediatricians being asked to calculate the post-test probability of a patient having pertussis after being given a clinical vignette, the pre-test probability, and other pieces of information. The correct answer was 0.18 (after Sox et al. 2009).

A study from 2006 (see Table 16.1) compared the statistical literacy of obstetricians, midwives, pregnant women, and companions who accompanied the women to a clinic (Bramwell et al. 2006). All of them were asked to estimate the probability that a positive screening test meant that a baby had Down syndrome. The participants were given information either as percentages or natural frequencies on how many babies have Down syndrome (1%), the chance that the test is positive if the baby does have Down syndrome (90%), and the chance that the test might be positive even if the baby does not have Down syndrome (1%). The answer is 0.476.

Most responses (86%) were wrong (Bramwell et al. 2006). Less than half (43%) of the obstetricians got the right answer, none of the midwives, 4 of the pregnant women, and 6 of their companions. People did better when the

Table 16.1 Asked to estimate the probability that a positive screening test meant that a baby had Down syndrome, four groups of participants rated the confidence of their answer. Responses are shown both as the percentage and actual number (in parentheses) of those who responded incorrectly in each group. Confidence rating ranges from 1 (not at all confident) to 6 (very confident). After Bramwell et al. (2006).

Group	Confidence Rating						No response
	1	2	3	4	5	6	
Pregnant women	21 (9)	23 (10)	23 (10)	9 (4)	14 (6)	7 (3)	2 (1)
Companions	13 (5)	13 (5)	18 (7)	25 (10)	13 (5)	18 (7)	3 (1)
Midwives	26 (11)	17 (7)	14 (6)	26 (11)	10 (4)	5 (2)	2 (1)
Obstetricians	5 (2)	10 (4)	12 (5)	24 (10)	20 (8)	29 (12)	0

information was presented as natural frequencies instead of percentages, but people's answers ranged widely. Perhaps most disturbingly, the percentage of the people who gave incorrect answers but who rated confidence above 4 (i.e., above mean-level of confidence) was 30% for patients, 56% for companions (mostly probably men), 41% for midwives, and 73% for obstetricians. In other words, a high proportion was wrong but still very confident that they answered correctly—a most particular and potentially dangerous form of wrongness.

High confidence among those who are wrong fits with the classic pattern shown by psychologists Justin Kruger and Jonathan Dunning; namely, those who are "unconsciously incompetent" do not even know how incompetent they are (Figure 16.2) (Kruger and Dunning 1999; see however Krueger and Mueller 2002). You need to become consciously incompetent and ultimately unconsciously competent.

All of the studies that I have found of health care professionals show the same pattern: most practitioners have a poor grasp of the statistical concepts underlying evidence-based health care. This is not surprising as most have had very limited training and simply do not make these explicit calculations when providing care. Indeed, although health professionals will undoubtedly have higher literacy levels than the general population, their statistical literacy may not be much better—as was shown in the study which asked obstetricians, midwives, pregnant women, and their companions to interpret a screening test for Down syndrome. We know that poor health literacy among patients is associated with poor health outcomes (Dewalt et al. 2004), but I have not found studies examining the effect of poor statistical literacy among health care professionals with outcomes. It seems unlikely that statistical illiteracy among health care providers could be beneficial and likely that it would be harmful.

I have also been unable to find studies of the statistical literacy of public health practitioners, commissioners of health care, or those who make health

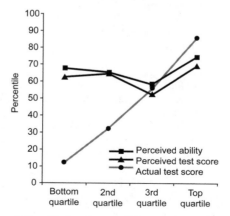

Figure 16.2   The relationship between actual score on a test of logical reasoning and perceived score and ability. After Kruger and Dunning (1999).

policy. Public health practitioners probably have a better grasp of statistical and epidemiological concepts than health care professionals working directly with patients, as they receive more training. Furthermore, they often work in teams that include statisticians and epidemiologists and in circumstances that allow time to access their skills. However, the work of public health practitioners overlaps with the work of commissioners of health and those who create health policy. These work in areas where the application of evidence is still more complex than the use of evidence in patient care. Many health care professionals are skeptical that evidence-based health care is much more than an aspiration, but evidence-based medicine seems to have much greater credence than evidence-based policy making.

Use of Research Evidence in the Commissioning of Health and Making of Health Policy

How evidence and what evidence is best used in the commissioning of health and the making of health policy is greatly contested. Enthusiasts for evidence-based medicine like Iain Chalmers have pushed hard the idea that similar methods might be used in setting policy (Chalmers 1995, 2003). Policy makers should use systematic reviews of "what works," preferably derived from randomized trials, to develop policy so as to avoid wasting resources on what will not work or worse implementing policies that will do more harm than good. This thinking may have reached its apotheosis in an article that Chalmers and I wrote with others on the evidence behind policies to reduce inequalities in health (Macintyre et al. 2001). We concluded that there was little systematic evidence on the effectiveness of the various policies.

Our narrow thinking was taken to task by George Davey Smith, Shah Ebrahim, and Stephen Frankel in an article subtitled "Evidence-based thinking can lead to debased policy making" (Davey Smith et al. 2001:184–185). The article was sarcastic about our "evaluation group":

> On the general question of what sort of evidence is useful to set policy in the public health domain, it is helpful to think back to earlier eras. During the first half of the 19th century, there were no "evaluation groups" to point out the lack of evidence from controlled intervention studies showing the health benefits of, for example, stopping children under 9 years of age from working in cotton mills, fencing off dangerous machinery, or reducing the number of hours children could work to only 10 per day. With an evaluation group, implementation of the Factory Acts could have been resisted. The factory owners were certainly keen on "evidence": the claim that working class children aged 5–10 had lower death rates than middle class children was used to suggest that factory labor was good for children under 10.

Huw Davies and colleagues, who have written extensively on how evidence can inform public services and policy making (Davies et al. 2000; Nutley et al. 2007), have written: "We have come to realize that evidence-based policy and evidence-based practice are overstated, hubristic even" (Davies et al. 2008:188). Martyn Hammersley, a social science researcher, has asked whether "the evidence-based practice movement [is] doing more good than harm" and taken Chalmers on directly, arguing that Chalmers fails to recognize the fallibility of evidence, that reliable evidence can come from sources other than research, and that using any evidence requires judgments about its validity and implications for particular contexts (Hammersley 2005).

There is a particular problem around the "hierarchy of evidence," which puts systematic reviews of randomized trials at the top, trials themselves next, and other forms of evidence lower. Most social scientists find this unacceptable and say that it is unhelpful for creating policy, where systematic reviews of randomized trials are rarely available and where many other forms of evidence must inevitably be considered. Interestingly, even some of the founders of evidence-based health care are moving in the same direction. For example, Alex Jadad and Murray Enkin have written in their thoughtful book on randomized trials: "Our main wish, from which all others stem, is that RCTs [randomized control trials] be taken off their pedestal, their exalted position at the top of an artificial evidence hierarchy, that all forms of evidence be appreciated for what they can offer" (Jadad and Enkin 2007:128). While chairing a session of the European Union Network for Health Technology Assessment, I was interested to learn that it thinks the same, and a Spanish politician speaking at the meeting said that his government found the hierarchy of evidence totally unacceptable.

In the creation of policy, Philip Davies (2004) proposes other types of research evidence which must be considered (Figure 16.3) and delineates some of the many interacting factors that influence policy making (Figure 16.4).

When it comes to setting policy, the implication for literacy in evidence-based practice is that literacy is needed in many forms of research evidence as

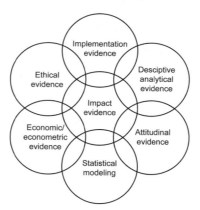

Figure 16.3 Types of research evidence that must be considered in the creation of health policy (Davies 2004).

well as in interpreting and incorporating other factors and forms of evidence that are not derived from research. It is difficult for one individual to possess all these competencies. Thus policy needs to be created by teams, not individuals.

Many practicing doctors, particularly general practitioners, insist that decision making in clinical practice is equally complex. Patients present with problems that have physical, psychological, and social components, and their objectives and values must be paramount in decision making, which may mean that systematic evidence from randomized trials counts for little.

But what about commissioning? The NHS has identified the competencies necessary for the pretentiously named "world class conditioning," and they include being strategic, thinking long term, being outcome driven and evidence-based, focusing on partnerships, and being clinically led and highly professional. Such competencies are, in other words, about much more than literacy in evidence; the evidence to be considered includes much more than systematic reviews and randomized trials.

This list of competencies is a wish list, and I see little evidence of commissioners in the United Kingdom having had much impact in reshaping health services. Most of the activity is at the margins—doing mostly a bit more or less of what was done in the previous year. Perhaps commissioners will improve with time, but they lack skills, data, resources for commissioning (as opposed to resources for provision), and high-level political will to make a real difference out of the fear of the many vested interests.

Anna Donald, one of the originators of evidence-based medicine, has argued that evidence can indeed be used most effectively in commissioning and policy making rather than just in clinical practice (Donald 2005:19). She states that "for the most part evidence needs to be put into practice upstream with policy makers, administrators, and procurers, leaving practitioners with only good options at their disposal."

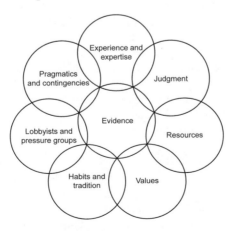

Figure 16.4   Factors that influence policy making in health care (Davies 2004).

Donald's argument arises from twenty years of experience in helping practitioners and policy makers use evidence in their work—mostly through founding and running a company, Bazian, which works with clinicians, publishers, commissioners, policy makers, and many organizations that want to use evidence effectively. Her starting point was the observation that most frontline practitioners are not equipped to analyze evidence by themselves: they don't have the time or the skills or often, it must be said, the inclination. Policy makers and commissioners are in a much better position to use evidence effectively because they have the time and access to people who can help them use evidence.

Like Phillip Davies, Donald also recognized the need for commissioners and policy makers to use a wide range of different sorts of evidence. She believes that a new speciality, "evidology," is needed as well as a new form of professional "evidologists." She bases this on an analogy from radiology: X-rays were discovered in 1895 but were not really used in medicine for forty years. Their effective use depended on the development of new machines, a new specialty, and a new way of working. She argues that it will be the same with evidence and that we are still far from knowing how to use evidence effectively.

Evidologists will be needed for the effective incorporation of evidence into all aspects of health practice, and their job will be to identify questions where evidence should be helpful, find and assess evidence dispassionately, commission evidence where necessary, and be a resource for policy makers, clinicians, and managers. They will not be searching simply for systematic reviews and randomized trials, but will use all forms of evidence. Perhaps the essence of their skill will be to be able to combine judiciously different sorts of evidence.

Causes in Providers: The Gap between Evidence and What Happens

A great portion of the preceding discussion considered the causes of illiteracy in evidence-based health care, particularly in the commissioning of health care and the creation of policy. I want now to return to the question of why health care practitioners do not do a better job of *using* evidence when treating patients. Their statistical illiteracy may be involved, but I suggest that this is not the most common reason why patients do not receive evidence-based interventions.

Paul Glasziou and Brian Haynes (2005), again some of the pioneers of evidence-based medicine, provide a particularly helpful analysis in this regard (Figure 16.5). Their argument is that there is a steady drop in potential effectiveness (a series of steps) that must be taken to provide optimal care; as there are seven steps, a 20% drop at each stage (which is probably conservative) leads to only around 20% of patients receiving the optimal care.

Their first step is awareness, but I see barriers before that step. These barriers are discussed in greater depth in other chapters, but I want to mention them here briefly. One problem is the bias prevalent in research that is undertaken: because of existing funding mechanisms there is, for example, a strong bias toward drug treatments and against non-drug treatments. Next, much of the research that is published is of low quality and relevance (Haynes 1993; Ioannidis 2005), which is not surprising as we grasp fully through studies of the complete inadequacy of peer review, the "quality assurance system" of journals and research funders (Smith 2006, 2009). In addition, the randomized trials that are published are mostly of drug treatments and known to be strongly biased in favor of the drug owned by the company funding the trial (Lexchin et al. 2003). A further, less recognized problem is that the major journals contain a collection of articles strongly biased toward the exciting, positive, sexy, and lucrative (N. S. Young et al. 2008). Those who read only these journals—probably the majority of practitioners who read any journals—receive a very distorted view of the world.

These constitute substantial problems, probably much more serious than is widely recognized. Systematic reviews that search for all relevant evidence can overcome some of the problems, but we are left with a deeply flawed evidence base that potentially undermines the whole concept of evidence-based health care and, more broadly, of practicing medicine using evidence effectively.

It is not surprising that health care practitioners are unaware of research evidence when hundreds of thousands of articles are published in tens of thousands of journals, and many attempts have been and are being made to bring the best evidence to the attention of practitioners (discussed further in the next section). An additional problem with awareness is that health care workers, particularly doctors, are targeted by drug companies and others to bring their attention to particular products. This is a billion dollar enterprise that far outweighs the resources put into creating and disseminating more evidence-based information—in the way that the spending on tobacco promotion dwarfs the funds spent on tobacco control. Manufacturers and advertisers have learned

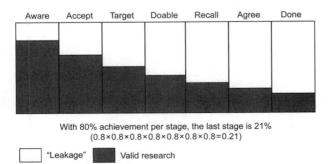

With 80% achievement per stage, the last stage is 21%
(0.8×0.8×0.8×0.8×0.8×0.8×0.8=0.21)

☐ "Leakage"   ■ Valid research

Figure 16.5 Steps that must be taken for research-based evidence to be used in managing a patient and the effect of "leakage" at each step (after Glasziou and Haynes 2005).

that "evidence based" sells and present their arguments on that basis to an audience largely incapable of seeing through what are often false arguments.

The second step is "acceptance." Health care workers may be aware of evidence that shows they should do something different from their routine practice but may refuse to accept and internalize the evidence for a whole variety of very human reasons. A fascinating study of why British general practitioners changed their prescribing patterns showed that (a) they rarely changed and (b) they hardly ever changed because of a change in evidence (Armstrong et al. 1996).

Applicability is the next step (Figure 16.5, "Target"). Health care practitioners may fail to identify the patients who stand to benefit from implementation of what the evidence shows. As Glasziou and Haynes (2005) wrote, "the relationship between diagnosis and treatment is rarely one to one." Practitioners have to balance the risks and benefits for individual patients in a way that we know they find hard to do. The patients seen by the practitioners may be different from the patients in whom the evidence was gathered, and perhaps the biggest problem here is comorbidity (Tinetti et al. 2004; Starfield et al. 2005). Most evidence is gathered in patients with single conditions and yet a very high proportion of the patients seen by doctors have multiple conditions—indeed, their chances of seeing a doctor increase exponentially with the number of conditions they have. We know that following guidelines designed for treating patients with single conditions may cause harm in patients with multiple conditions. This, it seems to me, is a huge problem for evidence-based health care that has not been adequately recognized, and it is not clear how best to respond. It simply is not possible to conduct trials in patients with every combination of conditions.

The fourth step is availability and ability (Figure 16.5, "Doable"). Drug treatment can be complicated, but interventions like spinal manipulation, cognitive behavioral therapy, or external cephalic version are much more complicated and may be beyond the competence of the health care practitioner—yet referral may be impossible or very slow. Alternatively, practitioners may lack equipment like ultrasonographic equipment or an expensive drug treatment may be simply unaffordable. Then the practitioner may simply fail to act. It's very human to fail to act, as the poet T. S. Eliot (1925, *The Hollow Men*) wrote:

> Between the idea
> And the reality
> Between the motion
> And the act
> Falls the Shadow.

This failure to act is particularly common with preventive interventions because there is not the urgency to act as there is with a very sick patient. (Ironically, the feeling of a need to act, "to do something," may in itself work against evidence-based practice because practitioners will act if there is no evidence. This is my hypothesis to explain why there seem to be so many interventions in intensive care that, when carefully examined, have proved to be more harmful rather than beneficial.)

The fifth step is recall, which means that the patient must be brought into the discussion and go through all the steps already taken by the clinician. The patient will have his or her own ideas, values, and opinions, and may reach very different conclusions from the physician. The patient's values must come first, and he or she may not want to proceed with the treatment.

The sixth step is for the patient to agree. Patients may analyze the evidence differently from the practitioner, or more likely they may have a whole host of reasons for declining the intervention. It may not fit with their values. They might be unwilling to accept the pain or the inconvenience of the treatment even though the practitioner judges it to be beneficial. In fact, the idea that it is for the clinician to process the evidence and then for the patient to "agree" or "disagree" with what the clinician suggests seems rather outdated. In a true clinician–patient partnership the two will process the evidence together.

The final step (Figure 16.5, "Done") identified by Glasziou and Haynes is adherence. Will the patient, for example, actually take the treatment, stop smoking, change diet, exercise more, or drink less alcohol. We know that less than 50% of drug prescriptions are followed exactly (Haynes et al. 1996), and people find it immensely difficult to change their lifestyles even if they agree that it is the right thing to do.

The analysis of Glasziou and Haynes concerns primarily a health care practitioner, probably a doctor, and a patient, but patient care takes place within an increasingly complex health care system. The system may include methods (e.g., reminders and incentives) that will make evidence-based care more likely, but the complexity of the system may make it less likely that patients receive evidence-based interventions. For example, we have strong evidence that giving patients who have had heart attacks thrombolytic treatment as quickly as possible is highly beneficial. However, many patients do not receive the treatment in good time because of delays in calling for help, calling the wrong number, ambulance delays, getting stuck in emergency rooms, delays in diagnosis, unavailability of staff, and many other reasons unique to each system. Improving systems is complicated and often does not happen, or is very slow to happen. Many people within health care are trained as if health care is an interaction primarily between individuals; they are not trained to improve systems.

Remedies for Providers to Increase the Likelihood that Patients Receive Evidence-based Interventions

The first remedy for providers to increase the likelihood that patients receive evidence-based interventions might be to improve the evidence base; that is, to make it more useful and less biased (see Schünemann et al. and Gray, both this volume).

There is every reason to work to improve the statistical and health literacy of both patients and clinicians, as described elsewhere in this volume, but I agree with Donald (2005) that most of the needed improvements will come not from concentrating on individual practitioners but from creating an environment for them where the evidence-based option is the easy option—or the only option. Perhaps the best example is the work of the National Institute for Health and Clinical Excellence (NICE) in the United Kingdom (Rawlins 2009). One of its functions is to decide which new interventions, often drugs, are not simply effective but cost effective and therefore should be made available within the NHS in England and Wales. These decisions are made in essence by combining evidence on what is cost effective, usually based on systematic reviews, together with the values of citizens and patients in a process that aspires to be transparent.

Unsurprisingly, NICE does not have a perfect process, and its decisions are often contested, particularly by pharmaceutical companies and patient groups. The process is slow and not fully transparent, and NICE's decisions often do not enter into what happens in the NHS—or do so only slowly. Then, deciding on the availability of new interventions can have only limited impact because most of the activity of the health service is concerned with long-established interventions. NICE does produce guidance on many aspects of public health and clinical practice and on implementing its guidance, but how much the guidance is followed and makes practice more evidence based is hard to assess.

NICE probably exerts most of its influence through health authorities and commissioners rather than directly on practitioners. One tool for influencing practice is the Quality and Outcomes Framework (QOF), which rewards general practices financially for achieving certain measures of quality (Roland 2004). The measures are based on evidence, often systematic reviews, and one of the general practitioners who negotiated the scheme with the government described it to me as "a machine for making practice more evidence based." He said that general practitioners would never accept measures to be introduced into the QOF unless they were evidence based.

Most practices score very highly on the QOF, which suggests lots of evidence-based practice. What is less clear, however, is whether QOF has actually encouraged evidence-based practice or whether it would have happened anyway. There was no baseline study and no control group in that it applies to every practice in the country, including Scotland and Northern Ireland. Some studies have suggested that the quality of care has improved more rapidly in those areas covered by the QOF than in other areas (Campbell et al. 2007), but a recent study suggests that quality in areas not covered has deteriorated (Campbell et al. 2009) illustrating well the problem of promoting evidence-based practice and the law of unintended consequences. In addition, the program has been enormously expensive for the British government (and lucrative for general practitioners), and whether the program has delivered value for money is debatable. Nevertheless, a similar program of incentivizing evidence-based practice in secondary care is now proposed.

Commissioners have considerable potential for promoting evidence-based practice by shifting resources to those activities firmly based on evidence and likely to produce maximum gains in health. There is, however, little evidence of this happening, perhaps because it is still too early or because the evaluation and publication of such results are not high on a commissioner's priority list. Still, a review of the effects of commissioning in Europe, New Zealand, and the NHS found little evidence of benefit (Ham 2008).

Turning to practitioners, the hope must be that training in the concepts of evidence-based practice, particularly for students, will eventually lead to more evidence-based practice. However, the original concept of evidence-based medicine—that practitioners would identify a clear question thrown up by treating a patient, systematically search published and unpublished evidence, assess the studies for quality, and combine the results of the studies, preferably quantitatively, to reach an answer—is clearly impossible. Practitioners do not have the time or the skills. There are problems at every stage—not least in failing to recognize the questions raised by encounters with patients (Smith 1996).

So if practitioners cannot do it for themselves, then summaries of systematically analyzed evidence must be provided. This enterprise began with journals, such as the *American College of Physicians Journal Club* and *Evidence-Based Medicine*, identifying new studies that were scientifically solid and relevant to practitioners and presenting them in a digestible form. These journals did not, however, reach many, and information on a new study is only of limited use: a practitioner needs something more complete that summarizes all available evidence.

The Cochrane Library, which is still perhaps the gold standard of evidence-based information, was one of the first information sources to attempt to present summaries of what the evidence says on particular topics to clinicians. It is, however, very patchy in its coverage, not available to everybody, and presented in a way that is not user friendly to clinicians. There is also a formidable, and largely unsolved, problem of updating the information.

The Cochrane Library was followed by information tools like Clinical Evidence, which attempted to present evidence-based information to practitioners in a more friendly and "actionable" format. There has also been an explosion of evidence-based guidelines. Whether and by how much these information tools have promoted evidence-based practice is unclear, but practitioners do not seem to use these tools much as they see patients. Applying the evidence to individual patients is hard because the questions that arise in practice are not usually "What is the best treatment for a patient with atrial fibrillation?" but rather "What is the best course of action in a 75-year-old woman who has atrial fibrillation, chronic obstructive pulmonary disease, mild dementia, drinks large amounts of alcohol, smokes, lives alone, and will attend the doctor only when pressured by her son to do so?" In reality, questions that arise in daily practice are much more often like the latter than the former (Smith 1996). Thus it is no wonder that applying evidence-based interventions is hard.

Another strategy for encouraging practitioners to practice in a more evidence-based manner is to provide a service that will provide an evidence-based answer to questions that arise during practice. There have been experiments with such services, but they have not become part of routine practice.

As practitioners do not tend to reach out for evidence-based information, it is a logical next step to try and deliver it to them as they see patients. Most general practitioners in Britain, for example, use a computer when consulting, and it is possible to provide evidence-based decision support to coincide with this. Doctors, however, do not seem to be very enthusiastic about decision support.

Conclusion

Many patients do not receive optimal care. Patients are treated within increasingly complex health systems, and there are reasons why patients do not receive optimal care. Their own statistical and health illiteracy as well as that of the clinicians treating them constitute part of the problem. There is every reason to work to improve the statistical and health literacy of patients and clinicians. However, the most effective response is likely to be to work "upstream" through policy makers and commissioners, to make it easier to use evidence-based treatments and harder to use those not based on evidence.

17

The Future of Diagnostics

From Optimizing to Satisficing

Henry Brighton

Abstract

In health care, our observations are shaped by interactions between complex biological and social systems. Practitioners seek diagnostic instruments that are both predictive and simple enough to use in their everyday decision making. Must we, as a result, seek a trade-off between the usability of a diagnostic instrument and its ability to make accurate predictions? This chapter argues that sound statistical reasons and evidence support the idea that the uncertainty underlying many problems in health care can often be better addressed with simple, easy-to-use diagnostic instruments. Put simply, satisficing methods which ignore information are not only easier to use, they can also predict with greater accuracy than more complex optimization methods.

Introduction

In the United Kingdom, 81% of costs in patient services result from hospital expenditure (Dept. of Health 2005). One way to reduce these costs is to improve health care management of people at high risk of hospital admission. Among older people, certain subgroups are at a particularly high risk. If these high-risk individuals can be identified early, and their health care managed more effectively, preventive care could mean financial savings (Wagner et al. 2006). This holds for many problems in health care. Thus, the identification of predictive diagnostic instruments relating variables to outcomes is a necessary goal, and observations will be used to guide this process.

Statistics provides tools for crafting sophisticated predictive models from observations. These observations are shaped by the interaction of complex biological and social systems. On the other hand, practitioners seek diagnostic instruments which are both predictive and simple enough to use in their everyday decision making. I will argue that this apparent dichotomy is false: There are sound statistical reasons, and evidence, supporting the idea that the complexity underlying the problems faced in health care can often be better addressed with simple, easy-to-use diagnostic models.

A bottom-up approach will be taken, starting with the identification of three forms of uncertainty that stand in the way of making accurate predictions. The remainder of the discussion will then contrast two broad perspectives on constructing diagnostic models. The first is optimization, which stresses the explicit attempt to conduct rationally motivated calculations over potentially complex models. Optimization attempts to find the most predictive model (or at least, approach it). The second perspective, satisficing, is less well-known, and seeks a good enough model by ignoring information. Satisficing tends to rely on simpler models and can consequently achieve greater predictive accuracy than "optimal" models.

The notion of robustness will be used to explain this counterintuitive relationship. A system is robust to the extent that its function is maintained when operating conditions change. In health care, uncertainty surrounds our models, observations, and context of use. Diagnostic instruments which attempt to "over-model" the problem can be less robust than those which ignore information. When designing and deploying diagnostic instruments, we should assume that changes in operating conditions will occur, even though their exact form may be hard or impossible to specify.

Fitting Models to Observations

By considering eight variables, such as a person's self-perceived health and their access to a caregiver, Wagner et al. (2006) considered the problem of predicting if older people will require hospital admission at some point during the following year. To develop a predictive model, they collected observations of older people. Each observation related the eight variables associated with the individual to a dependent variable detailing whether or not this individual required an overnight hospital admission at any point during a follow-up period of one year. Now, a good statistical model, one capable of improving health care management among older people, must somehow capture what is systematic in these observations. Once identified, these systematic patterns can be used to predict whether or not a previously unseen person will require hospital treatment in the future.

In health care, education, sociology, psychology, and beyond, a hugely diverse set of problems are framed in these terms. Despite this diversity, the statistical machinery employed is astonishingly uniform. The linear regression model rules in a methodological dictatorship. It has two components: an assumed linear relationship between the variables and the criterion, and the assignment of weights to these variables by the method of least squares. A raft of statistical add-ons can complement this basic machinery, but the basic properties of the machine remain the same. The methodological dictatorship is not the fault of the linear regression model, but the collective behavior of its users.

Often, the variables used in a linear model are referred to as "predictors." Predictors which "explain" a large amount of the variance are typically seen as informative. Similarly, when the linear model achieves a good fit to the data, the model is said to predict the data well. Additional manipulations, those which improve the fit of the model to the data further, are seen as a move in right direction, a step closer to the objective of capturing systematic patterns in the data. Stepping back from this statistical routine, it is worth considering exactly what has been predicted. The parameters of the model have been estimated from the observations. This parameterized model is then evaluated on its ability to "predict" these same observations. This is a process of post-diction, not prediction. The predictive ability of a model, under any meaningful definition of the term, refers to its ability to second guess properties on unseen data presented at some point of time in the future, after the model has been parameterized.

Faith in data fitting and abuse of the term prediction can, and often will, lead to faulty inferences from data (Pitt et al. 2002; Roberts and Pashler 2000). Because these inferences may inform policy, it is worthwhile pulling apart the conceptual distinction between post- and prediction. The following example provides a visual illustration. The temperature in London on a given day of the year is uncertain but nevertheless follows a seasonal pattern. Using the year 2000 as an example, Figure 17.1 plots London's mean daily temperature. On top of these observations, two polynomial models have been plotted; they

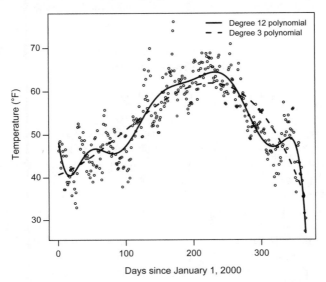

Figure 17.1 Mean daily temperature in London for the year 2000. Two polynomial models (a degree-3 and degree-12 polynomial) are fitted to this data.

both attempt to capture what is systematic in London's temperatures. The first model is a degree-3 polynomial (a cubic equation with four parameters), and the second is a degree-12 polynomial (which has 13 parameters). Comparing these two models, we see that the degree-12 polynomial captures monthly fluctuations in temperature, whereas the degree-3 polynomial captures a simpler pattern charting a rise in temperature that peaks in the summer, followed by a slightly sharper fall.

Now, which of these two models best captures London's mean daily temperatures? Outside idealized "laboratory" settings, data can be seen as containing both systematic and accidental patterns. A model which accurately captures both will describe the data closely and achieve a good fit. In the temperature example, the degree-12 model achieves a better fit to the data than the simpler degree-3 model for precisely this reason. However, accidental patterns, by definition, will not hold true of future data, and relying on these patterns to make predictions about the future will lead to errors. The key point here is that when judging models on the basis of their goodness-of-fit, one has no way of knowing if a good fit reflects the ability of the model to capture accidental patterns accurately, its ability to capture systematic patterns, or both.

Below, it will be demonstrated that the simpler degree-3 model provides a better model of the London's daily temperature even though it achieves a poorer fit than the degree-12 model. Before doing so, it is worth pointing out that, taken to an extreme, the policy of evaluating models exclusively on their ability to fit data implies that we only need one model. The best model is one which simply memorizes the list of observations. This model guarantees a perfect fit on all problems. Among the statistically trained, many are aware of the dangers of model fitting, but far fewer act to avoid them.

Out-of-Sample Prediction

Prediction is very difficult, especially if it's about the future.
—Niels Bohr (1885–1962)

Because the future is uncertain, how can we possibly evaluate the ability of a model to predict accurately whether an older person will require hospital admission or not in the future? Waiting is not an option. Recall that the objective is to identify systematic patterns governing the population given only a sample of observations. Because samples are likely to contain noise and accidental patterns, they will always provide an uncertain and potentially misleading view of the population. Several model selection criteria have been developed which provide principled alternatives to measuring the goodness-of-fit of a model to the data (e.g., Pitt et al. 2002). Cross-validation is one criterion, and it works by first fitting the model to a fraction of the available observations; thereafter it uses the remaining observations to measure the predictive ability of this fitted model (Stone 1974). This process is then repeated, each time partitioning the data randomly. The final estimate of predictive accuracy is the mean predictive accuracy with respect to many such partitions.

For example, if we sample the temperature in London on 50 randomly selected days in the year 2000, and then fit a series of polynomial models of varying degree to this sample, we can measure two quantities. The first measure is a familiar one, the goodness-of-fit of the models to the sample. The second measure is perhaps less familiar and considers how accurately these fitted models predict the temperature on those days of the year 2000, which were not observed. As a function of the degree of the polynomial model, Figure 17.2 plots the mean of these two measurements. Focusing on the goodness-of-fit of the models to the samples, we see that the more parameters the model has, the better the fit. This relationship reflects the point made above: Achieving a good fit to the data is trivial. Achieving high predictive accuracy is not so simple. The model with the lowest mean prediction error (with respect to many such samples of size 50) is a degree-4 polynomial. More complexity is not better. If we had relied on goodness-of-fit as an indicator of model performance, we would not have chosen this model.

Cross-validation estimates the out-of-sample predictive accuracy of the models, which is their accuracy in predicting outcomes for unseen observations drawn from the population when estimated from the samples of that population. Note that access to the population was assumed in the preceding example. This need not be the case. Cross-validation is usually applied to a

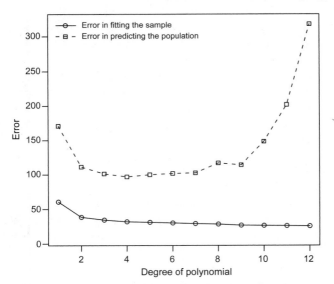

Figure 17.2   Model performance for London temperatures in 2000. For the same data, mean error in fitting the observed samples decreases as a function of polynomial degree. Mean error in predicting the whole population of the entire year's temperatures using the same polynomial models is minimized by a degree-4 polynomial.

sample of data, because we rarely (if ever) have knowledge of the population. For example, a fraction of the available observations of people's hospital admissions can be used to fit the model parameters, and then competing models can be judged on their ability to predict the remaining observations. Although the model parameters may be estimated from fewer observations, the idea is that this is a price worth paying if we can then estimate the predictive ability of the models.

The temperature example highlights two forms of uncertainty. First, a sample of observations provides an uncertain indicator of the population from which they are drawn. If the tape of experience were replayed, then we are likely to have a different sample with different characteristics. Second, there is uncertainty surrounding which model should be chosen to capture systematic patterns. In the temperature example, we do not know the functional form of data-generating function behind London's daily temperature. Similarly, we can be sure that when using a linear model to predict if a person will be admitted to hospital in the next year, this model will be a gross abstraction of the data-generating distribution. In both cases, the model is misspecified. Many of the issues raised thus far come into sharper focus when we examine the origins of linear regression.

Toward the end of the 18th century, Adrien-Marie Legendre and Carl Friedrich Gauss were both concerned with measuring the length of the meridian quadrant, the distance from the equator to the North Pole (Stigler 1986, 1999). Using error-prone observations of subsections of the arc measured at various points between Dunkirk and Barcelona, they faced the problem of how to integrate these observations. The accuracy of their estimates was important. The meter was to be defined as 1/10,000,000 of this arc. When tackling this problem, it appears that Legendre and Gauss independently developed the method of least squares. In contrast to the problem of estimating London's mean daily temperature, or estimating the number of future hospital admissions, Legendre and Gauss had the benefit of a precise geodesic model. There was little uncertainty surrounding this model, and the observations were used to estimate precise values for its parameters.

The problems that confronted Legrende and Gauss, such as measuring the length of the meridian quadrant or predicting the trajectory of a comet, can be seen as the antithesis of those we face in health care. Indeed, relative to our temperature example, Legendre and Gauss where almost certain where on the x-axis of Figure 17.2 they should be focused, which meant that they were not searching for the functional form of the data-generating model. Now, put in these terms, it is no surprise that choosing the best fitting model will lead to poor inferences. Without knowing the gross properties of the data-generating model, data fitting becomes the statistical equivalent of groping in the dark. Thus, the method of least squares is used, now as a matter of routine, in contexts which bear little resemblance to the context of its discovery. The key difference is the uncertainty surrounding our knowledge of the data-generating distribution.

Out-of-Population Prediction

In times of change learners inherit the earth; while the learned find themselves beautifully equipped to deal with a world that no longer exists.
—Eric Hoffer (1902–1983)

Thus far, it has been assumed that a sample is drawn from a population and that the properties of this population will determine the accuracy of our predictions. This is an idealization. One assumption underlying this belief is that the population will remain stationary over time. However, this is just one idealization among many. After finding a predictive model of future hospital admission among older people, this model could become standardized and used by doctors more widely. When used in a different hospital, city, region, country, or continent, the population will almost certainly change. Perturbations arise due to one or more of an endless list of factors (e.g., differences in the measurement techniques used, demographic and cultural changes affecting the health of individuals). Couched in terms of the weather example, a more realistic test of the models estimated from a sample of measurements is to consider how well they go on to predict the mean daily temperature in London on each day of, for instance, 2001. What we are predicting now lies outside the population used to estimate the model parameters. The two populations may differ because factors operating over longer time scales come into play, such as climate change.

To illustrate, Figure 17.3 examines how well the models estimated from samples of the temperatures in London in 2000 go on to predict the temperatures in 2001 and 2002. I have also plotted out-of-sample error for 2000 as a point of comparison, and, as we should expect, the error increases when we move from the out-of-sample problem to the out-of-population problem. Although there is more uncertainty in the out-of-population setting, much of the same pattern can be observed as before: A degree-4 polynomial yields the minimum mean error. This tells us that what we learned from the out-of-sample task transfers to the out-of-population task, since a degree-4 polynomial remains a good choice of model.

An additional change to the population that we wish to predict can be introduced by imagining that we want to use the temperatures in London to predict those observed in Paris. Paris lies 212 miles southeast of London, and Figure 17.3 shows how the prediction error suffers as a result of this geographical shift; however, the finding that degree-4 polynomials predict with the least error remains. Often, we will not be so lucky. This is an example of a robust model: The degree-4 polynomial models fitted to relatively small samples of observations remain, relative to the other models, accurate. The accuracy of the

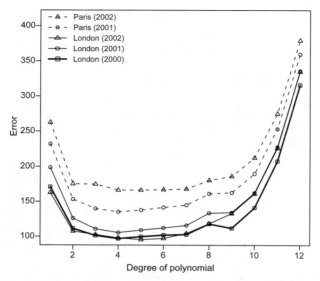

Figure 17.3 Out-of-population prediction. The models estimated from 50 samples of London's daily temperatures in 2000 can be used to predict the daily temperature for that entire year (thick line). This plot also shows how well these models go on to predict the daily temperature in London for 2001 and 2002, and in Paris for 2001 and 2002. Much the same pattern is observed across applications of the model, although the error increases due to greater uncertainty coming from changes in time and space.

model appears to be robust against several kinds of perturbation. The notion of robustness will be central to the remainder of the discussion.

Robustness to Uncertainty

Robust systems maintain their functioning when operating conditions change (Wagner 2005). The ability of diagnostic tool to make accurate predictions when the population changes is an example of a robust statistical model. The ability of the immune system to maintain a functioning organism despite continually evolving pathogens is an example of a robust biological system (Hammerstein et al. 2006). The ability of the flight control system of an aircraft to follow a course despite potentially severe atmospheric changes is an example of a robust human-engineered system (Kitano 2004). Some disciplines, such as biology, attempt to reverse-engineer robust design. Other disciplines, such as engineering, attempt to design robust systems. In diagnostics, too, we would like to engineer predictive instruments which remain predictive when operating conditions change. Which principles might guide the design of robust diagnostic instruments? Before examining this question, it is worth consolidating the three kinds of uncertainty discussed so far:

1. Model misspecification: The complexity of the processes that determine the content of our observations is such that our knowledge of the data-generating distribution will be uncertain. Consequently, we have no way of formulating a space in which the correct model is known to exist. Short of assuming certain knowledge of putative "natural laws" governing the observations, all models are misspecified and lead to error. Put simply, there is uncertainty surrounding our ability to formulate the data-generating distribution.

2. Model underspecification: Given a parameterized space of models, misspecified or not, observations are required to estimate the parameters of the model. Observations are finite in number and may be too few to estimate these parameters reliably. For example, even if we knew we were searching in the right space, a single observation will be insufficient to reliably select a good model, and errors result. Put simply, there is uncertainty surrounding the ability of the data to select the model parameters reliably.

3. Out-of-population prediction: Even with certain knowledge of the data-generating distribution, and therefore the "optimal" model, there is uncertainty surrounding the context in which this model is used to make predictions. Put simply, data-generating distributions can change for many reasons. You may, for example, have discovered the optimal model at the time of data collection, but this data-generating distribution is likely to have been perturbed by the time the model is used to make predictions.

All approaches to diagnostics must contend with these uncertainties. The substantive issue is how to design diagnostic instruments that are robust to the realities of model misspecification, model underspecification, and the uncertainty surrounding the problem itself. With these questions in mind, the remainder of this discussion will contrast two approaches to developing diagnostic systems: optimizing and satisficing.

From Optimizing to Satisficing

Optimizing is the process of seeking the optimal solution. What is the optimal solution? Consider a tin can manufacturer who attempts to reduce costs by minimizing the surface area of the cans produced. To package 12 ounces of soup, the manufacturer has calculated the height and width of the can which minimizes the amount of tin used. No other design uses less tin to package the same soup. This is an example of an optimal solution to a problem: From the space of candidate solutions, the optimal solution is the one which cannot be improved on. In this example, the relationship between variables and solution is certain. Solid geometry and the precision of our measurements ensure a close fit between our model and the real world. For most problems, including diagnostics, this kind of certainty will not exist. Optimization can nevertheless still be carried out, but in practice, one moves closer to the solution that is optimal only relative to a set of assumptions.

What characterizes the process of optimization? If we lacked knowledge of solid geometry, iteratively fine-tuning the tin can dimensions until the surface area is at a minimum would be a process of optimization. This process assumes that we can the measure the effect of changes to the parameters, and this measure serves as a proxy for performance. If we had knowledge of solid geometry, then we could derive the optimal solution directly. Both are examples of optimization. Broadly speaking, optimization is any process which (a) explicitly maximizes some criterion and (b) assumes that this criterion is monotonically related to performance. As a consequence, optimization methods have a strong tendency to assume that more computation leads to greater precision.

Everyday examples include the method of least squares, which minimizes the sum squared error between the model and observations. In Bayesian statistics, the aim is to select the model with the highest posterior probability, or perform model averaging to determine the most probable prediction. Underlying this approach is the view that the optimal model (or prediction) is "out there," and optimization provides a way of approaching it. Although these approaches are often given rational justification by appealing to probability theory, exact optimization methods are largely fictitious for real-world problems. The computational demands required to conduct the search are often too great. Instead, inexact and approximate methods are used. Thus, there is no single "process of optimization," since in practice additional assumptions often need to be made.

Satisficing, an approach first proposed by the Herbert Simon, offers an alternative to optimization (e.g., Simon 1990). Instead of attempting to maximize some criterion, a satisficer might ignore several factors seen as crucial to an optimizer and seek a good enough (or better) solution. As well as ignoring information, a satisficer will typically not attempt to maximize any criterion. Examples of satisficing include restricting attention to unit weights (either -1 or 1) in a linear regression (Dawes 1979; Einhorn and Hogarth 1975; Wainer 1976), ignoring covariation between cues (Langley et al. 1992), or simply relying on a single cue to make a decision (Gigerenzer and Goldstein 1996; Holte 1993). Strategies like these raise the following question: Why should we even entertain the idea of satisficing? After all, deliberately using impoverished models, such as unit weights, and deliberately curtailing search, as opposed to performing an exhaustive search, both seem potentially foolhardy policies. If these strategies seem ill-advised, then consider the examples given below. Keep in mind that these examples essentially pit two fictional statisticians, A and B, against each other. Statistician A, an optimizer, and statistician B, a satisficer, share the same knowledge of the problem, but they differ in how they approach the problem.

Optimizing versus Satisficing

First, consider how a retail marketing executive might distinguish between active and nonactive customers. Experienced managers tend to satisfice, by relying on a simple hiatus heuristic: Customers who have not made a purchase for nine months are considered inactive. Yet there are more sophisticated methods, such as the Pareto/NBD (negative binomial distribution) model, which considers more information and relies on more complex computations. When tested, however, these methods turned out to be less accurate in predicting inactive customers than the hiatus rule (Wübben and von Wangenheim 2008). Second, consider the problem of searching literature databases, where the task is to order a large number of articles so that the most relevant ones appear at the top of the list. In this task, a "one-reason" heuristic using limited search outperformed both a "rational" Bayesian model that considered all of the available information and PsychINFO (Lee et al. 2002).

Third, consider the problem of investing money into N funds. Harry Markowitz received the Noble Prize in economics for finding the optimal solution: the mean-variance portfolio. When he made his own retirement investments, however, he did not use his optimizing strategy, but instead relied on a simple heuristic: 1/N (i.e., allocate your money equally to each of N alternatives). Was his intuition correct? Taking seven investment problems, a study compared the 1/N rule with fourteen optimizing models, including the mean-variance portfolio and Bayesian and non-Bayesian models (DeMiguel et al. 2009). The optimizing strategies had ten years of stock data to estimate their parameters, and on that basis had to predict the next month's performance; after this, the ten-year window was moved one month ahead, and the next month had to be predicted, and so on until the data ran out. 1/N, in contrast, does not need any past information. Despite (or because) of this, 1/N ranked first (out of 15) on certainty equivalent returns, second on turnover, and fifth on the Sharpe ratio, respectively. Even with their complex estimations and computations, none of the optimization methods could consistently earn better returns than this simple heuristic.

Now, after being informed of these results, statistician A (the optimizer) might raise the following objection: These examples fail to provide an argument against optimization because, quite clearly, the "optimization" models are suboptimal. Statistician A is correct, but his argument is irrelevant. Recall that there is no single process of optimization, and it will always be possible to find an alternative optimization model, after the fact, which outperforms the satisficing method proposed before the future was observed. Obviously, this is an entirely different question unrelated to the substantive issue of designing a diagnostic instrument which predicts well in the face of uncertainty, before the future has been observed.

Why Satisfice?

There are two reasons to satisfice. First, as the examples given above illustrate, satisficing methods can predict with greater accuracy than optimizing methods, particularly when facing real-world uncertainties. Indeed, this discussion would be incomplete without mentioning a diverse collection of analytic results and arguments in support of satisficing. Over several decades, research into judgment and decision making has provided support for the robustness of unit weighing schemes and simple cognitive heuristics (Gigerenzer and Brighton 2009). In data mining and knowledge discovery, Domingos (1999) lists numerous cases in which methods that restrict search (a key concept in satisficing) can outperform methods that attempt to optimize formal measures of simplicity. In pattern recognition and machine learning, the naïve Bayes classifier ignores information by assuming variables are conditionally independent. Despite this, the naïve Bayes classifier often outperforms more sophisticated methods which consider these dependencies, even when these dependencies are known to exist (Domingos and Pazzani 1997). In statistics, Hand (2006) questions the assumed progress associated with evermore sophisticated optimizing methods by invoking some of the arguments presented here, as well several others. In forecasting, Makridakis and Hibon (1979) questioned the common assumption that simple models often pay the price of reduced predictive accuracy. They compared 22 forecasting models and found that a simple model which ignores observations outperformed more complex models on 111 problems. Each of these contributions supplies pieces of an emerging picture, where satisficing, and related concepts, provide principles for engineering robust diagnostic instruments.

The second reason to satisfice is that the resulting models tend to be easier to use and understand. The examples given above included a simple rule which can be used to predict inactive customers, a single criterion which can be used to search for documents, and a simple method for allocating money to a collection of funds. To take another example, when a patient arrives at hospital with acute chest pain, a doctor must decide if the patient should be admitted to coronary care unit or a regular bed. Pozen et al. (1984) developed the Heart Disease Predictive Instrument (HDPI) to help doctors make this decision. HDPI is based on a logistic regression and requires doctors to consider seven variables and then conduct a series of calculations with the aid of a chart and pocket calculator. HDPI improved decision making, but doctors found it difficult to use. Green and Mehr (1997) went on to shown that, after withdrawing the HDPI, doctors continued to make better decisions, rather than revert to their original performance levels. How can this finding be explained? Green and Mehr hypothesized that the doctors had learned which variables were relevant, and then applied a simple cognitive strategy to make decisions using this subset of these variables. Investigating further, Green and Mehr developed the simple decision tree, shown in Figure 17.4 (based on the take-the-best heuristic; Gigerenzer and Goldstein 1996), to replace the HDPI. This tree poses a short series of yes/no questions, enabling doctors to make decisions without carrying out any additional calculations or looking up numbers in a chart. Crucially, this decision

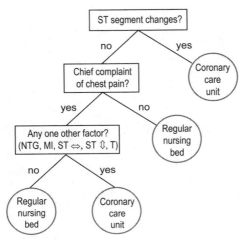

Figure 17.4 A simple "fast and frugal" decision tree used in coronary care unit alloca-tion. ST ↔: flattening of ST segment; ST ↑↓: elevation or depression of ST segment; NTG: nitroglycerin; MI: myocardial infarction; T: T-wave.

tree proved to be more accurate in providing patients the appropriate care, and was far easier to use.

Problems in health care are shaped by immensely complex interactions be-tween biological and social systems. Traditionally, there has been a tendency to believe that the best response is to develop statistical models and diagnostic systems which respond, in kind, by combating complexity with complexity. Satisficing offers an alternative viewpoint and suggests that the complexity of optimization is better suited to simple problems where we can be sure that we are optimizing the correct criterion. For complex problems involving high degrees of uncertainty, our assumptions will often fail to hold and operating conditions will change in unexpected ways. Satisficing can simultaneously of-fer a more robust response to such perturbations and simpler, easier to use, diagnostic instruments.

18

Direct-to-Consumer Advertising

Status Quo and Suggestions to Enhance the Delivery of Independent Medication Information

Wolf-Dieter Ludwig and Gisela Schott

Abstract

Direct-to-consumer advertising (DTCA) of prescription drugs has become a focus of public policy concern and academic research. Through it, pharmaceutical companies influence major parts of the health system, including the drug trials upon which DTCA is based. Advocates emphasize its potential in educating the public about health conditions and treatment options, but evidence supporting this argument is sparse. Critics highlight potential risks, such as encouraging the use of new drugs with unknown safety profiles—a view supported by some data.

The literature is analyzed to characterize the data on approved drugs currently available on the market. Arguments for and against DTCA are given and an outline is presented of the current regulatory system in the United States, New Zealand, Canada, and Germany. Thereafter, appropriate ways of informing patients are discussed.

Neither the central regulatory system in the United States nor the voluntary self-regulations in New Zealand and Canada have been able to ensure compliance with standards of acceptable advertising practice for DTCA. Therefore, the ban on DTCA in Europe is justified and should be maintained. To communicate the benefit-risk ratios of drugs to patients, evidence-based, independent, and neutral information is necessary and must be supported.

Introduction

Pharmaceutical companies and providers of medical devices use DTCA to promote medications and medical devices to the public through many media forms—newspapers, magazines, billboards, television, radio, and the Internet (Wilkes et al. 2000). Additional forms (e.g., patient brochures and videos) are often made available in doctor's offices or designed to be given to patients by medical professionals or patient groups.

DTCA is just one example of the marketing and public relation efforts by drug companies to promote brand-name prescription drugs. More subtle forms of direct and indirect drug promotion, however, also take place, such as "disease awareness advertising" (i.e., bringing attention to a particular disease or "help-seeking" promotional campaigns run without naming a specific drug). This type of advertising encourages consumers to seek the advice of their health care practitioner about a diagnosis, a new treatment, or the prevention of a disease or condition. Reference is often provided to an outside source for further information, one that names individual branded products or specific programs. Other examples include articles placed in journals and newspapers as well as the financial support of patients' organizations.

Doctors and other health care professionals are also target audiences of marketing and public relation efforts. Activities such as advertising in medical journals, the placement and promotion of favorable studies in medical journals, the visits of sales representatives to doctors, reprints, the provision of free drug samples to doctors to pass on to patients, gifts for doctors, and subsidized "educational" events and conferences are commonplace and have been, from the industry's perspective, very successful.

For prescription drugs, DTCA methods differ from all other advertising in two main ways: First, consumers (i.e., patients) must consult a physician for a prescription before obtaining the product. Second, DTCA of prescription drugs is regulated, as is the advertising of other products deemed to have potentially harmful effects on human health.

Currently, DTCA of prescription drugs is legal in only two industrialized countries: the United States and New Zealand. In Canada, it is prohibited. However, due to proximity, a considerable portion of the population is exposed to DTCA via the U.S. media. The collective experiences from these countries will serve as a basis to evaluate the situation in Europe (in particular, Germany) where DTCA is also prohibited, but where there is recurrent pressure to have it introduced.

To inform the discussion of communicating accurate drug information to the public, we analyze data on approved drugs currently available on the market and highlight arguments for and against DTCA. The current regulatory system of DTCA in the United States, Canada, and New Zealand is outlined and recommendations made to inform patients effectively.

Drug Information Available at Market Authorization: Rhetoric and Reality

The development of effective medicines has contributed significantly to the welfare of patients, especially over the last fifty years. Medicines can offer enormous health benefits if treatment choices are made rationally; that is, when they are the appropriate treatment for a condition, are used in the right dose, at the right time(s), and for the right duration. Clearly, the irrational prescription and use of medicaments not only harms people's health, it creates problems in health systems and wastes limited available financial resources.

Any medicine progresses along a continuum "from bench to bedside" over a period of many years: from the initial development in the laboratory, through clinical testing, licensing, promotion to doctor, patient, and consumer, and final prescription. The rationale for the very existence of major pharmaceutical companies is to bring new and useful drugs to market (House of Commons 2005). A drug innovation is generally defined as the discovery, development, and bringing to market of a new molecular entity (NME). Drug discovery involves trying to match the understanding of disease with an NME that might promise some therapeutic effect. Following initial drug discovery, NMEs undergo several phases of development from (a) preclinical studies including chemical, pharmacological, and toxicological studies in human cells, animal tissues, and whole animals to (b) clinical stages of research involving humans. The latter stage is traditionally separated into four phases:

- Phase I trials involve healthy participants or patients (e.g., phase I cancer trials) and are performed to determine the relevant pharmacokinetic and pharmacodynamic parameters of drugs in humans, frequent side effects, and target organs for toxicity (relationship to dose and schedule). They establish the maximal tolerated dose (MTD) and gain early evidence of efficacy.
- Phase II trials involve individuals affected by the target condition. They are designed to determine the safety and efficacy of a new drug in the relevant patient group. If the drug proves acceptably safe and efficacious in 200–500 individuals who take part in this phase of testing, tests are undertaken in a larger group of patients in subsequent trials.
- Phase III trials involve larger groups of patients (approximately 2,000–3,000 individuals), although cohort size depends on the condition, as some rarer diseases may necessitate a smaller group of patients. Trials at this stage determine safety and efficacy of the product on a larger scale and compare the product either to a drug already on the market to treat the target condition or to a placebo. These trials form the basis of the drug approval application.
- Phase IV trials are post-marketing studies designed to gain additional information, including the drug's risks, benefits, and optimal use over the long term and in routine clinical practice (NIH 2009a; House of Commons 2005).

Preclinical studies and phase I to III studies in humans are driven primarily by industrial priorities and the fulfillment of regulatory requirements, rather than by a conceptual framework designed to address issues arising from medical practice (Figueras and Laporte 2003). Regulatory authorities in the European Community have set out in detail the information required to apply for a drug to be manufactured, sold, supplied, or promoted. Under the International Conference on Harmonization of Technical Requirements for Registration of Pharmaceuticals for Human Use, standards have been established that are binding throughout the European Union, as well as between the United States, the European Union, and Japan (Abraham 2002). Accordingly, drug companies are required to provide impartial information about their products to health care professionals and patients: summaries of product characteristics (SPC), packaging and labeling details, and patient information leaflets. This material has legal status and is mainly controlled by regulatory authorities. However, because this information refers solely to the accompanying product, it does not contain a comparison to other medicines or nondrug treatments, and thus has inevitable limitations. Moreover, SPCs can fall short of their objective by offering clinical advice that is unclear or impractical.

The current process of drug regulation has many flaws, and serious concerns have been raised as to whether it is adequate enough to protect public health (Ray and Stein 2006). Both the U.S. Food and Drug Administration (FDA) and the European Medicines Agency (EMA) approve medications based on clinical studies of limited duration and which include relatively small numbers of patients, who are often healthier than the target population for the new drug. Thus, several, yet crucial effects of new drugs will be unknown at the time of licensing: the safety, the effects of long-term exposure, the frequency of rare adverse effects, the effects in special populations or for indications not studied before marketing, the efficacy of a new drug with respect to clinical (as opposed to surrogate) end points, and the efficacy of the new drug relative to others for the same indication (Ray and Stein 2006). To date ample evidence exists to suggest that these deficiencies pose a serious threat to patient safety, to the effectiveness of therapy, and to the credibility of the regulatory process (Hugman and Edwards 2006).

In addition, one of the most important categories of information that patients want to know about a new drug they are taking is the likelihood or probability of adverse effects. However, currently, this information is not being delivered by patient information leaflets (e.g., in the United Kingdom; Carrigan et al. 2008) or by DTCA.

A call for global reform on the safety of medicines has been made to ensure that the welfare, safety, and concerns of patients are at the absolute center of all thinking, planning, and operations. Known as the Erice Manifesto, this reform specifies the challenges that must be addressed to ensure the continuing development and usefulness of science. In particular, it prescribes the active involvement of patients and the public in the core debate about the risks and benefits of medicines, and emphasizes the necessity of developing new ways to collect, analyze, and communicate information about the safety and effectiveness of medicines (Drug Safety 2007).

The approval, prescribing, and safety surveillance of prescription drugs entail a complicated mix of science, regulatory law, clinical judgment, business, and politics (Avorn 2007). As a rational basis for treatment decisions, however, physicians ultimately need clinical drug studies that provide sound data on the relative effectiveness of a new drug by comparing its clinical efficacy, toxicity, convenience, and costs with available alternatives.

This need, however, conflicts with current practice; namely, that clinical studies are driven primarily by industrial priorities and interests. Recent studies have comprehensively explored the extent of the financial relationships between industry, scientific investigators, and academic institutions; its effects on research as well as how it influences the prescribing; and the ultimate consequences for patients (Bekelman et al. 2003; Moynihan 2003a, b). Guidelines to manage these conflicts of interest have been developed which give priority to the patients' welfare at all levels of interaction between doctors and industrial sponsors (Ludwig et al. 2009).

An increasing body of evidence shows a clear association between industry support and the publication of pro-industry results (Bekelman et al. 2003; Lexchin et al. 2003). Recent results demonstrate the various ways that pharmaceutical companies are able to influence a drug trial: from the design of the protocol to the concealment of adverse drug reactions (Schott et al. 2010a,b). Moreover, the influence (both direct and indirect) of pharmaceutical companies in drug selection and acquisition throughout health care systems has increased, as has public awareness of the imbalance between true innovations and promotional activities.

Although the primary function of drug companies is to develop and market drugs, the industry spends more time and resources generating, gathering, and disseminating information (Collier and Iheanacho 2002). According to recent estimates of pharmaceutical promotion expenditures in the United States, pharmaceutical companies spend almost twice as much on promotion as they do on research and development (Gagnon and Lexchin 2008). Because of the inherent importance to the business interests of companies, any generated data are considered commercially sensitive, and thus remain confidential and are protected by law.

The Pros and Cons of Direct-to-Consumer Advertising

Arguments in Favor

There is little actual evidence to support the claims that DTCA has a beneficial effect on health outcomes. Proponents of DTCA (PhRMA 2008), however, argue that it benefits public health in the following ways:

- increases awareness about disease,
- educates patients about treatment options,

- motivates patients to contact their physicians and to engage in a dialog about health concerns,
- increases the likelihood that patients will receive appropriate care for conditions that are frequently underdiagnosed and undertreated, and
- encourages adherence to prescription drug treatment regimens.

Proponents argue that consumers should have the ability to be informed not only by governmental organizations, which often aim to reduce health care costs, but also by the pharmaceutical industry, which possesses the best data on medicines produced (Bonaccorso and Sturchio 2002). They argue that it is paternalistic to deny patients access to information provided by the pharmaceutical industry (Gold 2003). Another argument refers to the placebo effect that pharmaceutical advertising may induce, which might increase the clinical effectiveness of the advertised products (Almasi et al. 2006). Through the placebo effect, it is argued, DTCA may potentially reduce the amount of treatment requested or required and could improve patient adherence and outcomes.

Advocates of DTCA regret that the pharmaceutical industry in Europe has been limited in how it contributes to the public awareness of disease and the benefits of modern medicine (Bonaccorso and Sturchio 2002).

Arguments against Its Use

Critics argue that DTCA provides incomplete and biased information, leads to inappropriate prescribing, increases health care costs due to the added costs of advertising, and takes up valuable time in the physician–patient encounter (Parnes et al. 2009). These claims are supported by some evidence, as reviewed below.

Increased Requests for Specific Drugs and Increased Prescription of Advertised Products without Documented Health Outcome Benefits

Most data show a positive correlation between the amount of money spent on DTCA and prescriptions written for an advertised drug (Gilbody et al. 2005; Zachry et al. 2002; Law et al. 2008), but there is also evidence of an opposite effect (Zachry et al. 2002; Law et al. 2008).

A systematic review of robust evaluations of the negative and positive impact of DTCA was conducted by Gilbody et al. (2005): From 2853 citations, only 4 studies (6 publications) met the inclusion criteria. One of them, a controlled study, examined the impact of DTCA in the United States compared to Canada using a cross-sectional survey of physicians and patients (Mintzes 2002; Mintzes et al. 2003). This study found that patients in the United States were more likely to request DTCA drugs, and that physicians in both settings were more likely to acquiesce to these requests despite ambivalent feelings about prescribing the advertised drug. Two studies found a significant increase in the prescribing volume of drugs that had been the subject of DTCA campaigns (Zachry et al. 2002; Basara 1996). The effect of DTCA appears to have increased the number of conditions diagnosed as well as the proportion of prescriptions specifically for the advertised drug. For example, Zachry et al. (2002) found that for every US$1000 spent advertising cholesterol drugs, approximately 32 extra people were diagnosed with hyperlipidemia and 41 advertised cholesterol-lowering drugs were prescribed. However, Zachry et al. (2002) also showed a negative correlation between the amount of money spent on advertising an antihistamine and the resulting number of prescriptions (Zachry et al. 2002).

A variable impact of DTCA on drug use was also observed in a controlled longitudinal study in Canada (Law et al. 2008). Prescriptions rates for etanercept (for rheumatoid arthritis) and mometasone (for allergies) did not increase in English-speaking provinces relative to French-speaking controls in Canada after the start of DTCA in the United States. In contrast, for the same regions, tegaserod prescriptions (for irritable bowel syndrome) increased 42% (0.56 prescriptions/10,000 residents, 95% confidence interval 0.37–0.76) immediately after the start of a DTCA campaign in the United States. This increase did not persist over time, despite continuing advertising, and tegaserod was eventually removed from the market because of concerns about safety (Giacomini et al. 2007).

In Colorado, an investigation of primary care practices (Parnes et al. 2009) found that patient inquiries for prescription medications were uncommon (58 of 1647 patient encounters, 3.5%). The rate of patient inquiry for advertised products was even lower (2.6%). No studies were found that examined the influence of DTCA on patient satisfaction with care, health outcomes, or the cost effectiveness of DTCA (Gilbody et al. 2005).

In the Netherlands, an "awareness campaign" for a fungal nail condition (onychomycosis) was associated with an increase in new prescriptions as well as a greater market share of the company's specific antifungal agent (terbinafine) ('t Jong et al. 2004). The authors point out that several campaigns like this could deleteriously impact the workloads of general practitioners, taking away time from those patients who need care for more serious problems and increasing overall health care system costs. In addition, terbinafine appears to be of limited efficacy. In a randomized controlled trial of 306 patients, only 25% were completely cured at the end of 18 months (Erin et al. 2005). Furthermore, there is a rare but serious risk of liver toxicity associated with terbinafine (FachInfo 2010).

In a randomized trial using standardized patients (SPs; persons mostly with professional acting experience assigned to different roles), DTCA was found to influence requests for the advertised antidepressants. The SPs were randomly assigned to make 298 unannounced visits to 152 family doctors; they were to show symptoms of a major depression or an adjustment disorder and make a brand-specific drug request, a general drug request, or no request in approximately one-third of visits (Kravitz et al. 2005). For major depression,

302   W.-D. Ludwig and G. Schott

prescription rates of antidepressants were 53%, 76%, and 31% for SPs who made brand-specific, general, and no requests, respectively. Minimally acceptable initial care (any combination of an antidepressant, mental health referral, or follow-up within two weeks) was offered to 98% of SPs in the major depression role who made a general request, 90% of those making a brand-specific request, and 56% of those making no request. Kravitz et al. (2005) found that patient requests have a profound effect on physicians' prescribing decisions in major depression and adjustment disorder, and that DTCA may have competing effects on quality, potentially both averting underuse and promoting overuse.

An analysis of a large administrative database in the United States showed that cost-sharing strategies were limited by DTCA. When consumers do not directly pay for their medicines, they are especially likely to be influenced by advertising (Hansen et al. 2005; WHO/HAI 2009).

Little Educational Value in Direct-to-Consumer Advertising

Several studies have shown that drug advertisements directed toward physicians (e.g., in medical journals) are often inaccurate (Santiago et al. 2008; Kaiser et al. 2004). In several surveys, little educational value was found in drug ad material to consumers. For example, an analysis of 320 advertisements for 101 drug brand names in 18 popular U.S. magazines from 1989–1998 showed that virtually all advertisements (95%) gave the name of the condition treated by the promoted drug, and that a majority (60%) provided information about the symptoms of that condition. However, the advertisements seldom provided information about the drug's mechanism of action (36%), its success rate (9%), treatment duration (11%), alternative treatments (29%), and behavioral changes that could enhance the health of affected patients (24%) (Bell et al. 2000). These results suggest that comparative information does not reach the public through DTCA.

Analysis of 23 television prescription drug advertisements, aired in 2001, showed that consumers were given more time to absorb facts about benefits than about risks (Kaphingst et al. 2004). Furthermore, the authors found that reference to additional product information was given only in text, thus casting doubt on whether these ads make "adequate provision" for dissemination of detailed product information. Insufficient presentation of risk information was also found in another analysis of DTCA via television (Macias et al. 2007).

Limited educational value was also found in DTCA in oncology. A content analysis of DTCA in print media showed that all of the text was difficult to read: description of benefits as well as risks or adverse effects (Abel et al. 2007). Another content analysis and expert evaluation of advertising claims in DTCA for bleeding disorder products showed that, on average, approximately twice the amount of text was devoted to benefits compared with risks or adverse effects, and the latter was more difficult to read (Abel et al. 2008). Only about two-thirds of the advertising claims were considered by a majority of the experts to be based on at least a minimal level of quality evidence. Abel et al. (2008) conclude that print media DTCA for bleeding disorders does not fulfill the FDA's standards of truth and fair balance.

Concern about a particular unbalanced advertisement was raised by the World Health Organization (Quick et al. 2003): A disease awareness campaign promoted cholesterol testing by showing the tagged toe of a corpse. Fear of death was the technique used to sell a medicine. Other important risk factors that contribute to heart disease (e.g., smoking, obesity, sedentary lifestyle) were left unmentioned (WHO/HAI 2009).

Still, a study that analyzed DTC prescription drug web sites found that a majority is meeting fair balance and adequate provision criteria (Macias and Lewis 2005). Compared to print media, most web sites included brief summaries or prescribing information.

In conclusion, these studies indicate that DTCA aims to persuade rather than to inform. Efficacy is oversold, whereas known and unknown risks and harms are generally omitted or minimized. The studies show that people believe that only safe medicines are allowed to be advertised to consumers. This unrealistic public understanding is especially problematic (WHO/HAI 2009).

Medicalization

Medicalization is a "process by which nonmedical problems become defined and treated as medical problems, usually in terms of illnesses and disorders" (Kawachi and Conrad 1996). Moynihan et al. (2002) propose that some forms of medicalization can be better described as "disease-mongering" and they identify various examples. Pharmaceutical manufacturers, doctors, and patient groups use the media to portray conditions as being widespread and severe. Ordinary problems or ailments (e.g., baldness) are often classified as medical problems or mild symptoms that will lead to serious disease (e.g., irritable bowel syndrome). Disease mongering can also include treating personal problems (e.g., shyness) as medical ones (social phobia) or conceptualizing risks as diseases (osteoporosis).

DTCA is likely to expand drug treatment in healthier populations. This can occur through broader disease definitions, promotion of drugs for disease prevention, and prescription drug use for symptoms previously treated with over-the-counter remedies or nondrug approaches (e.g., lifestyle changes). In the United States it has also been observed that older drugs are substituted for newer ones among patients already being treated (Mintzes 2002).

Direct-to-Consumer Advertising Is Often Used for
New Drugs with Unclear Benefits and Harms

Even critics agree that DTCA could be useful if it was used to promote well-studied, generally safe drugs proven effective for serious undertreated conditions, such as statins for cardiovascular disease (Nature Reviews Drug Discovery 2008). However, drugs that are advertised to consumers are predominantly new drugs used to treat chronic diseases. In the United States, the five top medicines, ranked according to DTCA spending from January to November 2004 (Arnold 2005), were:

- Nexium® (esomeprazole) for ulcer/reflux (US$226.0 million),
- Crestor® (rosuvastatin) for lipid lowering (US$193.2 million),
- Cialis® (tadalafil) for impotence (US$152.6 million),
- Levitra® (vardenafil) for impotence (US$142.0 million) and
- Zelnorm® (tegaserod) for irritable bowel syndrome (US$122.0 million).

For 17 out of the 20 drugs with the highest spending on DTCA in 2005, serious advertising campaigns began within a year after FDA approval (Donohue et al. 2007). This, however, poses serious issues to overall patient health, for when it comes to medicines, "newer" does not necessarily equate to being better (WHO/HAI 2009). When a drug is approved, and for a period of time thereafter, little is actually known about a drug's rare, adverse, or long-term side effects. An analysis of all drugs approved in the United States between 1975 and 1999 found that half of drug safety withdrawals occurred within the first two years of marketing (Lasser et al. 2002). More recently, drugs with significant levels of advertising in the United States have needed to be withdrawn for safety reasons, including cerivastatin (Lipobay®) and rofecoxib (Vioxx®). These withdrawals contradict the assumption that consumers benefit from hearing about new drugs and, consequently, the American College of Physicians has issued a call to restrict DTCA for two years after approval (ACP 2009).

In 2008, 29 new drugs were approved in Germany. A new active principle proposed 12, but 5 of these did not show additional benefits to existing therapies. Seven of the 29 new drugs had an improved pharmacodynamic or pharmacokinetic; 10 were "me-too" drugs[1] (Schwabe and Paffrath 2009). Recently, the independent drug journal, *La Revue Prescrire*, a member of the International Society of Drug Bulletins (ISDB), examined 120 new products from 2008 and found that nearly half (n = 57) offered no significant advantages over existing options (Prescrire International 2009). New drugs rarely represent major therapeutic advances by showing clear evidence of an advantage over existing therapies. In fact, evidence from clinical outcomes is often inadequate at the time a drug first enters the market and the lack thereof can lead to false interpretations.

In November 2007, a new era for medical DTCA began when viewers of the nationally televised Thanksgiving Day football game between the Dallas

---

[1] "Me-too" drugs are structurally very similar to those already in existence and differ in only minor ways. There is a negative connotation associated with the term; however, me-too products may create competition to drive down prices.

Cowboys and the New York Jets witnessed the launch of the first DTCA campaign for percutaneous transluminal coronary angioplasty. The commercial "Life Wide Open" advertised Cypher™, the sirolimus-coated stent produced by the Cordis division of Johnson and Johnson. This commercial did not, however, include sufficient information for patients on the risks and benefits of a complex therapeutic issue—one that even specialists continue to debate (Boden and Diamond 2008).

Higher Health Care Costs

Advertising can influence both prescription use and shifts to higher-priced drugs (Gilbody et al. 2005). From 1996–2004, the total amount spent by manufacturers on advertising increased annually; thereafter it declined in 2004–2005 (from US$11.9–11.4 billion), rose in 2006 to US$12.0 billion, and fell in 2007 to US$10.4 billion. The share directed toward consumers decreased from US$4.8 billion in 2006 to US$3.7 billion in 2007, while the share directed toward physicians decreased during the same time period from US$7.2–6.7 billion (Kaiser Family Foundation 2008).

Focusing on the ratio of money spent for advertising versus research and development, Gagnon and Lexchin (2008) calculate that in 2004, US$57.5 billion was spent on promotion in the U.S. market, compared to US$31.5 billion spent on research and development. This figure is conservative, as some promotion methods (e.g., ghost writing, illegal off-label promotion, seeding trials, or educational grants) were not able to be included in the analysis.

Individual brands of prescription drugs have substantial advertising budgets. For example, in 2003, Pfizer spent US$100 million annually on Viagra®, while Bristol-Myers Squibb spent US$70 million on Plavix® (Thomaselli 2004).

By increasing the use of expensive drugs and raising the incidence of adverse effects from newly released drugs, DTCA results in higher costs to the taxpayer, insurance companies, and individuals.

International Experiences with Direct-to-Consumer Advertising

United States

In its history, the United States has never had legislation specifically prohibiting the advertising of prescription drugs to the public. Under the 1938 Federal Food, Drug, and Cosmetic Act, which outlined the requirements for pharmaceutical companies seeking product approval, the FDA has the statutory authority to regulate the entry of prescription drugs into the market. The Consumer Bill of Rights (1962) expanded its mandate to include the regulation of prescription drug labeling and advertising, including DTCA. In 1969, the FDA issued final regulations which postulated that drug advertising materials must be accurate and not misleading, that claims must be supported by substantial evidence, that they reflect a balance between risks and benefits, and that they are consistent with appropriate FDA labeling and do not promote medicines for off-label usage (U.S. GAO 2006). All advertising materials must contain a "true statement" of information, including a brief summary of side effects, contraindications, and the effectiveness of a drug. In 1997, restrictions on broadcast advertising were loosened: details about risks were no longer required in the actual advertisement, so long as the product's major risks were stated and detailed information was made available elsewhere (e.g., on web sites or printed ad material). The relaxing of information requirements induced an increase of full product ads on U.S. television. The number of broadcast ads grew from 293 in 1999 to 486 in 2002 (Mintzes 2006).

The Department of Health and Human Services—the principal agency created to protect the health of all Americans and provide essential human services, of which the FDA is a subagency—regulates the promotion and advertising of prescription drugs. This includes the regulation of DTC materials as well as materials directed to medical professionals. Oversight is carried out by the Division of Drug Marketing, Advertising, and Communications (DDMAC) within FDA's Center for Drug Evaluation and Research. Regulations require that pharmaceutical companies submit final advertising materials to FDA at the time they are first published. Sometimes pharmaceutical companies submit blueprints of advertising material to the FDA for comment prior to public dissemination (U.S. GAO 2006).

If violations are found (e.g., the depiction of risks and benefits is not properly balanced), the agency may issue a regulatory letter. In these letters, drug companies are directed to take a specific action, such as stopping the dissemination of the advertisement. If the violation is judged to be eminently serious, the drug company is directed to run another advertisement to correct misleading impressions left by the violating advertisement. For example, Bayer was recently required to run an ad to correct misleading impressions about the indication of the contraceptive pill Yaz® (FAZ 2009).

Regulatory letters are drafted by the DDMAC (U.S. GAO 2006). Since 2002, letters sent out by the FDA to pharmaceutical manufacturers, notifying them of regulatory violations for prescription-drug advertising, are checked by its legal department prior to distribution. As a direct result, the frequency of regulatory actions dropped sharply. From 1997 to 2006 the number of violation letters fell from 142 to only 21. During the same period, the proportion of letters that raised concern about DTCA actions increased from 15.5% of all letters in 1997 to 33.3% in 2006. Main points of concern were that ads either minimized risks, exaggerated effectiveness, or both (Donohue et al. 2007).

To minimize any inaccurate impression of a drug caused by a misleading advertisement, the FDA established a goal of issuing regulatory letters "within 15 working days of review" at the legal department (U.S. GAO 2006). FDA reviews only a small portion of the DTC materials it receives. Since the review group (seven people) was established in 2002, the number of DTC materials received per year has almost doubled, and the effectiveness of FDA's regulatory letters has been limited. From 2004–2005, 19 regulatory letters were actually issued, on average eight months after the materials in question were first disseminated to consumers. In that time, drug companies had already discontinued use of more than half of these advertising materials.

The FDA was advised to establish formal criteria for prioritizing DTC materials under review, systematically apply its criteria to materials it receives, and track which materials it reviews (U.S. GAO 2006). Recently, the U.S. Senate has considered legislation prohibiting DTCA during the first two years after the release of a new drug (Shuchman 2007).

In addition to governmental regulation, the Pharmaceutical Research and Manufacturers of America, which represents America's leading pharmaceutical research and biotechnology companies, has developed guidlines to "provide accurate, accessible and useful health information to patients and consumers" (PhRMA 2008). Under these guidelines, DTCA, which is termed "DTC communications," is supposed to comply with the regulations of the FDA.

Many violation examples exist, ranging from inadequate communication of risks, to an overstatement of benefits, and a lack of fair balance between presentation of benefit and risk communication. In addition, safety and efficacy claims are not always supported by proper scientific studies. Repeat violations are common (Lexchin and Mintzes 2002; U.S. GAO 2006). Litigation has resulted in drug companies being made to pay high sums because of illegal off-label promotion (Mello et al. 2009).

New Zealand

In New Zealand, DTCA is regulated under the Medicines Act of 1981 and the Medicines Regulations of 1984 (Ministry of Health 2006). This legislation prohibits false or misleading claims or branding, as well as endorsements by health practitioners. The Medicines Act sets out the sort of information that must be included in an advertisement for a medicament: the name of the advertiser, the ingredients, authorized uses of the product, and details about contraindications to usage and appropriate precautions for using the medicine. The penalty provision in the Medicines Act offers only limited disincentives against unbalanced or inappropriate DTCA: NZ$500 plus up to NZ$50 per day for the continued dissemination of a non-conforming advertisement (Ministry of Health 2006).

Regulation of DTCA relies on legislation and, primarily, industry codes of practices. Pharmaceutical companies and associations, advertisers, and publishers have developed a self-regulatory system to ensure that advertisements making therapeutic claims meet standards of social responsibility and comply with legislative requirements. No formal framework is in place, however, to supervise adherence. The Advertising Standards Authority (ASA) and the

Researched Medicines Industry (RMI) administer the self-regulatory component of the co-regulatory model for DTCA. ASA has developed a code for therapeutic advertising that covers all advertisements making therapeutic claims and which applies to all media forms (ASA 2005). The requirements of the code are broadly consistent with the requirements of the Medicines Act. The RMI code of practice (RMI 2006) also needs to be taken into account.

Advertisements have to be pre-vetted via a system known as the Therapeutic Advertising Pre-vetting System (TAPS) (ANZA 2007). Mainstream media agree not to accept an advertisement for publication unless it has been preapproved by TAPS. A complaints and appeals system, which has the ability to require an advertisement to be withdrawn, is maintained by ASA. The complaints and appeals board includes independent members of the medical profession and consumer representatives. The voluntary scheme is entirely funded by industry (Ministry of Health 2006). During 2004, TAPS approved 1596 advertisements for therapeutic products. During the same time, three complaints were received concerning prescription medicines advertised to consumers, one of which related to a product by a pharmaceutical company. The complaint was upheld.

There are several weaknesses in this self-regulatory system. The pre-vetting and complaint response systems are not independent of the advertising and pharmaceutical industries. There is no independent technical review, at the pre-vetting stage, to assess the completeness or balance of efficacy and risks. Detailed criteria for content and presentation of efficacy, risk, and cost information in advertising are lacking. A deterrent penalty is also missing. In addition, the complaints board reviews grievances about all advertised products—not just those specific to drug advertisements (Toop et al. 2003).

Canada

In Canada, DTCA is prohibited. However, due to proximity, a considerable portion of the population is exposed to DTCA via the U.S. media. For example, around 30% of English-speaking Canadians watch television programs from U.S.-based networks (Mintzes et al. 2009).

In 2000, Canadian policy was changed to allow help-seeking advertisements and reminder advertising of prescription drugs. Reminder advertising states the brand name without health claims. In the United States, reminder advertising is forbidden for drugs with a black box warning, the strongest U.S. regulatory warning of serious harmful effects. Unfortunately, Canada does not have a system that issues black box warnings.

The task of regulating pharmaceutical advertising in Canada has been largely delegated to three organizations: the Marketing Practices Review Committee of Canada's Research-based Pharmaceutical Companies (R&D); Advertising Standards Canada (ASC), an advertising industry association; and the Pharmaceutical Advertising Advisory Board (PAAB), a multi-stakeholder group. Health Canada, the responsible federal department, directly processes complaints about DTCA, including complaints sent to ASC or PAAB. However, there are no published guidelines for submission or handling of complaints about DTCA (Mintzes 2006).

From 1996–2006, the pharmaceutical industry spent over CAN$90 million on branded advertising in Canada (Mintzes et al. 2009). Almost all of the spending (88%) occurred after the change of regulation. In television and radio advertisements, a sharp increase was noted. Celebrex® (celecoxib), which carries a U.S. black box warning and was subject to three safety advisories in Canada, was the most heavily advertised drug on Canadian television in 2005 and 2006. Of 8 brands with advertising costs greater than CAN$500,000, 6 were subject to Canadian safety advisories and 4 had black box warnings. This demonstrates that regulators in Canada have failed to prevent the advertising of products with a serious potential for harm (Mintzes et al. 2009).

Germany

Legal Basis

As for all products, the Gesetz gegen den unlauteren Wettbewerb [law against unfair competition] applies to marketing of drugs. To protect consumers, the Gesetz über die Werbung auf dem Gebiete des Heilwesens (Heilmittelwerbegesetz or HWG) [law regulating the advertisement of medicaments] was legislated in 1965 and has since been amended (HWG 2006). In §10 HWG, the advertising of prescription drugs is limited to doctors, pharmacists, and persons who legally dispense drugs.

On an European level, the advertising of drugs is regulated by the Directive 2001/83/EG (European Parliament 2001). As in the HWG, DTCA for prescription drugs is forbidden (Article 88, 1st indent). In contrast to the HWG, information about health and diseases are explicitly allowed (Article 86). An attempt to overturn the ban of DTCA was firmly rejected by the European parliament in 2002.

In 2007, another attempt was made to change the rules, even though the European Commission denied any intention of removing the ban on DTCA (Velo and Moretti 2008). The proposal was brought forth by the EC's Pharmaceutical Forum, which is chaired by the EC's Vice-President, Günter Verheugen (who is also responsible for enterprise and industry within the commission), and is dominated by industry representatives. A first public consultation on the provision of information to patients on medicinal products was published by the EC in 2007. Despite the negative comments received by the commission, a new consultation on "Legal Proposal on Information to Patients" was launched in February 2008. The aim of the EC proposal was to ensure "good-quality, objective, reliable and non-promotional information on prescription-only medicinal products to citizens and to harmonize the existing situation in member states in this area" (EC 2008). This proposal would have enabled the pharmaceutical industry to "inform" patients directly about prescription drugs via the Internet, television, radio, printed material actively distributed, etc: It included a proposed structure to monitor and sanction offenders, to be carried out by national co-regulatory bodies, national competent authorities, and an EU advisory committee.

The EC claimed that the relaxation of the ban on prescription-only medicines would permit informed choices and promote the rational use of medicinal products. This stance, however, does not take into account that patients, as every human being, are subject to a multitude of rationality deficits. Informed decisions do not depend on the *quantity* but rather on the *quality* of the available information (Buchner 2009).

The public consultation received a total of 192 responses (ESIP 2008). Although there was agreement on the need to provide patients with understandable, objective and high-quality information on drugs, nearly all comments were opposed to removing the ban of DTCA in Europe. An alliance of five international organizations—Health Action International (HAI), ISDB, the European Consumers' organization, the Medicines in Europe Forum, and the Association International de la Mutualité—claimed, as did others, that pharmaceutical companies have an inherent conflict of interest which renders them unable to provide the information patients need in an unbiased manner (AkdÄ 2008; ISDB et al. 2008).

The Council of the European Union also expressed concerns about the proposed provision of information by marketing authorization holders. There was consensus on the need to improve the dissemination of information to the general public on prescription-only medicinal products. However, many delegations feared that the suggested system would be overly cumbersome to competent authorities without significantly improving the quality of information provided to patients. In addition, many did not find the distinction between "information" and "advertising" sufficiently clear and therefore feared that the prohibition of advertising of prescription-only medicinal products to the general public could be easily circumvented (CONSILIUM 2009).

As in the United States, pharmaceutical alliances in Germany have set rules, which their members are obliged to obey (FSA 2008).

Existence of Direct-to-Consumer Advertising

Even though DTCA is officially prohibited in Germany, "undercover" advertising practices do exist. For example, in May 2009, an oral contraceptive that uses estradiolvalerat instead of ethinylestradiol came onto the market. In the lay media, this was announced as the "first anti-baby-pill with natural hormones" or even as the "first pill without hormones" and an "alternative to hormonal contraception" (Strappato 2009; Frauen Zimmer 2010). The manufacturer, Bayer Schering, advertises it openly on its web site as "Pill with a Q"

(Bayer Health Care 2010). Despite ongoing public claims for transparency, a detailed list of adverse drug reactions is missing from the web site and has not even been published or made available to experts (arznei-telegramm 2009).

Another example is the heavy campaign for the human papillomavirus vaccination, which was run in the media, especially on television. Neither a product name nor a drug company was mentioned, but there are only two products on the market with this indication in Germany. In the commercials, celebrities were emotionally appealing to the audience to vaccinate their daughters. Substantial information about risks and benefits of the vaccination was irresponsibly not given. In the United States, the vaccine manufacturer also provided educational grants to professional medical associations concerned with adolescent and women's health and oncology, which encouraged the creation of educational programs and product-specific speaker's offices to promote vaccine use. However, much of the material used did not provide balanced recommendations on risks and benefits (Rothman and Rothman 2009).

Requirements for Valuable Patient Information

Suggestions for the response to patient requests for advertised medicines have been made (WHO/HAI 2009). One strategy is to shift the discussion away from the medicine to patients and their symptoms, as well as to explain the range of drug and nondrug treatments, including the likely outcome with no treatment. The motives of pharmaceutical advertisers could be discussed. Where available, patients should be directed to reliable information sources.

There has been increased interest in the use of decision aids, which provide information about options and help clarify personal values. These adjuncts range from leaflets, face-to-face methods (e.g., coaching or counseling), to interactive multimedia web sites. Elwyn, O'Connor et al. (2009) have developed an instrument to measure the quality of patient decision support technologies.

The role and value of written information for patients has been evaluated in several analyses (Grime et al. 2007; Nicolson et al. 2009). A recent Cochrane Review assessed the effects of providing written information about individual medicines on relevant patient outcomes in relation to prescribed and over-the-counter medicines; there is some evidence that this can improve knowledge (Nicolson et al. 2009).

Another systematic review showed that patients value drug information tailored to their condition. Not all patients want written information, but those who do want sufficient detail to meet their needs, which vary over time and between patients (Grime et al. 2007).

Criteria for evidence-based patient information have been presented (Steckelberg et al. 2005) and some will be highlighted here. In terms of content (e.g., the aim of the procedure), the course of the disease without intervention and the probability for risks and benefits should be included. References and conflicts of interest should be stated. End points relevant to the patient should also be considered. If there is no evidence, this needs to be stated. Of equal importance is the framing of data; knowledge about the comprehensible presentation of numbers, such as using absolute risk reduction instead of relative risk reduction, must be taken into account. Also, formatting aspects of layout must be considered. When developing patient information material, it is crucial to include the input from patients (Steckelberg et al. 2005).

To improve comprehensibility of written patient information, recommendations include the use of short familiar words, brief sentences, short headings that stand out from the text, and a familiar style of prose. In terms of layout, the use of large typeface size and bullet points to organize texts has been proposed (Raynor and Dickinson 2009). To judge the quality of written consumer health information in treatment choice, Charnock et al. (1999) developed an instrument, and discussion of further requirements to improve the value of patient information is currently in progress.

From March to April 2008, the EMA conducted a survey to find ways of improving the information it provides on the benefits and risks of medicines (EMA 2009). Patients and health care professionals recommended that benefits and risks must always be communicated together, and that the benefits and risks must be clearly explained. The participants also recommended that concise, easy-to-read summaries of the benefits and risks of medicines should be presented alongside more comprehensive scientific data. A paragraph about essential information should be included in the summary of product characteristics and the package insert of drugs (Kommission der EU Gemeinschaften 2008a, b).

Initiated by the Deutsches Netzwerk Evidenzbasierte Medizin [German network for evidence-based medicine], a group of scientists presented criteria for good health information (Klemperer et al. 2009):

- Information for citizens and patients should be characterized by a systematic search, election, and critical evaluation of data.
- The best available evidence should be considered.
- If no evidence is available, this must be stated.
- Health information should be understandable and relevant to the target group.
- Users or concerned persons should be involved in its production.
- Information about the treatment of diseases should mention morbidity, mortality, quality of life, and circumstances of treatment.
- The treatment should be compared with other treatment options, including a strategy of non-treatment.
- Information material should be worded without giving preference to one approach.
- Probabilities should be mentioned when good data exists and should be represented as an absolute risk reduction.

- For the communication of risks, the natural history of disease should be the basis. A combined presentation of absolute risk, relative risk, the number needed to treat, a graphic, and a comparison to risks of daily life is necessary.

Clearly, authors and providers of patient information should avoid conflicts of interest. Commercial interests are hardly compatible with the principles of good health information.

DTCA has been criticized for not providing valuable information about the benefits and harms of drug therapies. In addition, Davis (2007) has shown that consumers prefer detailed, readily accessible risk information. To meet these demands, brief summaries in DTCA could be replaced by "drug facts boxes," which have been shown to improve consumer knowledge and judgments of drug benefit and side effects (Schwartz and Woloshin, this volume; see also Schwartz et al. 2007, 2009; Schwartz and Woloshin 2009). The use of drug facts boxes has resulted in better choices between drugs for current symptoms and has corrected the overestimation of benefit in the setting of prevention. The FDA's Risk Advisory Committee has recommended adoption of the drug facts box as the standard for their communications.

Discussion and Recommendations

"Senior managers, most of whom came up through the ranks of R&D or sales organizations, often lack insight into consumer behavior and don't understand what it takes to get people off their sofas and into the offices of their physicians, preferably with the names of specific drugs in mind" (Aitken and Holt 2000:82–91). This quote, meant as a critique of pharmaceutical companies and expressed by two managers from McKinsey, clearly reveals the goal of DTCA for prescription drugs.

DTCA cannot be adequately controlled. Neither the central regulatory system in the United States nor the voluntary self-regulations in New Zealand and Canada have been able to ensure compliance with standards of acceptable practice. As a result, advertisements that contain partial, incorrect, or unbalanced information continue to mislead the public. DTCA overstates the efficacy of drugs and suppresses potential adverse effects. Furthermore, the high cost of DTCA gets passed on to the medical system and results in higher drug prices.

These findings confirm that the ban of DTCA in Europe is justified and should be maintained. However, national borders are not always sufficient to protect the public fully in the current global pharmaceutical market. The Internet has increasingly come to be used as a source for medical information or advice, and thus the regulation of information dissemination on a national level is often inadequate (Mackenzie et al. 2007). In addition, it is difficult to differentiate advertising from other forms of influence, such as launched articles in magazines and newspapers or support of patient groups.

To be effectively engaged and actively participate in health care, the public needs better information about health, diseases, treatments, and medicines—information that must be independent, accessible, reliable, accurate, appropriate, consistent, evidence-based, unbiased, updated, comparative, transparent, and understandable (BEUC 2007). The requirements for drug information are very complex and highly individual; thus, it is essential for policy makers and health professionals to specify these specific needs and respond accordingly. Over time, developing trust in information sources is crucial.

Organizations with strong concerns about the future of patient information on drugs in Europe—including the Medicines in Europe Forum, Health Action International Europe, and ISDB as well as several consumers' organizations, such as the Bureau Européen des Unions de Consommateurs and the European Consumer Consultative Group—have suggested concrete policy options to improve information to patients within the existing legal framework:

- Ensure the transparency of medicine regulatory agencies to guarantee access to drug evaluation data and pharmaco-vigilance data.
- Grant public access to drug trial results and share patient data among researchers (Kaiser 2008).
- Foster the role of the EMA as a central and impartial source of information of medicines.
- Improve the visibility of some trusted web sites, such as the EMA and EU health portal web sites (which are currently very difficult to find through a normal web search) and exploit synergies between them.
- Require pharmaceutical companies to fulfill their obligations in terms of packaging and improving package information leaflet content and relevance as an information tool.
- Provide better education to health care professionals about drug and device promotion (Mintzes 2005; Mansfield et al. 2006; WHO/HAI 2009).
- Develop and reinforce good sources of health information.
- Implement health education programs in schools.

The ISDB has developed a program of activities to promote independent information (ISDB 2006).The call on WHO and other regulatory agencies to assure full transparency on conflicts of interest and the access to data on adverse drug reactions (housed at the WHO Uppsala center) makes important points. Furthermore, the ISDB committee campaigns for nonprofit research and independent continuous medical education based on ISDB bulletins. ISDB and its members commit themselves to the active monitoring and critical appraisal of guidelines, which are often influenced by the pharmaceutical industry. ISDB has also begun to collaborate with consumer organizations on campaigns to advance the interests of consumers. ISDB bulletins are invited to translate their "technical" content into language that is easy to understand for the general public. The journal, *Gute Pillen – Schlechte Pillen* [good pills – bad pills], published by ISDB is an example of independent consumer information, aimed at improving the interaction between patients and prescribers and intended to make better use of drugs, and thus ensure better health and economic outcomes.

In conclusion, the role of pharmaceutical companies in the production of good quality information for patients and consumers should be limited to clear labeling and informative patients' leaflets. Competitiveness could be increased through the development of drugs offering real therapeutic advantages, which would be recognized as such and thus not require expensive marketing. Patient information should be the purview of independent organizations which should work together to produce evidence-based, reliable, and comparative information, free from the influence of drug companies.

Acknowledgment

We thank Bradley Hunter and Henry Pachl for their support in preparing this article.

Overleaf (left to right, top to bottom):
Heather Buchan, Martin Härter, Norbert Schmacke
Holger Wormer, France Légaré, David Davis
Kai Kolpatzik, Wolfgang Gaissmaier, Ralph Hertwig
Evening discussions

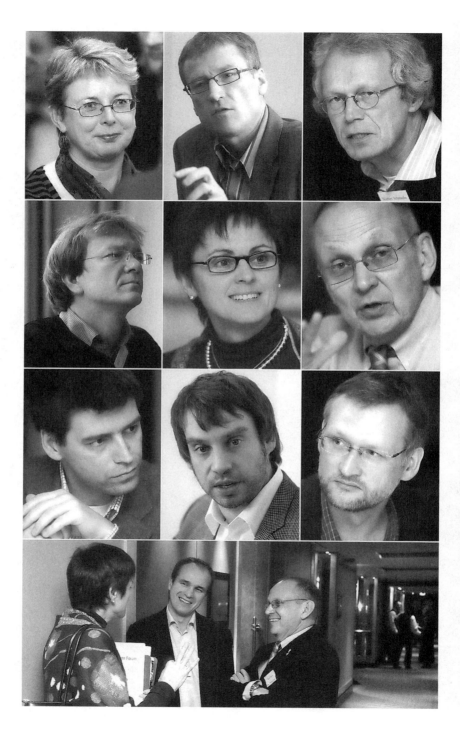

19

How Will Health Care Professionals and Patients Work Together in 2020?

A Manifesto for Change

Ralph Hertwig, Heather Buchan, David A. Davis,
Wolfgang Gaissmaier, Martin Härter, Kai Kolpatzik,
France Légaré, Norbert Schmacke, and Holger Wormer

Abstract

How can we accelerate the shift to a new paradigm of patient-centered health care? In this report, a manifesto for change is put forth, while acknowledging that health care systems are highly complex systems for which there is no simple solution. The starting premise is that one needs to launch and reinforce positive developments among both clinicians and patients. To this end, a vision is offered to transform medical schools into health professional schools; specific ways of leveling the knowledge playing field between clinicians and patients are described to empower patients to ask more questions and dissuade clinicians from "avoidable ignorance." The Wennberg three-step action plan is proposed to demonstrate how a patient-centered health care paradigm can work for important process and outcome measures. To foster patients' engagement within the health care system, an existing model that teaches health literacy to children in primary schools is described and possibilities are proposed to foster the delivery of quality health care information via the media and online communities, with the Internet being *the* technology that is most likely to complete the change in the dynamic of doctor–patient interaction. The 21st century is viewed as the century during which reform ushers in an adult conversation between patients and doctors.

Introduction

Immediately after the election of Barack Obama and in the midst of the worst economic recession since the Great Depression, the President Elect's newly designated chief of staff, Rahm Emanuel, pronounced what has since become known as the Emanuel Principle: "Rule one: Never allow a crisis to go to waste. They are opportunities to do big things" (Zeleny 2008). Stigler's (1983) law of eponymy has it that a great idea is never named after the person who had it first. Corroborating this law, Emanuel's observation echoed the advice of Niccolo Machiavelli in *Il Principe:* "Never waste the opportunities offered by a good crisis" (Machiavelli 1513).

We are indeed in the middle of a good crisis. Except in a few countries, health care systems in the industrialized world suffer from rising costs which, if not radically reformed, could soon bankrupt governments. The most glaring example is the system in the United States. Over the past few decades, U.S. health care costs have risen at a consistent 2.5 percentage points above the growth rate of the economy. If this trajectory were to continue until 2050, it is reckoned that Medicare and Medicaid (the government programs that insure the elderly and the poor, respectively) would together consume 20% of America's GDP, almost as much as today's entire federal budget (Economist 2009). Moreover, many experts expect that the health care reform that was finally passed in March 2010 will not reign in the drivers of America's roaring health care costs (Economist 2010) and, according to a RAND analysis (based on the U.S. Senate version of the bill), will further increase America's overall health care spending, relative to status quo projection (Ringel et al. 2010). America, of course, is not alone in this pickle. According to the Organisation for Economic Co-operation and Development (OECD), health expenditures grew rapidly in many countries between 2000 and 2003, with an annual average OECD growth rate of 6.2% over that period. In 2008, the highest health expenditures as a share of GDP were found in the United States (16.0%), followed by France (11.2%), Switzerland (10.7%), and Austria and Germany (10.5%). Health care costs have simply spiraled out of control.

As Muir Gray expressed at the start of this Forum: "The last 40 years have been fantastic" for public health, with ever-increasing resources, the development of sophisticated research methodologies and treatment procedures, and the build-up of modern infrastructure. The once-full coffers are emptying, however, and we are entering a new period of scarce resources precisely as economic demands on the health care system are increasing. These demands include, for example, expenditures on long-term care for an aging population and on the consequences of climate change, which is expected to worsen virtually every health problem known, from heart disease and heatstroke to salmonella and insect-borne infectious diseases (Brahic 2009).

Financial necessity, however, is not the sole driver of change. Change is also needed for ethical and clinical reasons. There is ample evidence that the 21st century Moloch—the medical–pharmaceutical complex, the modern rival of what President Eisenhower once called the industrial–military complex—makes systematically faulty (but profit-maximizing) assumptions about patients' preferences. Treatment has become supply-centered rather than

patient-centered. Supply-centered medical treatment means that the care ordered for patients—such as diagnostic tests, hospital admissions, operations,
specialist visits, and home nursing—is frequently driven by the financial, legal,
and related needs of the providers, or by unresolved patient needs rather than
by the medical needs of the patients. More care, however, is not appreciably
better, and by some measures, it is worse than less care (see the various analyses reported in the Dartmouth Atlas of Health Care 2010). The crisis of the
health care system is thus not just a financial one; it is also a troubling ethical
one. A Moloch is so called for a reason. This Moloch keeps asking for costly
sacrifices, forcing societies to neglect other important tasks (e.g., maintaining
vital infrastructures such as schools or bridges), and damaging, for example,
the global competitiveness of American businesses.

Taken together, there is a strong case to be made for change. The starting
premise of this group report is that progress will occur: First, there will be
efficient mechanisms and guidelines to enforce the complete and transparent
reporting of research results. Second, future generations of medical students
and health professionals will no longer suffer from statistical illiteracy but be
trained to deal with, interpret, and communicate risk and uncertainty to their
patients. Third, efficient ways of communicating unbiased evidence to health
professionals and patients will be designed and implemented, enabling them to
make shared decisions. All's well that ends well—except that we are not there
yet. Before these new mechanisms can take full effect—and that is our second
premise—we need to take action to foster change as quickly and as effectively
as possible. How do we curtail this revolutionary period in which the old guard
may want to retain the reigning paradigm and resist change as long as possible? Or, to use Thomas Kuhn's (1962) phrase of paradigm shift, how do we
accelerate the shift into a new paradigm of patient-centered health care, how do
we speed up the reform of the old system, and how do we render it likely that
2020 will not be a replay of 2010?

There are many actual and perceived barriers to implementing more patient-
centered care. Table 19.1 lists the most prominent ones.[1] In this chapter, we
address some of these barriers and ignore others. This is not a reflection of
their importance (or lack thereof) but of our decision to focus on the health care
professional (in particular, on the clinician) and the patient as units of analysis,
rather than on the health care system per se. By treating both of these players
separately, we do not mean to imply that they are separate. They are two key
players tied up in the context of a larger system. Pulling the strings of one
affects the movements of the other, and the parameters of the system that en-
closes them affect both. Therefore, any analysis of one player says something
about the other. In our prescription for change, we aimed to be bold rather than
timid. Yet, in highly complex systems like the health care system one cannot

---

[1] This table was inspired by, but is not identical to, a list of barriers to implementing shared decision making in clinical practice by Légaré et al. (2008).

Table 19.1.   Barriers to implement more patient-centered care.

Overarching barriers:

- Evidence about risks, benefits and outcomes lacking for many complex conditions or where people have multiple health problems.
- Diseases associated with aging in industrialized societies may require lifestyle interventions rather than medical care.
- Concern of policy makers that patient-centered care will increase health care demands and costs.

Patient level barriers:

- Lack of confidence about ability to make judgments about information on potential benefits and risks.
- Emotions about illness lead to preference for external decision maker.
- Lack of understanding of potential role in decision making.
- Lack of understanding of treatment options and potential impact on health and well-being.
- Health status precludes active role.
- Multiple decisions may be required.
- May be seeking complementary or alternative care and not want to share details with health professional.

Health professional level barriers:

- Lack of time to explore patient preferences.
- Lack of skills to explore patient preferences.
- Unconvinced that patient-centered care/shared decision making is appropriate or provides the best outcomes.
- Preference for role of "benevolent patriarch/matriarch" rather than "patient-centered facilitator."
- Unaware that patient values can differ from those of the health professional.
- Lack of knowledge, skills or capacity to provide social support and care rather than health care.

Organizational/system level barriers:

- Lack of awareness that behaviors of multiple care providers may interact and adversely affect patients.
- Lack of a single designated coordinator of care for the patient.
- System designed for acute care rather than ongoing management of chronic illness.
- Care required may be social support rather than health care and health system not well constructed to provide this care.
- Reimbursement systems may not be well aligned with the type of care that is required/chosen.

Interactional barriers:

- Relationship between patient and health professional not well established.
- Poor communication between patient and health professional.
- Patient may be receiving care from multiple providers who are unaware of or do not communicate with each other.

---

simply press a reboot button; one needs to launch and reinforce the positive developments. Our approach was to work subversively within the system rather than to blow it up. After all, our manifesto for change has been written by a bunch of academics rather than health care "revolutionaries."

How to Change Clinicians

We derived three tactics to spur change in clinicians. The first action targets medical education. We spell out a new kind of school and then propose to build on pockets of excellence that embody bits and pieces of this vision. The following fictitious report, describing the opening day of the new Strüngmann School for Health Professionals, introduces us to this vision. The second action aims to alter the dynamic between patients and clinicians by increasing the latter's risk of looking, well, incompetent. The third action calls for a concerted research effort that paves the way for establishing informed patient choice in preference-sensitive conditions.

𝔉rankfurter 𝔊lobe

Late Edition	26 October 2020

New School for Health Professionals Opens

It is a sunny, fall Monday morning—the first day of the brand-new Strüngmann School for Health Professionals.

Opening in several primary care locations and other acute care settings across the inner city, it is not your usual medical school. No tall towers, no ivy-covered buildings; this school exists in a dispersed fashion, its faculty members also primary care clinicians and specialists, and other health professionals. It is heavily linked by videoconference and Internet connectivity, and it is difficult to tell the doctor from the nurse, from the student or other trainee. And another difference: some patients are considered "faculty." They sit on curriculum advisory panels, giving direction and shaping the curriculum.

This is *interesting*, I think.

It took me several minutes to find the dean's office for my interview. Other medical leaders I have interviewed in the past have entertained me in their large corner offices with couches, corner-window views, and served coffee. This one is different: somewhere down a long hallway, the dean sits in her family physician consultant's office. Her computer, I notice, sits on a small swivel stand and has two screens—more about that later. She is pleasant, though business-like, and reminds me of her time constraints. We start right away.

How and why did the school get started? She laughs. "That question alone would take 30 minutes to answer," she says. "It's a pretty long list, beginning, I think, with patient dissatisfaction. Not that patients didn't like their own physician, but there was general unhappiness with the health care system, its overall impersonal nature and sense of 'not being in the patient's control.' There were also other elements such as the ability of physicians to have time with their patients, their lack of understanding of what was happening to them—and yes, the occasional, perhaps more than occasional, physician who treated the patient as an object, not a person."

I had read that the school spends a large amount of time on admissions and asked if that is so. "Yes," she replied. "Studies demonstrate that there are qualities we look for in clinicians which are modified, if not driven, by personality—elements of altruism, self-awareness, the ability to accept and respond to negative feedback, lifelong learning skills, an openness to teamwork, and collaboration. While we think that these are teachable and modifiable skills, we've developed a list of attributes which we seek with great diligence through our long admissions process. We think it pays off. The saying 'An ounce of prevention is worth a pound of cure' holds true in medical education as well."

"Oh," she adds, "and we look for smart kids, too." Science background? Well, yes and no; there are lots of smart science and math grads. "We're looking for those abilities plus others. And, at least so far, we haven't been disappointed."

What's your curriculum like? Looking at the clock, she answers, "Roughly, we've divided it into three parts: they are overlapping to a certain extent but there is a degree of mastery at each level before the learner can advance to the next. First there is the basic, core material—anatomy, physiology, pathophysiology of disease, biochemistry, pharmacology, epidemiology—the usual, but there are other things that we consider absolutely basic: ethics and communication—the two-way kind. These are very important, of course, even critical, but only the first of many building blocks. We also include an important core stream on quality improvement, teamwork, and change management. Some students can sail through the modules— all of them are online—passing each step as they go; some take longer to progress. Some of the modules require small group discussion; others require live, interactive

learning to give the learners a chance to role-play."

"Once they've demonstrated mastery of the core, they move to the second phase: the applied phase. Here, the student learns to work through problems to apply what he or she has demonstrated in the mastery phase. This is accomplished with standardized or real patients—real patient problems right here and elsewhere in the system. In fact, there are virtually no classrooms—all 'lectures,' you might call them, are online. We use patient experiences—real, videotaped, simulated, and paper problems—to emphasize the application of learning. We also use patient feedback extensively—very important for faculty development. Something new that we're trying is the patient–instructor, especially useful in chronic disease management. To accomplish this we have had to add a formal structure committed to teaching patients to be better advocates, to understand at some level the use of evidence to weigh options, and to be more assertive, true partners in their care. This cannot include all patients, of course, but we are privileged to be able to call on a select group of them as associate faculty members. By this and other means, students learn to apply skills of communication, shared decision making,"—strangely, she pats her computer at this point—"evidence and its application, formats of updating, and other issues."

"How long does this phase last?" I ask.

"As long as it takes," she replies. "Once the learner has passed all the competency measures here in the real-world setting— as judged by patients, by other staff members, by their peers—they then go to the third stage."

This third stage, I learn, is called "improvement"—and she hesitates here because we are almost out of time. Because of the hesitation, I think to ask her to explain why she touches her computer, intrigued by the small gesture.

"I am glad you asked, because this simple tool," she says, pointing to the two screens, "has made so much possible. The patient gets to see her lab results, her graphs, her risk tables—anything that I can see—so that we can talk about it. I can print off important resources from web sites for her, have her interact with me here in the office, show her how her test results now conform to the benchmark (or not), how she might proceed (or not) with hip surgery, and much more— or we can do it later in her own home by email or on my CareBook page. It's just a tool, you know, but I really like it: it enables us to share in decisions, takes a great burden off of me. I become much more the knowledge broker and facilitator—the patient, in many ways, then becomes her own care provider, just as she can provide feedback to, and therefore help teach, me and my students."

And what of the third phase of the health professional school, I ask, thinking that I might steal a few minutes more.

"Oh that," she says, getting up and holding the door open for me. "That's called improvement; it begins with demonstrated mastery in all these competencies and, well, never really ends. That's

why we call this the 'health professional school without walls.' It has to do with practice-based learning, working in systems, patient safety, teamwork, constantly updating our knowledge base. So you see, I am a learner here, too. Here's a trick we learned years ago: a big part of the development of the new school hinged on the functional merger of traditional continuing education with quality improvement and patient safety as well as with faculty's professional development. We began to see how it might work when we dedicated ourselves to patient safety and reduced variations in care—that was our 'quality improvement phase.' But, we realized how important this merger was when we began to appreciate the full impact of the 'hidden curriculum.' We would discuss altruism or teamwork, or quality improvement in undergraduate years, test for it, and then learned that these traits had diminished by the time students were exposed to jaded clinicians, and tired, overworked residents. Our faculty includes our patients, patient experiences, and my colleagues."

And the students?

"The students teach us as well. Aren't we lucky?" she asks.

Back to Reality

We realize that our model school is not just around the corner. The envisioned changes are unlikely to be fully integrated into the continuum of health professional education by 2020. Nonetheless, there are many examples of excellence in basic health professional education:

- Evidence-based health care curricula exist in many medical (e.g., McMaster), nursing (e.g., University of York), and other health-allied professionals' basic or undergraduate training programs (e.g., University of Hamburg or the Center for Evidence Based Physiotherapy at the University of Minnesota).
- Patient-centered care is being used to drive the curriculum of some medical schools (e.g., University of Western Ontario);
- There are examples of interprofessional care in undergraduate nursing, medical, and other health professional educational programs (e.g., University of Minnesota);

- Patient decision support education has been incorporated into an undergraduate nursing curriculum (e.g., University of Ottawa).
- Innovative patient engagement strategy has been implemented at the Dartmouth–Hitchcock Medical Center's Center for Shared Decision Making in Lebanon, New Hampshire.

We would strongly urge others to build on these successes, and to do something further: bring these elements together to form a more integrated curriculum, focusing on and developing evidence-based health care, patient-centered care, interprofessional care, and patient decision support. In addition to changes in undergraduate medical and health professional education, we note the development of several features of residency training that offer examples of best practices: the increasing emphasis on evidence-based medicine, patient-centered care, collaborative care models, practice-based learning and improvement, and shared decision making.

Given the long pipeline that produces physicians and other health professionals, however, continuing professional development or medical education (CPD or CME) demonstrates the potential to become a vehicle for change. In this regard, we view continuing education as a natural lifelong process, incorporating, but not using exclusively, conferences, courses, and workshops. Additionally, viewing CME or CPD as an accumulation of patient experiences, feedback, group discussion, teamwork, information at the point of care, and many other elements, we see progress toward more shared decision making being made on several dimensions, based on best evidence.

1. Regulatory changes in the United States and Canada have decreased the reliance on commercial support for CME activities, reducing if not entirely eliminating degrees of bias in presentation and messages to clinicians.
2. Movements in revalidation and recertification based on performance rather than just a simple accumulation of hours of credit can lead to performance measures related to shared decision making.
3. The increased emphasis on comparative effectiveness studies in the United States and on similar health technology and government- or insurance-funded comparative studies elsewhere can create content for clinicians to be used in shared decision making.
4. There are studies of incorporation of shared decision making into CPD activities that are promising from both practical and research perspectives.

Although not entirely conclusive, results from a Cochrane Review of interventions to improve the adoption of shared decision making by health care professionals suggest that multifaceted interventions (educational meetings, distributing educational materials to physicians, plus audit and feedback) may be the most effective method for implementing it in clinical practice (Légaré et al. 2010).

When will we expect to see these changes? Perhaps we will see them in the smaller changes described above. Perhaps we will see them at the end of the new health professional school. To get there, however, we need to recognize that we are all in the same spaceship and that collaboration is necessary, hopefully enjoying the ride together, seeking what humankind has best to offer: well-being through a network of meaningful and respectful relationships.

Leveling the Knowledge Playing Field: Open Access and Dr. Google

Starting with Arrow (1963), the relationship between clinician and patient has been seen as a paradigmatic example of an agency relationship (e.g., Behrens et al. 2010). There are many situations in which one person, called the principal, delegates decision-making authority to another, called the agent. In medicine, the patient is the principal and the physician is the agent. The health of the patient depends crucially on the performance of the physician, and the patient faces myriad uncertainties: Is my physician capable and knowledgeable? Will she act unselfishly and on my behalf? Will she do everything medically possible to help me? Faced with these questions, the principal has two choices: try to employ a contract to bind the agent to perform as desired or else rely on trust.

Over the past few decades, the dependable and trust-inspiring Marcus Welby medical care system (Dranove 2001) has disappeared, if it ever existed. *Marcus Welby M.D.* was a popular television show in the early 1970s. The TV doctor "was everyone's favorite primary care physician....He was wise, kind, and one of the most trusted members of his community" (Dranove 2001:7). According to Dranove, the primary care physician in the era of Marcus Welby medicine would make a house call, spend as much time as necessary to make an initial diagnosis, make a carefully described prescription, if necessary, and might even phone later to check on the recovery. If the patient was seriously ill, the physician would make a referral to a specialist. The doctor remained a staunch advocate for the patient throughout treatment, and the patient could trust him. The Marcus Welby medical system no longer exists. In the new medical world, built-in conflicts of interest between doctors and patients abound, rendering the heuristic just to trust the white coat no longer adaptive (Wegwarth and Gigerenzer 2010b). Unfortunately, the other choice available to the patient to respond to the principal–agent dilemma is not a good one either: Economists have outlined various limitations of contracting, rendering contracts "less than ideal for use in medicine" (Dranove 2001:15), including the problem that contracts can hardly cover all possible contingencies of the medical care process as well as the problem of hidden actions and hidden information.

With nowhere to go—because patients cannot unconditionally trust any longer and cannot employ contractual solutions—what can patients do? How can they level the playing field? To avoid misunderstandings: Physicians spend four to five years in medical school and another four to six years in residency training, and have many additional years of experience. Patients cannot catch up on this medical expertise. Outside of sending patients to medical schools, however, numerous things can be done to make physicians' "avoidable ignorance" (Albert Mulley, pers. comm.) untenable. Our rationale is the following: Anything that increases clinicians' perceived risk of losing face by being unable to answer patients' questions should foster their willingness to work toward avoiding their avoidable ignorance. How? Here are some concrete proposals:

1. Open access: Patients should have access to the same data as the clinicians (interpretation of lab reports, systematic reviews, individual research report, medical file). Remember the two-screened monitor in the new school for health professionals. Another form of open access is to render accessible medical knowledge and recent evidence not only to health care professionals but also to patients, patient advocates, relatives, and, more generally, citizens. Tools to provide this access are, for instance, that of the "patient university" in Hannover or Jena, Germany (MHH 2010; GU 2010).

2. Do not waste education opportunities: Provide learning opportunities for patients. For example, the British health care system sends out 1.5 billion letters (e.g., communications with the patients about invitations to screenings, reminders) but misses hundreds of millions of opportunities to educate patients, for example, by offering additional information about the screening, risk information, decision aids, or links to decision aids (see, e.g., the Ottawa Hospital Research Institute's A–Z inventory of decision aids [OHRI 2010]).

3. Wisdom of the crowd: Are there ways to foster communication among patients, so that patients can benefit from the experience of others and vicariously learn what the important questions are? Let us introduce the patient to the patient (using Internet portals such as patientslikeme, healthtalkonline, krankheitserfahrungen), and link patients to the current 20,000-plus medical web sites on the World Wide Web.

Let us not be naïve, however. The Internet can empower patients but will not replace the traditional doctor–patient relationship anytime soon. Nor is the information provided by medical web sites necessarily objective or even correct. To make matters more complex, different web sites may give conflicting information, and the resulting confusion may become a major headache for physicians. But let us also not get on a high horse: By Ioannidis' (2005) calculations, most published research findings are false, and according to an analysis carried out by *Nature, Wikipedia* comes close to *Britannica* in terms of the accuracy of its science entries (Giles 2005; see also Nature 2006).

The rationale behind our proposed actions is to enable patients to pose questions and eventually to ask better questions when communicating with their health care providers. Admittedly, this may not always work. Some patients may turn into smart alecks, and some doctors may become obstinate when challenged. Also, a little knowledge can be a dangerous thing. But differing from Alexander Pope's original meaning, unpredictable knowledge on the part of patients can be a dangerous thing to the clinicians: Nobody wants to keep looking incompetent.

Let us not end without bringing up a truly cherished resource beyond knowledge that the Internet offers—time. For clinicians, time is the final constraint, and a widespread perception is that doctors spend less time with their patients, relative to the past. In contrast to this perception, studies show that the average length of consultations in the United Kingdom and the United States actually increased in the 1990s (Mechanic 2001; Mechanic et al. 2001). Clinicians' perception that less time is being spent with patients may stem from the need to do more during a patient visit (e.g., provide preventive care), from raised patient expectations (e.g., more information), and from the growing complexity of health care. For patients, time is less of a severely limited resource because they typically only need to worry about themselves rather than a host of other patients. A patient, therefore, has more time than a clinician to search for information, read, and reflect, and as of now this resource has mostly been untapped. With the help of the Internet, this resource could be harnessed, for instance, by no longer narrowing the consultation to face-to-face time with the doctor. Figure 19.1 illustrates an expanded consultation using a patient's concern about breast cancer. By involving patients in the process of information search and decision making, doctors may be able to use the face-to-face consultation more meaningfully and more satisfactorily—for themselves and patients. The expanded consultation, however, does expect the patient to prepare for the visit at the doctor's office. Such preparations and follow-up work can range from becoming acquainted with anatomical and medical terms or taking a family history to assess a risk to using a decision support web site to reflect on the information and treatment options discussed during the face-to-face consultation.

The Proof of the Pudding Is in the Eating

According to Kuhn's (1962) analysis of scientific revolutions, a paradigm shift is more likely to occur when the new paradigm offers concrete solutions to scientific anomalies. Without a concrete solution, no scientist will be persuaded to switch to a new paradigm. To the extent that Kuhn's analysis generalizes to paradigm shifts in health care systems, we can take advantage of his "demonstrate-to-me-that-it-works" heuristic to foster a shift to the new health care paradigm of patient-centered care and shared decision making. Admittedly, this heuristic is only one of several strategies toward persuading clinicians (see

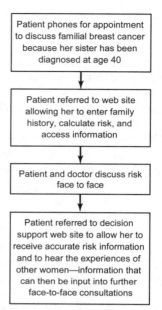

Figure 19.1 Stages of an expanded consultation that uses web-based tools to redesign the model of traditional clinical practice (courtesy of Muir Gray).

Cialdini 2001). Yet, it would be ironic if a community devoted to the utility of evidence were not betting on this heuristic. Table 19.2 spells out an action plan—courtesy of John Wennberg—to get research on the potential efficacy of informed and shared decision making off the ground, with the goal of demonstrating its benefits, and ushering in a new health care paradigm by the year 2020. Key components of this research endeavor—the measurement of preferences (e.g., Sepucha and Ozanne 2010) and patient decision aids (e.g., Elwyn, Frosch et al. 2009)—are already in place.

It is possible that the "demonstrate-to-me-that-it-works" heuristic could work across a range of variables, such as decision quality, patient satisfaction (e.g., more compliance, fewer complaints, fewer law suits), clinician satisfaction, and, possibly, costs. The last one, of course, will be particularly crucial for policy makers, and many appear to operate under the assumption that if patients have more say in the decision-making process that they will inevitably demand more costly treatment. In fact, the opposite may be true. Initial evidence suggests that people, once comprehensively and transparently informed about the costs and benefits of treatment options, tend to prefer the more conservative course of action (e.g., not taking hormone replacement therapy; O'Connor et al. 2009); similarly, the more (and the better) patients were informed about the costs and benefits of screening for prostate cancer with PSA tests, the less likely they were to partake in screening (Frosch et al. 2001). More generally, shared

Table 19.2 The Wennberg three-step action plan for change.

Goal: To establish informed patient choice as the standard for determining medical necessity for treatments for selected preference-sensitive conditions by the year 2020.

Step 1. Years 2010–2014

1. Undertake pilot projects (and build on existing ones) for selected conditions to test implementation strategies in shared decision making using decision aids. Include various clinical centers, emphasizing primary care sites but not excluding surgical specialty sites.
2. Develop decision quality measures designed to evaluate patient knowledge of relevant facts and concordance between individual patient concerns about treatment outcomes and the treatment choice the individual makes.
3. Evaluate and improve upon implementation of pilot strategies, decision quality measures, and patient decision aids (see Elwyn, Frosch et al. 2009).
4. Funding for these projects—from payers.

Step 2. Years 2015–2018

1. Broadly implement successful models with costs paid for by payers.
2. Measure continuously decision quality to evaluate shared decision-making processes.
3. Reward primary care physicians (and specialists) who successfully implement shared decision making (i.e., good scores on decision quality).
4. Promote advocacy of the ethic of informed patient choice by primary care physicians as the cornerstone of their professional responsibility.

Step 3. Year 2019–2020

1. Based on success of above, payers establish informed patient choice as a standard of practice and a requirement for payer willingness to pay for selected discretionary surgery and diagnostic screening tests.
2. As a result of research and development, extend the list of preference-sensitive conditions.

List of priority preference-sensitive conditions for inclusion in the pilot project:

Conditions	Treatment options
Silent gall stones	Surgery vs. watchful waiting
Chronic stable angina	Percutaneous coronary intervention vs. surgery vs. other methods
Hip and knee arthritis	Joint replacement vs. pain medication
Carotid artery stenosis	Surgery vs. aspirin
Herniated disc	Back surgery vs. other strategies
Early prostate cancer	Surgery vs. radiation vs. waiting
Enlarged prostate	Surgery vs. other strategies
Mental health (depression)	Antidepressants vs. psychotherapy
Breast cancer	Lumpectomy vs. mastectomy

decision making appears to be effective in lowering overuse (e.g., Evans et al. 2005) and raising underuse (O'Connor, Bennett et al. 2007).

We end with a question to which there is both an ideal and a pragmatic answer: Which of two strategies should be pursued in realizing patient-centered care? Should each clinician eventually aspire to be a good communicator and learn the ABCs of shared decision making, or should a team environment with a designated decision coach (Stacey et al. 2008) compensate for undeniable interindividual differences in communication skills and plain empathy (e.g., Wagner's Chronic Care Model discussed in Bodenheimer et al. 2002a, b)? Although the second approach appears to be more pragmatic, it carries the risk that the decision-making process is rated second or third, relative, say, to the heroic skills of a surgeon. Remunerating the decision coach as highly as or more than the surgeon, however, would quickly disrupt the old regime's hierarchy.

How to Change Patients' Engagement
with the Health Care System

The title of this Forum stipulates a controversial concept, namely, that of "better" patients. Although proponents of shared decision making can probably agree on what constitutes a better doctor, the concept of a "better" patient is much more controversial. Disagreement centers on the question of the extent to which patients can and should be expected to take responsibility in the process of making decisions. To appreciate the difference in views, let us describe two opposing positions: The first begins with the assumption of patient heterogeneity and takes the position that not every patient can be expected to live up to our lofty ideals of shared decision making. According to this view, patients ought to be empowered to define their own goals but cannot be expected to do so under all circumstances. Take, for example, a working mother who has two teenage children and an abusive alcoholic for a husband. She has just received the dreadful news that she has breast cancer. The psychological reality for this patient—and many other patients who have just received news of a life-threatening disease and are in the grip of fear, confusion, and depression—may be that she simply does not have the mental resources to define her values and ponder which of the treatment options meets them best.

According to the second view, there are limits to a patient's autonomy in the following sense: People have no right to futile care. Specifically, if the available treatment options require a discretionary choice involving trade-offs, then patients have an *obligation* to get involved. From this premise follows, for example, that an elective surgical procedure will not be offered to a person who does not want to get involved.

The positions just outlined represent two somewhat opposing views (of course, more and less extreme variants of these views exist) in this necessary debate concerning the ethical implications of shared decision making for patients. We ourselves did not achieve agreement as to which of the two positions is more appropriate. We did, however, agree that future patients are likely to be patients who will make different demands of their doctors. That is, it is less likely that health care professionals will be able to restrict their role to that of interventionists curing specific medical conditions. Instead, the management of change will become increasingly more important, and therefore patients and their health care providers will devote more of their shared decision-making process to lifestyle changes: to preempt medical conditions, to attenuate them, and to render it possible to adapt to them.

Moving beyond a clarification of the controversial concept of a better patient, let us turn to how we aim to nudge the patient to make informed and better decisions. Our action plans are focused on the following domains: early education, health care in the media, and ways to enlist the environment.

Becoming Health Literate: The Earlier the Better

Thinking about our health and practicing a healthy lifestyle should not wait until our first serious encounter with the medical repair shop. The long-term benefit of *early* health education could be spectacular: acquiring a skill that people will be able to draw on throughout their lives. Just as children learn to read and write, they should also learn how to understand frequencies and probabilities, thus equipping them, for example, to evaluate risks accurately. Before learning the mathematics of uncertainty, younger children could experience the psychology and biology of health (e.g., Why do I get goose bumps? Why am I ticklish? What happens to the food I eat?). Early health literacy could be the foundation upon which adults make sounder lifestyle decisions throughout their lives.

A health curriculum is not a lofty idea. Successful models already exist. One example is a program called ScienceKids—Kinder entdecken [children explore]. Its goal is to create interest in health-related topics among children during primary school education (age six to ten years). The program has been developed by the AOK Baden-Württemberg, a branch of the largest German public health insurance company, in cooperation with the Department of Culture and Education in the state of Baden-Württemberg (AOK Baden-Württemberg 2010). The program is embedded in the curriculum of primary schools and its main goals are:

1. Find answers, using an exploratory approach, to (sometimes delicate) questions that are linked to the function of the body, nutrition, exercise, sports, and well-being.
2. Teach children the meaning, relevance, and joy of pursuing a healthy lifestyle.
3. Build a foundation for improved health competence by enabling children to experience and figure out their own body.
4. Raise parents' awareness of health-related topics and offer specific support.
5. Establish an activity-based sustainable health education.

6.   Develop a concept for improving health literacy and creative skepticism.

The modular structure of the curriculum is flexible enough to be implemented in classrooms, in workshops, and as part of extracurricular activities. As Figure 19.2 illustrates, first-hand experience takes the place of moralistic exhortations. Children are treated as scientists, thus harnessing their natural curiosity and joy in experimenting with the world. Each school participating in the program is offered a mini-laboratory, which can accommodate up to 30 students and enables teachers to conduct experiments during regular lessons. If children are empowered to search for answers to their questions—what happens to the food that I eat; what are my body's needs; what does it take to feel good— chances are that their newly gained competence and knowledge will have a longer-term impact on their health behavior.

How was the curriculum designed? At the outset and using the children's magazine of the AOK, children were asked to submit their questions concerning diet, exercise, and health. Based on this "raw material," experts in the field of nutrition science, sports, and didactics of science developed the instructional material. During a week at a summer science camp, nearly 50 children, scientists, and students then jointly vetted the material. Subsequently, the curriculum was pilot-tested in 70 schools, with experts further optimizing the program and tailoring it to the primary school setting. To boost its reach, the program has since then been incorporated into the teachers' training, and ScienceKids multiplicators offer to train teachers and schools in this curriculum. Last but not least, the web site (AOK Baden-Württemberg 2010) offers teachers up-to-date information and additional background material to teachers.

Although the benefits of using schools as a conduit to health literacy are obvious, introducing another topic into what is already a packed curriculum

(a)   (b)

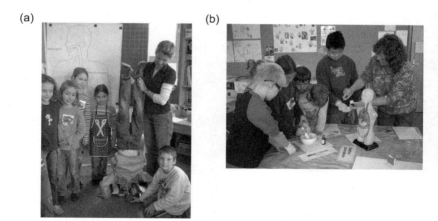

Figure 19.2   Children in the ScienceKids program learn through hands-on experience about their body. (a) Can one drink while doing a handstand? (b) How does our digestive system work? (Used with permission; © AOK Baden-Württemberg)

is a tough sell. Advocates for extending this program nationwide and into secondary schools' curricula[2] will need to enlist opinion leaders, parents and teacher organizations, and payers to lobby for a *health and risk school* (see Bond 2009). We believe one key to persuading not only these stakeholders in children's health literacy but also school boards and policy makers lies in the power of the "demonstrate-to-me-that-it-works" heuristic. The ScienceKids program represents a bold and inspiring step in this direction.

Nudging the Public

There are at least two routes to changing people's behavior. One is to target them directly by, for example, educating them. Another is to target the environment of which their behavior is a function. Herbert Simon (1992:156) stressed that if "people were perfectly adaptable, psychology would need only to study the environments in which behavior takes place" to understand how they think and function. He illustrates this with the example of predicting the shape of a gelatin dessert: Would you stand a chance of correctly guessing its shape by understanding the internal properties of gelatin? Probably not; looking at the shape of the mold it was poured into, however, will do the job.

Let us illustrate the power of the environment using the thorny problem of organ donation. Since 1995, some 50,000 people have died waiting for a suitable organ donor (Johnson and Goldstein 2003; for a more general treatment, see Thaler and Sunstein 2008). Although many people assert that they approve of organ donation, relatively few sign a donor card: only about 28% in the United States (Johnson and Goldstein 2003). So why don't more sign up as potential donors? Do they lack empathy for the suffering of others? Or are they concerned that, should an emergency room doctor discover that they are potential donors, the doctor may not work as hard to save them? In light of these concerns, why then are 99.9% of the French or Hungarians potential donors? The striking difference in the rates of potential donors between countries makes lack of empathy or fear unlikely to explain the big picture. A simple heuristic could explain such striking differences in the rate of potential donors across countries (Gigerenzer 2008). The default heuristic's policy states: "If there is a default, do nothing about it." The default heuristic leads to different outcomes because environments differ. In explicit-consent societies such as the United States, Germany, and the Netherlands, the law prescribes that nobody is a donor unless they choose to be a donor. In presumed-consent societies such as France and Hungary, the default is the opposite: Everyone is assumed to be a donor, unless they choose not to be a donor. From a rational choice perspective, the default should be toothless because people are assumed to disregard it if it

---

[2] A curriculum of health literacy for secondary schools has recently been developed and pilot-tested (Steckelberg et al. 2009).

conflicts with their preference; that is, in an explicit-consent environment they should opt in, whereas they should opt out in a presumed-consent environment.

Regardless of whether one believes that a presumed-consent environment promotes a public good or heightens the risk of overusing a costly technology, the organ donation example illustrates the power of the environment to effect a target behavior.

For another illustration, take the endemic problem of poor diet and physical inactivity—a problem that, according to Mokdad et al. (2004), will soon be the leading cause of mortality in the United States. As in the organ donation example, it is instructive to compare different societies. The proportion of obese U.S. Americans (22.3%) is about three times as high as that of the French population (7.4%; see Rozin et al. 2003). Why is that? After all, French cuisine is not renowned for its caloric asceticism. The lower obesity rate in France is likely to result from a multitude of factors, but one powerful environmental factor appears to be crucial: portion size. Rozin and colleagues compared average portion sizes in restaurants, supermarkets, and cookbook recipes, and found that, on average, French portion sizes were substantially smaller, relative to U.S. portion sizes. This was even the case within the same global chain of fast food restaurants: a medium portion of French fries at a McDonalds restaurant in France was 90 g, relative to 155 g in Philadelphia.

Our environment—in terms of mundane properties, such as the frequency of convenience stores or the neighborhood's walkability—affects what and how much we eat (Story et al. 2008) and the scope of our physical activities (Saelens et al. 2003). These and many other examples illustrate that health care professionals, policy makers, and citizens should co-opt the environment as a powerful ally in nudging ourselves toward healthier behaviors and shared decision making (e.g., by changing representations of risk and uncertainty; see Gigerenzer et al. 2007).

How to Get Better Information to the Patients

Currently, the mass media (e.g., newspapers, TV, magazines, the Internet) are likely to be the most important sources of health knowledge for the general public (and, in some cases, even for the physician). Can we foster higher-quality information in the media (see Wormer, this volume)? We realize that media products are produced to be sold and that the laws of the market will not change anytime soon. Yet, one could try to nudge the media toward presenting higher-quality information. Here is a simple but admittedly time-consuming approach. Volunteers of a scientific society or institution (such as the EBM network) could monitor, for example, the prime-time news of the four most important TV stations (e.g., on German TV: ARD, ZDF, SAT1, RTL) and/or some of the nationwide daily newspapers (e.g., in Germany, the *Süddeutsche Zeitung, Frankfurter Allgemeine Zeitung*, and *Die Welt*) for a specified period. Rather than fuming in their ivory towers over glaring mistakes, the experts could routinely submit a letter to the editors-in-chief of these media outlets, explaining mistakes and pointing out how information could have been presented in a more reader-friendly way. Be polite and not condescending, and hook the editor by focusing on the audience and its attraction to a newspaper article or a TV show that enables them to understand the uncertainties of the modern world. Of course, some in the media industry may not care, or may perceive the experts' interference as an act of self-promotion; however, others may see a niche for their product in a highly competitive environment. One outcome of this endeavor could be that "friendly monitoring" becomes a media issue, calling attention to the importance of the public's right to high-quality information. Additionally, media houses themselves may invite experts (or their students) to editorial conferences ("our embedded uncertainty expert") or teach statistical reasoning courses to journalists (in-house seminars or in journalism schools).

In the future, which already began yesterday, a major source of health-related information will be online communities. They represent both opportunities and risks (discussed above). Let us focus on the risks for the moment. The Internet allows each user to spread even the most nonsensical health myths. This can happen without any evil intent, as individuals share personal experiences and their interpretations thereof. Such personal case reports can be biased and biasing in any direction: They can also impact on people's decisions more than statistical information (e.g., Fagerlin et al. 2005). Online communities, of course, are also easy targets for those who intentionally want to spread misinformation. Sneaking into patient forums, for example, and claiming to have been cured by whatever method is an obvious way for people with a commercial interest to do this.

Notwithstanding these risks, online communities grant experts a wide window onto patients' reasoning and concerns. Moreover, experts—as in the case of newspapers—can help to foster high-quality information. They can, for example, train a few members of the community to operate as a "chief medical officer." Community-based glossaries and wikis, such as *Wikipedia*, could be regularly monitored and—if necessary—improved (the German Wikipedia, for instance, appears to fail important criteria of evidence-based patient and consumer information; see Mühlhauser and Oser 2008).[3] Debates of, for instance, new treatment options in online communities may also foreshadow future questions that doctors will be asked during regular visits (thus allowing the medical community to prepare Q&As). Finally, some online communities, when systematically studied, may even reveal pertinent information to medical researchers about target patients' attitudes, beliefs, behaviors, and outcomes. In fact, this information is already being harnessed, for instance, by various web

---

[3] Based on its search engine ranking and page view statistics, the English version of Wikipedia has already surpassed other online health information providers (e.g., MedlinePlus) as a source of online health information (Laurent and Vickers 2009).

sites (PatientsLikeMe 2010). Clearly, public health experts cannot afford to ignore this information marketplace in the Internet.

Conclusion

Our manifesto for change aims for better doctors *and* patients. To nudge doctors to change, we envision evolving medical schools into health professional schools. We spell out existing clusters of excellence that can provide parts of a blueprint for such a new educational institution. We suggest concrete ways of leveling the knowledge playing field between clinicians and patients, thus empowering patients to ask ever-better questions. Fearing those questions, the clinician should no longer be able to afford the luxury of "avoidable ignorance." People are creatures of habit. However, if one can demonstrate that the new health care paradigm works on important process and outcome dimensions, this may help break such habits. To this end, we propose the Wennberg three-step action plan for change (see Table 19.2).

How can we change patients' engagement with the health care system? We propose bringing health literacy into high school curricula and describe an existing model of teaching health literacy to children in primary schools. We also remind others and ourselves not to overlook the environment as an important ally for change. Engineering a smart environment can complement the approach of empowering people to learn, reason, and decide for themselves. In the future, the visit to the doctor will no longer mark the beginning of patients' opportunity to learn about their ailments. Their reasoning will begin prior to the visit and will last beyond (Figure 19.1). The Internet and web-based resources such as online communities will completely change the dynamic of the doctor–patient interaction. We propose a few pragmatic ways in which health care providers can help to foster good information in these new realms of knowledge.

Ostensibly, our manifesto for change ignored numerous key barriers to change, some of which are listed in Table 19.1. Possibly, our most glaring omission is that we did not—at least not explicitly—speak about the levers of change. Although we, for instance, spelled out a vision of the health professional school of the future, we did not name the levers that could be pushed to bring about the desired institutional changes. We can imagine several of these—accreditation standards, increased training of faculty, government and social imperatives—but are reluctant to pinpoint precise levers of change because there is no single cross-country solution. Deciding which combination of levers—including economic incentives (e.g., fee-for-service system versus fee-for-health system), regulations and laws, education and information, appeal to the idealistic streak in health care professionals, and, of course, evidence—seems appropriate must hinge on the players and institutions in question. It will depend on how the virtuous goals (including moving toward patient-centered care, curbing costs, or extending coverage) are prioritized, and which go in tandem or are in conflict. It will also depend on the historically evolved idiosyncrasies of the health care system in question, and so on. Thus, our reticence to talk explicitly about leverage points is owed to the lack of a silver bullet, and we did not want to replace it with platitude.

The 20th century was the century of fantastic progress in medical research, the implementation of a rich health care infrastructure, and ever-increasing resources that societies devoted to health care. However, those golden days are over. We expect that scientific progress will continue at a staggering rate, but more will have to be achieved with fewer resources. Care in the 21st century needs to become patient-centered and the patient lobbyist can help to spur a new culture of decision making, transparency, communication, and patient participation in the world of health care. A pinnacle of individual freedom is the freedom of choice. In the act of choosing, individual freedom unfolds (e.g., Schwartz 2004). The litmus test for a society's commitment to freedom and democracy is the degree to which its citizens can choose between religious beliefs (including the belief to disbelieve), political parties, opinions, and sexual orientation. The litmus test for a democratic health care system is the degree to which patients are empowered to choose, based on transparent information. The 21st century should be the century during which the wind of change ushers in an adult conversation between patients and doctors.

Abbreviations

AAMC	Association of American Medical Colleges
AAUW	American Association of University Women
ABIM	American Board of Internal medicine
ACE	Angiotensin-Converting Enzyme
ACGME	Accreditation Council for Graduate Medical Education
ACP	American College of Physicians
AGREE	Appraisal of Guidelines for Research and Evaluation
AIDS	Acquired Immune Deficiency Syndrome
AIFA	Agenzia Italiano del Farmaco (Italian Medicines Agency)
ALLHAT	Antihypertensive and Lipid-Lowering Treatment to Prevent Heart Attack Trial
AMA	American Medical Association
AOK	Allgemeine Ortskrankenkasse (Germany) [universal medical insurance]
ARR	Absolute Risk Reduction
ASA	Advertising Standards Authority (New Zealand)
ASC	Advertising Standards Canada
BPH	Benign Prostatic Hyperplasia
CanMEDS	Royal College of Physicians and Surgeons of Canada
CATIE	Clinical Antipsychotic Trials in Intervention Effectiveness
CDER	Center for Drug Evaluation and research
CE	Continuing Education
CHSR	Coalition for Health Services Research
CI	Confidence Interval
CIHR	Canadian Institutes of Health Research
CME	Continued Medical Education
COGS	Conference on Guideline Standardization
CONSORT	Consolidated Standards of Reporting Trials
COREQ	Consolidated Criteria for Reporting Qualitative Research
CPD	Continuing Professional Development
CT	Computer Tomography
DALY	Disability-Adjusted Life Year
DDMAC	Division of Drug Marketing Advertising and Communications (part of the FDA)
DTCA	Direct-To-Consumer Advertising
DUET	Database of Uncertainties about the Effects of Treatment
EC	European Commission
ELISA	Enzyme Linked Immunosorbent Assay
EMA/EMEA	European Medicines Agency
EQUATOR	Enhancing the Quality and Transparency of Health Research
EU	European Union
FDA	Food and Drug Administration
FOBT	Fecal Occult Blood Test
FP7	Seventh Framework Program (EU)
GDP	Gross Domestic Product

GNOSIS	Guidelines for Neuro-Oncology: Standards for Investigational Studies
GRADE	Grading of Recommendations Assessment Development and Evaluation
HCI	Hospital Care Intensity
HDPI	Heart Disease Predictive Instrument
HIV	Human Immunodeficiency Virus
HTA	Health Technology Assessment
HWG	Heilmittelwerbegesetz (Germany) [law regulating the advertisement of medicaments]
ICMJE	International Committee of Medical Journal Editors
ICU	Intensive Care Unit
IOM	Institute of Medicine
IPDAS	International Patient Decision Aids Standard
IPE	Interprofessional Education
IQWiG	*Institut für Qualität und Wirtschaftlichkeit im Gesundheitswesen* (Germany) [Institute for Quality and Efficiency in Health Care]
ISDB	International Society of Drug Bulletins
IV	Intravenous
MCAT	Medical College Admission Test
MEDLINE	Medical Literature Analysis and Retrieval System Online
MHRA	Medicines and Healthcare Products Regulatory Agency
MIAME	Minimum Information about a Microarray Experiment
MOOSE	Meta-Analysis of Observational Studies in Epidemiology
MRI	Magnetic Resonance Imaging
MTD	Maximal Tolerated Dose
MUMM	Managed Uptake of Medical Methods
NCI	National Cancer Institute
NCTM	National Council of Teachers of Mathematics
NHMRC	National Health and Medical Research Council (Australia)
NHS	National Health Service (U.K.)
NICE	National Institute for Health and Clinical Excellence (U.K.)
NIH	National Institutes of Health (U.S.A.)
NIHR	National Institute for Health Research (U.K.)
NME	New Molecular Entity
NNR	Number Needed to Read
NNT	Number Needed to Treat
NSABP	National Surgical Adjuvant Breast and Bowel Project
ORION	Outbreak Reports and Intervention Studies of Nosocomial Infection
PAAB	Pharmaceutical Advertising Advisory Board
PORT	Patient Outcomes Research Teams
PRISMA	Preferred Reporting Items for Systematic Reviews and Meta-Analyses
PROMIS	Patient-Reported Outcome Measurements Information System
PSA	Prostate Specific Antigen
QOF	Quality and Outcomes Framework
QUORUM	Quality of Reporting of Meta-Analyses
R&D	Research and Development

REMARK	*Reporting Recommendations for* Tumor Marker Prognostic Studies
RMI	Researched Medicines Industry
RRR	Relative Risk Reduction
SARS	Severe Acute Respiratory Syndrome
SBU	Scientific Council on Health Technology Assessment (Sweden)
SDP	Shared Decision-Making Program
SEER	Surveillance, Epidemiology and End Result Program for Prostate Cancer
SII	Social Insurance Institution (Finland)
SP	Standardized Patient
SPC	Summary of Product Characteristics
SQUIRE	Standards for Quality Improvement Reporting Excellence
STARD	Standards for Reporting of Diagnostic Accuracy
STREGA	Strengthening the Reporting of Genetic Association
STROBE	Strengthening the Reporting of Observational Studies in Epidemiology
TAPS	Therapeutic Advertising Pre-vetting System
TREND	Transparent Reporting of Evaluations with Non-randomized Designs
WHCA	World Health Communication Associates
WHO	World Health Organization

Glossary

Absolute risk reduction (ARR)   Measure of the efficacy of a treatment in terms of the absolute number of people saved (or lost, in the case of an *absolute risk increase*). For instance, if a treatment reduces the number of people who die of a disease from 6 to 4 in 1,000, then the absolute risk reduction is 2 in 1,000, or 0.2 percentage points, while the *relative risk reduction* is 33% (see below). Absolute risk reductions are transparent, while relative risk reductions tend to mislead people.

Basic numeracy   Ability to understand simple percentages, absolute numbers, and chance.

Bias   A systematic error in the design, conduct, or the analysis of a study.

Citizen   A native or inhabitant of a particular place; used synonymously with "person" or "member of society." Usage is not meant to exclude on the basis of nationality or citizenship.

Conditional probability   The probability that an event A occurs given event B, usually written as p(A|B). An example of a conditional probability is the probability of a positive screening mammogram given breast cancer, which is around .90. The probability p(A), for instance, is not a conditional probability. Conditional probabilities are notoriously misunderstood, in two different ways. One is to confuse the probability of A *given* B with the probability of A *and* B; the other is to confuse the probability of A given B with the probability of B given A. This confusion can be reduced by replacing conditional probabilities with *natural frequencies*.

Decision support interventions or decision aids   Tools designed to help people make informed health care decisions. They provide information about the options and outcomes and assist in the clarification of personal values. Decision aids are designed to complement, rather than replace, counseling from a health practitioner.

Drug bulletins   Periodicals that report on issues related to drug therapy. They are produced independently of the pharmaceutical industry and aim to provide balance to the large number of journals that depend on advertising by manufacturers.

False positive rate   The proportion of positive tests among individuals who do not have a disease (or condition). It is typically expressed as a conditional probability or a percentage. For instance, mammography screening has a false positive rate of 5–10% depending on age; that is, 5–10% of women without breast cancer receive nevertheless a positive test result. The false positive rate and the specificity (power) of a test add up to 100%. The rates of the two possible errors, false positive and false negatives (misses), are dependent: decreasing the false positive rate of a test increases the false negative rate, and vice versa.

Health literacy   The degree to which individuals can obtain, process, and understand basic knowledge about diseases, causes, prevention, diagnostics, treatment, and services they need to make appropriate health decisions.

Health system literacy   The degree to which individuals understand how the health system works, including knowledge about the incentives within it, such as the widespread practice of defensive medicine as a reaction to the threat of litigation.

Illusion of certainty Belief that an event is absolutely certain, even though it may not be. For instance, people tend to believe that the results of modern technologies (e.g., DNA fingerprinting) or medical tests (e.g., HIV testing) are certain, that is, is error-free. The illusion can have benefits, such as reassurance, but it also has costs, such as suicide after a false positive HIV test. Its origin is not simply cognitive, but often social. For instance, with respect to political or religious values, the illusion of certainty may be a requirement for being accepted by a social group, fostering social control.

Meta-analysis A statistical technique used to combine the results from several studies that address a shared research hypothesis.

Mismatched framing Practice of reporting benefits and harms of treatments differently: benefits are exaggerated, whereas harms are downplayed. This can be done in various ways, one of which is to frame the benefit as a relative risk reduction (big numbers) and the harms as an absolute risk increase (small numbers).

Natural frequencies A transparent form of risk communication. While conditional probabilities (such as sensitivity and false positive rate) make it difficult for most physicians to infer the positive predictive value of a test, natural frequencies make it easy. For instance, consider a disease with a prevalence of 4%, a test with a sensitivity of 80%, and a false positive rate of 5%. What is the probability that a patient has the disease, given a positive test result? Few physicians understand how to calculate the answer (40%) using Bayes's rule. Representing the same information in natural frequencies, however, fosters insight. Think of 1,000 people: 40 are expected to have the disease, and 32 of these will correctly test positive. From the other 960 without the disease, 48 will also test positive. Thus, a total of 80 (32 + 48) are expected to test positive, but only 32 actually have the disease, which is 40%. Natural frequencies correspond to the way human beings encountered information before the invention of books and probability theory.

Number needed to treat (NNT) Number of people who need to take a treatment over a specified period of time before 1 person shows a benefit. Example: a study showed that among every 1,000 patients who used a drug, 3 died of a heart attack within 10 years, while among 1,000 patients who used a placebo, 5 died of a heart attack in the same time period. The NNT is 500; the absolute risk reduction is 1 in 500; and the relative risk reduction is 40%. In other words, 499 out of every 500 patients do not benefit in terms of mortality reduction. NNT is also used to measure the harm of a treatment. Example: if 1 in 7,000 women who take oral contraceptives get a thromboembolism, then the number needed to harm 1 woman is 7,000. In other words, 6,999 do not show this side effect.

Outcome reporting bias The selection of a subset of the originally recorded outcome variables; selection is made on the basis of results and thus reporting is incomplete. Outcome reporting bias is a major reason for producing results that cannot be replicated.

Positive predictive value Probability that a person has the disease (or condition) if the test result is positive.

Relative risk reduction (RRR)   Measure of the efficacy of a treatment in terms of the relative number of people saved or lost. For instance, if a treatment reduces the number of people who die from 6 to 4 in 1,000, then the relative risk reduction is 33.3%. Reporting relative risks is popular because the numbers are larger and thus appear more impressive than the absolute risk reduction (which would be 2 in 1,000 or 0.2%) or NNT (which would be 500). Relative risks do not convey how large, in absolute terms, the risk is. For instance, if a treatment reduces the number of people who die from 6 to 4 in 10,000, the relative risk reduction is still the same (33.3%), although the absolute risk reduction has decreased to 0.02%. Reporting relative risk reductions without absolute risks is incomplete and potentially misleading.

Sensitivity   The proportion of positive tests among individuals who have a disease (or condition). Formally, the sensitivity is the conditional probability p(positive| disease) of a positive test result given the disease. Sensitivity is also called hit rate.

Specificity   The proportion of negative tests among individuals who do not have a disease (or condition). Formally, specificity is the conditional probability p(negative| no disease) of a negative test result given no disease. Specificity and the false positive rate add up to 100%. Specificity is also called the power of a test.

Statistical illiteracy in health   Inability to understand health statistics, including concepts such as 5-year survival rates and false positive rates; lack of basic competencies in understanding evidence and knowing what questions to ask.

Statistical literacy   Ability to understand basic concepts, relations, and facts about uncertain evidence.

Supply-sensitive care   Frequency of treatment is to a substantial degree determined by the resources that are locally available (e.g., the number of medical specialists or hospital beds per person).

Bibliography

Note: Numbers in square brackets denote the chapter in which an entry is cited.

AACN. 2009. Lifelong learning in medicine and nursing: Final conference report. Washington, D.C.: American Association of Colleges of Nursing. http://www.aamc. org/meded/cme/lifelong/macyreport.pdf (accessed 15 June 2010). [15]

AAMC. 1998. Report II. Contemporary issues in medicine: medical informatics and population health. Washington, D.C.: Association of American Medical Colleges. https://services.aamc.org/publications/showfile.cfm?file=version88.pdf&prd_id= 199&prv_id=240&pdf_id=88 (accessed 14 June 2010). [15]

————. 2001. Report V. Contemporary issues in medicine: Quality of care. Washington, D.C.: Association of American Medical Colleges. https://services.aamc.org/publications/showfile.cfm?file=version91.pdf&prd_id=202&prv_id=243&pdf_id=91 (accessed 18 June 2010). [15]

————. 2008. Report X. Contemporary issues in medicine: Education in safe and effective prescribing practices. Washington, D.C.: Association of American Medical Colleges. https://services.aamc.org/publications/showfile.cfm?file=version115.pdf &prd_id=234&prv_id=284&pdf_id=115 (accessed 14 June 2010). [15]

Abel, G. A., S. J. Lee, and J. C. Weeks. 2007. Direct-to-consumer advertising in oncology: A content analysis of print media. *J. Clin. Oncol.* **25**:1267–1271. [18]

Abel, G. A., E. J. Neufeld, M. Sorel, and J. C. Weeks. 2008. Direct-to-consumer advertising for bleeding disorders: A content analysis and expert evaluation of advertising claims. *J. Thromb. Haemost.* **6**:1680–1684. [18]

Abraham, J. 2002. The pharmaceutical industry as a political player. *Lancet* **360**:1498–1502. [18]

Access Economics. 2008. Exceptional Returns: The Value of Investing in Health R&D in Australia, vol. 2. Canberra: Australian Society for Medical Research. [5]

ACGME. 2010. Accreditation Council for Graduate Medical Education. http://www. acgme.org (accessed 14 June 2010). [15]

ACP. 2009. Improving FDA Regulation of Prescription Drugs: Policy Monograph. Philadelphia: American College of Physicians. http://www.acponline.org/advocacy/ where_we_stand/policy/fda.pdf (accessed 18 June 2010). [18]

Adams, J. 2000/1765. The Revolutionary Writings of John Adams. Indianapolis: Liberty Fund. [1]

Addis, A., and F. Rocchi. 2006. Drug evaluation: New requirements and perspectives. *Recenti Progr. Med.* **97**:618–624. [5]

Agenzia Italiana del Farmaco. 2003. Bando di assegnazione di finanziamento per la ricercaindipendente sui farmaci. http://www.agenziafarmaco.it/allegati/bando_acc_ programma.pdf (accessed 2 June 2010). [13]

Aitken, M., and F. Holt. 2000. A prescription for direct drug marketing. *McKinsey Q.* **5**:82–91. [18]

AkdÄ. 2008. Stellungnahme: Konsultationspapier der Europäischen Kommission zur Patienteninformation über Arzneimittel. Berlin: Arzneimittelkommission der deutschen Ärzteschaft. http://www.akdae.de/46/40/20080407.pdf (accessed 10 April 2010). [18]

ALLHAT Collaborative Research Group. 2002. Major outcomes in high-risk hypertensive patients randomized to angiotensin-converting enzyme inhibitor or calcium channel blocker vs. diuretic: The antihypertensive and lipid-lowering treatment to prevent heart attack trial (ALLHAT). *JAMA* **288**:2981–2997. [1, 13]

Almasi, E. A., R. S. Stafford, R. L. Kravitz, and P. R. Mansfield. 2006. What are the public health effects of direct-to-consumer drug advertising? *PLoS Med.* **3**:e145. [18]

Alper, B. S., J. A. Hand, S. G. Elliott, et al. 2004. How much effort is needed to keep up with the literature relevant for primary care? *J. Med. Libr. Assoc.* **92(4)**:429–437. [12]

Als-Nielsen, B., W. Chen, C. Gluud, and L. L. Kjaergard. 2003. Association of funding and conclusions in randomized drug trials: A reflection of treatment effect or adverse events? *JAMA* **290(7)**:921–928. [6]

Altman, D. G. 1994. The scandal of poor medical research. *BMJ* **308**:283–284. [7]

———. 1996. Better reporting of randomised controlled trials: The CONSORT statement. *BMJ* **313**:570–571. [7]

Altman, D. G., and J. M. Bland. 1991. Improving doctors' understanding of statistics. *J. R. Stat. Soc. Ser. A* **154**:223–267. [2, 9, 12]

Anderson, J. G., and S. J. Jay. 1997. Dynamic computer simulation models. *J. Contin. Educ. Health Prof.* **17**:32–42. [15]

Andriole, G. L., E. D. Crawford, R. L. Grubb III, et al. 2009. Mortality results from a randomized prostate-cancer screening trial. *N. Engl. J. Med.* **360(13)**:1310–1131. [1, 2, 9]

Angell, M. 2004. The Truth about the Drug Companies. New York: Random House. [1, 12]

Angell, M., and J. Kassirer. 1994. Clinical research: What should the public believe? *N. Engl. J. Med.* **331**:89–190. [11]

Annan, R. 2009. Draft CIHR Strategic Plan: Targeted Research with End-users. Ottawa: Canada Research Funding Org. http://canadaresearchfunding.org/2009/05/ (accessed 27 April 2010). [5]

Antes, G. 2008. Die Qualität wissenschaftlicher Arbeiten: Eine Bewertungshilfe für Journalisten. In: WissensWelten: Wissenschaftsjournalismus in Theorie und Praxis, ed. H. Hettwer et al., pp. 89–107. Gütersloh: Verlag Bertelsmann Stiftung. [11]

ANZA. 2007. TAPS: Therapeutic Advertising Pre-vetting Systems. Auckland: Association of New Zealand Advertisers Inc. [18]

AOK Baden-Württemberg. 2010. ScienceKids: Kinder entdecken Gesundheit. http://www.sciencekids.de/116-0-Impressum.html (accessed 10 June 2010). [13, 19]

Appleton, D. R. 1990. What statistics should we teach medical undergraduates and graduates? *Stat. Med.* **9**:1013–1021. [9]

Armstrong, S. D., H. Reyburn, and R. Jones. 1996. A study of general practitioners' reasons for changing their prescribing behaviour. *BMJ* **312**:949–952. [16]

Arnold, K. 2008. Qualität im Journalismus: Ein integratives Konzept. *Publizistik* **53(4)**:448–508. [11]

Arnold, M. 2005. Changing channels. *Med. Mark. Media* **40(4)**:34–39. [18]

Arora, N., J. Ayanian, and E. Guadagnoli. 2005. Examining the relationship of patients' attitudes and beliefs with their self-reported level of participation in medical decision making. *Med. Care* **43**:865–872. [4]

Arriba. 2010. http://www.arriba-hausarzt.de (accessed 10 June 2010). [13]

Arrow, K. J. 1963. Uncertainty and the welfare economics of medical care. *Am. Econ. Rev.* **53**:941–973. [19]

arznei-telegramm. 2009. Qlaira: Eine Pille ohne Chemie? *Arznei Telegramm* **40**:62–63. [18]

ASA. 2005. Therapeutic Products Advertising Code. http://www.asa.co.nz/code_therapeutic_products.php (accessed 1 February 2005). [18]

Assman, S. F., S. J. Pocock, L. E. Enos, and L. E. Kasten. 2000. Subgroup analysis and other (mis)uses of baseline data in clinical trials. *Lancet* 355:1064–1069. [7]

Auerbach, S. 2001. Do patients want control over their own health care? A review of measures, findings, and research issues. *J. Health Psychol.* 6:191–203. [4]

Avorn, J. 2007. Keeping science on top in drug evaluation. *N. Engl. J. Med.* 357:633–635. [18]

AWA. 2009. Allensbacher Markt und Werbeträgeranalyse: Reichweiten, Kaufzeitungen. http://www.awa-online.de (accessed 27 May 2010). [11]

Bachmann, L. M., F. S. Gutzwiller, M. A. Puhan, et al. 2007. Do citizens have minimum medical knowledge? A survey. *BMC Med.* 5:14. [1]

Bacon, F. 1620. Novum Organum Scientiarum. Londinii: J. Billium. [13]

Badenschier, F., and H. Wormer. 2010. Issue selection in science journalism: Towards a special theory of news values for science news? In: Sociology of the Sciences Yearbook, ed. P. Weingart. Heidelberg: Springer, in press. [11]

Baines, C. J. 1992. Women and breast cancer: Is it really possible for the public to be well informed? *CMAJ* 142:2147–2148. [2]

Bandura, A. 1986. Social Foundations of Thought and Action: A Social Cognitive Theory. Englewood Cliffs: Prentice-Hall. [15]

Barry, M. J. 2009. The PSA conundrum. *Arch. Intern. Med.* 166:7–8. [1]

Barry, M. J., F. J. Fowler, Jr., A. G. Mulley, Jr., J. V. Henderson, Jr., and J. E. Wennberg. 1995. Patient reactions to a program designed to facilitate patient participation in treatment decisions for benign prostatic hyperplasia. *Med. Care* 33(8):771–782. [3]

Barry, M. J., A. G. Mulley, Jr., F. J. Fowler, and J. E. Wennberg. 1988. Watchful waiting vs. immediate transurethral resection for symptomatic prostatism: The importance of patients' preferences. *JAMA* 259(20):3010–3017. [3]

Basara, L. R. 1996. The impact of a direct-to-consumer prescription medication advertising campaign on new prescription volume. *Drug Inf. J.* 30:715–729. [18]

Bayer Health Care. 2010. Die Pille mit Q. http://www.pille-mit-q.de (accessed 21 June 2010). [18]

Beaver, K., K. Luker, R. Owens, et al. 1996. Treatment decision making in women newly diagnosed with breast cancer. *Cancer Nurs.* 19:8–19. [4]

Behrens, J., W. Güth, H. Kliemt, and V. Levati. 2010. Games that doctors play: Two-layered agency problems in a medical system. In: Dimensionen Öffentlichen Wirtschaftens. Festschrift in honor of Prof. R. Windisch, ed. A. Mehler and U. Cantner. Jena: University of Jena. [19]

Bekelman, J. E., Y. Li, and C. P. Gross. 2003. Scope and impact of financial conflicts of interest in biomedical research: A systematic review. *JAMA* 289:454–465. [13, 18]

Bell, R., R. L. Kravitz, and M. S. Wilkes. 1999. Direct-to-consumer prescription drug advertising and the public. *J. Gen. Intern. Med.* 14:651–657. [14]

Bell, R., M. S. Wilkes, and R. L. Kravitz. 2000. The educational value of consumer-targeted prescription drug print advertising. *J. Fam. Pract.* 49:1092–1098. [14, 18]

Berger, B., A. Steckelberg, G. Meyer, J. Kasper, and I. Mühlhauser. 2010. Training of patient and consumer representatives in basic competencies of evidence-based medicine: A feasibility study. *BMC Med. Educ.* 10:16. [12]

Bergsma, L. J., and M. E. Carney. 2008. Effectiveness of health-promoting media literacy education: A systematic review. *Health Educ. Res.* 23:522–542. [13]

Bernstam, E. V., M. F. Walji, S. Sagaram, et al. 2008. Commonly cited website quality criteria are not effective at identifying inaccurate online information about breast cancer. *Cancer Nurs.* 112:1206–1213. [11]

Bero, L. A., and D. Rennie. 1996. Influences on the quality of published drug studies. *Intl. J. Technol. Assess. Health Care* 12:209–237. [13]

Berwick, D. M., H. V. Fineberg, and M. C. Weinstein. 1981. When doctors meet numbers. *Am. J. Med.* 71:991–998. [1]

BEUC. 2007. Consumers need better information. Brussels: Bureau Européen des Unions de Consommateurs. http://ec.europa.eu/health/ph_overview/other_policies/pharmaceutical/docs/R-032_en.pdf (accessed 21 June 2010). [18]

Billett, S. 1996. Towards a model of workplace learning: The learning curriculum. *Stud. Cont. Educ.* 18(1):43–45. [15]

Biondi-Zoccai, G. G. L., M. Lotrionte, A. Abbate, et al. 2006. Compliance with QUOROM and quality of reporting of overlapping meta-analyses on the role of acetylcysteine in the prevention of contrast associated nephropathy: Case study. *BMJ* 332:202–209. [7]

Black, N. 2006. The Cooksey review of UK health research funding: The art of being all things to all people. *BMJ* 333:1231–1232. [5]

Blanchard, C., M. Labrecque, J. Ruckdeschel, and E. Blanchard. 1988. Information and decision making preferences of hospitalized adult cancer patients. *Soc. Sci. Med.* 27:1139–1145. [4]

Blöbaum, B., and A. Görke. 2006. Quellen und Qualität im Wissenschaftsjournalismus: Befragung und Inhaltsanalyse zur Life-Science-Berichterstattung. In: Medien-Qualitäten: Öffentliche Kommunikation zwischen ökonomischem Kalkül und Sozialverantwortung, ed. S. Weischenberg et al., pp. 307–328. Konstanz: UVK Verlagsgesellschaft. [11]

Blümle, A., G. Antes, M. Schumacher, H. Just, and E. von Elm. 2008. Clinical research projects at a German medical faculty: Follow-up from ethical approval to publication and citation by others. *J. Med. Ethics* 34(e20). [8]

Boden, W. E., and G. A. Diamond. 2008. DTCA for PTCA: Crossing the line in consumer health education? *N. Engl. J. Med.* 358:2197–2200. [18]

Bodenheimer, T., E. H. Wagner, and K. Grumbach. 2002a. Improving primary care for patients with chronic illness, Part 1. *JAMA* 288:1775–1779. [19]

———. 2002b. Improving primary care for patients with chronic illness: The chronic care model, Part 2. *JAMA* 288:1909–1914. [19]

Bonaccorso, S. N., and J. L. Sturchio. 2002. For and against: Direct to consumer advertising is medicalising normal human experience. *BMJ* 324(7342):910–911. [18]

Bond, M. 2009. Risk school. *Nature* 461:1189–1192. [11, 12, 19]

Bossuyt, P. M., J. B. Reitsma, D. E. Bruns, et al. 2003. Towards complete and accurate reporting of studies of diagnostic accuracy: The STARD Initiative. *Ann. Int. Med.* 138(1):40–44. [6]

Bower, B. 1991. Teenage turning point. *Science News* 139:184–186. [10]

———. 1997. Null science. *Science News* 151:356–357. [10]

Boykoff, M. T., and J. M. Boykoff. 2004. Balance is bias: Global warming and the US prestige press. *Glob. Environ. Change* 14:125–136. [11]

Braddock, C. H., K. A. Edwards, N. M. Hasenberg, T. L. Laidley, and W. Levinson. 1999. Informed decision making in outpatient practice: Time to get back to basics. *JAMA* 282:2313–2320. [2]

Brahic, C. 2009. Climate change diagnosed as biggest global health threat. *New Scientist*, May 14. [19]

Bramwell, R., H. West, and P. Salmon. 2006. Health professionals' and service users' interpretation of screening test results: Experimental study. *BMJ* 333:284–286. [9, 16]

Braun, D. 1994. Structure and Dynamics of Health Research and Public Funding: An International Comparison. Dordrecht: Springer. [5]

Brenner, D. J., and E. J. Hall. 2007. Computed tomography: An increasing source of radiation exposure. *N. Engl. J. Med.* 357:2277–2284. [1]

Brodie, M., E. C. Hamel, D. E. Altman, R. J. Blendon, and J. M. Benson. 2003. Health news and the American public 1996–2002. *J. Health Polit. Policy Law* 28:927–950. [11]

Brosius, H. B. 1995. Alltagsrationalität in der Nachrichtenrezeption: Ein Modell zur Wahrnehmung und Verarbeitung von Nachrichteninhalten. Opladen: Westdeutscher Verlag. [11]

Brown, R., P. Butow, M. Boyer, and M. Tattersall. 1999. Promoting patient participation in the cancer consultation: Evaluation of a prompt sheet and coaching in question asking. *Br. J. Cancer* 80:242–248. [4]

Brumfiel, G. 2009. Science journalism: Supplanting the old media? *Nature* 458:274–277. [11]

Bucher, H. J., and K. D. Altmeppen, eds. 2003. Qualität im Journalismus: Grundlagen, Dimensionen, Praxismodelle. Wiesbaden: Westdeutscher Verlag. [11]

Buchner, B. 2009. The pharmaceutical package of the European Commission: Empowerment for patients? *Eur. J. Health Law* 16:201–206. [18]

Bunge, M., A. Steckelberg, and I. Mühlhauser. 2010. What constitutes evidence-based patient information? Overview of discussed criteria. *Patient Educ. Couns.* 78:316–328. [2, 12]

Burgers, J. S., B. Fervers, M. Haugh, et al. 2004. International assessment of the quality of clinical practice guidelines in oncology using the appraisal of guidelines and research and evaluation instrument. *J. Clin. Oncol.* 22(10):2000–2007. [6]

Burke, M. A., and S. A. Matlin, eds. 2008. Monitoring Financial Flows for Health Research 2008: Prioritizing Research for Health Equity. Geneva: Global Forum for Health Research. [5]

Cabot, R. C. 1903. The use of truth and falsehood in medicine: An experimental study. *Am. Med.* 5:344. [3]

CAHPS. 2010. Survey and tools to advance patient-centered care. https://www.cahps.ahrq.gov/default.asp (accessed 21 June 2010). [13]

CAIPE. 1997. Interprofessional Education: A Definition. London: CAIPE. [15]

Campbell, S., D. Reeves, E. Kontopantelis, et al. 2007. Quality of primary care in England with the introduction of pay for performance. *N. Engl. J. Med.* 357:181–190. [16]

Campbell, S., D. Reeves, E. Kontopantelis, B. Sibbald, and M. Roland. 2009. Effects of pay for performance on the quality of primary care in England. *N. Engl. J. Med.* 361:368–378. [16]

Carrigan, N., D. K. Raynor, and P. Knapp. 2008. Adequacy of patient information on adverse effects: An assessment of patient information leaflets in the UK. *Drug Safety* 31:305–312. [18]

Casscells, W., A. Schoenberger, and T. Grayboys. 1978. Interpretation by physicians of clinical laboratory results. *N. Engl. J. Med.* 299:999–1000. [1, 9]

Cassileth, B., R. Zupkis, K. Sutton-Smith, and V. March. 1980. Information and participation preferences among cancer patients. *Ann. Int. Med.* 92:832–836. [4]

Cegala, D., D. Post, and L. McClure. 2001. The effects of patient communication skills training on the discourse of older patients during a primary care interview. *J. Am. Geriatr. Soc.* **49**:1505–1511. [4]

Chalmers, I. 1990. Underreporting research is scientific misconduct. *JAMA* **263(10)**:1405–1408. [6]

———. 1995. What do I want from health research and researchers when I am a patient? *BMJ* **310**:1315–1318. [16]

———. 2003. Trying to do more good than harm in policy and practice: The role of rigorous, transparent, up-to-date evaluations. *Ann. Am. Acad. Pol. Soc. Sci.* **589**:22–40. [16]

Chalmers, I., and M. Clarke. 1998. Discussion sections in reports of controlled trials published in general medical journals: Islands in search of continents. *JAMA* **280**:280–282. [7]

Chalmers, I., and P. Glasziou. 2009. Avoidable waste in the production of reporting research evidence. *Lancet* **374**:86–89. [7]

Chalmers, I., and R. Matthews. 2006. What are the implications of optimism bias in clinical research? *Lancet* **367**:449–450. [7]

Chan, A.-W., and D. G. Altman. 2005a. Epidemiology and reporting of randomised trials published in PubMed journals. *Lancet* **365**:1159–1162. [7]

———. 2005b. Identifying outcome reporting bias in randomised trials on PubMed: Review of publications and survey of authors. *BMJ* **330**:753. [7]

Chan, A.-W., A. Hrobjartsson, M. T. Haahr, P. C. Gøtzsche, and D. G. Altman. 2004. Empirical evidence for selective reporting of outcomes in randomized trials: Comparison of protocols to published articles. *JAMA* **291(20)**:2457–2465. [6]

Charles, C. A., A. Gafni, and T. Whelan. 1997. Shared decision-making in the medical encounter: What does it mean? *Soc. Sci. Med.* **44**:681–692. [4]

Charney, E., and H. Kitzman. 1971. The child-health nurse (pediatric nurse practitioner) in private practice: A controlled trial. *N. Engl. J. Med.* **285(24)**:1353–1357. [15]

Charnock, D., S. Shepperd, G. Needham, and R. Gann. 1999. DISCERN: An instrument for judging the quality of written consumer health information on treatment choices. *J. Epidemiol. Comm. Health* **53**:105–111. [11, 18]

Chew, F., S. Palmer, and S. Kim. 1995. Sources of information and knowledge about health and nutrition: Can viewing one television programme make a difference? *Public Underst. Sci.* **4**:17–29. [11]

Chin, T. 2002. Drug firms score by paying doctors for time. *Am. Med. News* **45(17)**. [12]

Christensen, C. M., R. Bohmer, and J. Kenagy. 2000. Will disruptive innovations cure health care? *Harv. Bus. Rev.* **78(5)**:102–112, 199. [15]

CHSR. 2009. Federal Funding for Health Services Research. Washington, D.C.: Coalition for Health Services Research. http://www.chsr.org/coalitionfunding2008. pdf (accessed 18 May 2010). [5]

Cialdini, R. B. 2001. Influence: Science and Practice, 4th ed. Boston: Allyn and Bacon. [19]

CIHR. 2004. Finding a Balance in Federal Health Research Funding, Cat. No. MR21-55/20004E. Ottawa: Canadian Institutes of Health Research. [5]

———. 2009a. Health Research Roadmap: Creating Innovative Research for Better Health and Healthcare. CIHR's Strategic Plan 2009/10–2013/14 draft. Ottawa: Canadian Institutes of Health Research. [5]

———. 2009b. Research with Impact, Cat. No. MR1-2009E-PDF. Ottawa: Canadian Institutes of Health Research. [5]

Clark, F., and D. L. Illman. 2006. A longitudinal study of the *New York Times* science times section. *Science Comm.* **27**:496–513. [11]

Clarke, M., P. Alderson, and I. Chalmers. 2002. Discussion sections in reports of controlled trials in general medical journals. *JAMA* **287**:2799–2801. [7]

Clarke, M., S. Hopewell, and I. Chalmers. 2007. Reports of clinical trials should begin and end with up-to-date systematic reviews of other relevant evidence: A status report. *J. R. Soc. Med.* **100**:187–190. [7]

Club Penguin. 2010. http://www.clubpenguin.com (accessed 25 May 2010). [12]

CMSG. 2010. What is a systematic review? Cochrane Musculoskeletal Group. http://www.cochranemsk.org/cochrane/review/default.asp?s=1 (accessed 7 June 2010). [7]

Cohn, V. 1989. Reporters as gatekeepers. In: Health Risks and the Press: Perspectives on Media Coverage of Risk Assessment and Health, ed. M. Moore. Washington, D.C.: The Media Institute. [11]

Colhoun, H., D. Betteridge, P. Durrington, et al. 2004. Primary prevention of cardiovascular disease with atorvastatin in type 2 diabetes in the collaborative atorvastatin diabetes study (CARDS): Multicentre randomised placebo-controlled trial. *Lancet* **364**:685–696. [14]

Collier, J., and I. Iheanacho. 2002. The pharmaceutical industry as an informant. *Lancet* **360**:1405–1409. [18]

CONSILIUM. 2009. Press release: 2947th Council meeting on employment, social policy, health and consumer affairs. Luxembourg: Council of the European Union. http://www.consilium.europa.eu/uedocs/cms_data/docs/pressdata/en/lsa/108380.pdf. [18]

CONSORT. 2010. Transparent reporting of trials. http://www.consort-statement.org/home/ (accessed 28 April 2010). [6]

Cooksey, D. 2006. A Review of UK Health Research Funding. London: Stationery Office. [5]

Coomarasamy, A., and K. S. Khan. 2004. What is the evidence that postgraduate teaching in evidence based medicine changes anything? A systematic review. *BMJ* **329**:1017. [9]

Coulter, A. 1997. Partnerships with patients: The pros and cons of shared clinical decision making. *J. Health Serv. Res. Policy* **2**:112–121. [4]

Coulter, A., and P. D. Cleary. 2001. Patients' experiences with hospital care in five countries. *Health Affairs* **20(3)**:244–252. [13]

Coulter, A., and C. Jenkinson. 2005. European patients' views on the responsiveness of health systems and healthcare providers. *Eur. J. Public Health* **15**:355–360. [12]

Coulter, A., and H. Magee. 2003. The European Patient of the Future. Philadelphia: Open Univ. Press. [4]

Covey, J. 2007. A meta-analysis of the effects of presenting treatment benefits in different formats. *Med. Decis. Making* **27**:638–654. [2, 9]

Cram, P., M. Fendrick, J. Inadomi, et al. 2003. The impact of a celebrity promotional effect on the use of colon cancer screening. *Arch. Intern. Med.* **163**:161–165. [5]

Current Care. 2010. Evidence-based treatment guidelines for the Finnish Medical Society, Duodecim. http://www.kaypahoito.fi/web/english/home (accessed 23 May 2010). [12]

Cvengros, J., A. Christensen, S. Hillis, and G. Rosenthal. 2007. Patient and physician attitudes in the health care context: Attitudinal symmetry predicts patient satisfaction and adherence. *Ann. Behav. Med.* **33**:262–268. [4]

Dartmouth Atlas of Health Care. 2010. http://www.dartmouthatlas.org (accessed 27 April 2010). [3, 19]

Davey Smith, G., S. Ebrahim, and I. S. Franke. 2001. How policy informs the evidence. *BMJ* 322:184–185. [16]

Davidoff, F., P. Batalden, D. Stevens, G. Ogrinc, and S. Mooney. 2008. Publication guidelines for improvement studies in health care: Evolution of the SQUIRE project. *Ann. Int. Med.* 149(9):670–676. [6]

Davies, H., S. Nutley, and I. Walter. 2000. What Works? Evidence-based Policy and Practice in Public Services. Bristol: Policy Press. [16]

———. 2008. Why "knowledge transfer" is misconceived for applied social research. *J. Health Serv. Res. Policy* 13:188–190. [16]

Davies, P. 2004. Is evidence-based government possible? Jerry Lee Lecture 2004. Washington, D.C.: Campbell Collaboration Colloquium. http://www.nationalschool. gov.uk/policyhub/downloads/JerryLeeLecture1202041.pdf (accessed 15 June 2010). [16]

Davis, D., M. Evans, A. Jadad, et al. 2003. The case for knowledge translation: Shortening the journey from evidence to effect. *BMJ* 327:33–35. [12, 15]

Davis, D., P. E. Mazmanian, M. Fordis, et al. 2006. Accuracy of physician self-assessment compared with observed measures of competence: A systematic review. *JAMA* 296:1094–1102. [15]

Davis, D., M. A. Thomson O'Brien N. Freemantle, et al. 1999. Impact of formal continuing medical education: Do conferences, workshops, rounds and other traditional continuing education activities change physician behavior or health care outcomes? *JAMA* 282:867–874. [15]

Davis, J. J. 2007. Consumers' preferences for the communication of risk information in drug advertising. *Health Affairs* 26:863–870. [18]

Dawes, R. M. 1979. The robust beauty of improper linear models in decision making. *Am. Psychol.* 34:571–582. [17]

DeAngelis, C. D., J. M. Drazen, F. A. Frizelle, et al. 2004. Clinical trial registration: A statement from the International Committee of Medical Journal Editors. *JAMA* 292:1363–1364. [13]

Deber, R. B., and A. O. Baumann. 1992. Clinical reasoning in medicine and nursing: Decision making versus problem solving. *Teach. Learn. Med.* 4:140–146. [4]

Deber, R. B., N. Kraetschmer, and J. Irvine. 1996. What role do patients wish to play in treatment decision making? *Arch. Intern. Med.* 156:1414–1420. [4]

Decision Laboratory. 2010. http://www.decisionlaboratory.com (accessed 22 May 2010). [12]

Degner, L., and J. Sloan. 1992. Decision making during serious illness: What role do patients really want to play? *J. Clin. Epidemiol.* 45:941–950. [4]

DeMiguel, V., L. Garlappi, and R. Uppal. 2009. Optimal versus naive diversification: How inefficient is the 1/N portfolio strategy? *Rev. Financ. Stud.* 22:1915–1953. [17]

Dentzer, S. 2009. Communicating medical news: Pitfalls of health care journalism. *N. Engl. J. Med.* 360(1–3). [10]

Dept. of Health. 2005. Departmental Report 2005: The Health and Personal Social Services Programmes. Norwich: Stationery Office. [17]

Des Jarlais, D. C., C. Lyles, N. Crepaz, and the TREND Group. 2004. Improving the reporting quality of nonrandomized evaluations of behavioral and public health interventions: The TREND statement. *Am. J. Public Health* 94(3):361–366. [6]

Deutsche Krebshilfe. 2009. Brustkrebs: Ein Ratgeber für Betroffene, Angehörige und Interessierte: Die blauen Ratgeber. Bonn: Deutsche Krebshilfe e.V. [1]

Dewalt, D. A., N. D. Berkman, S. Sheridan, K. N. Lohr, and M. P. Pignone. 2004. Literacy and health outcomes: A systematic review of the literature. *J. Gen. Intern. Med.* **19**:1228–1239. [16]

Deyo, R. A., D. C. Cherkin, J. Weinstein, et al. 2000. Involving patients in clinical decisions: Impact of an interactive video program on use of back surgery. *Med. Care* **38(9)**:959–969. [3]

Dierks, M., and G. Seidel. 2005. Gleichberechtigte Beziehungsgestaltung zwischen Ärzten und Patienten: Wollen Patienten wirklich Partner sein? In: Gemeinsam Entscheiden: Erfolgreich Behandeln. Neue Wege für Ärzte und Patienten im Gesundheitswesen, ed. M. Härter et al., pp. 35–44. Köln: Deutscher Ärzteverlag. [4]

DISCERN. 2010. Quality criteria for consumer health information. http://www.discern.org.uk (accessed 9 June 2010). [11]

Dobbs, M. 2007. Rudy wrong on cancer survival chances. *Washington Post*, Oct. 30. http://blog.washingtonpost.com/fact-checker/2007/10/rudy_miscalculates_cancer_surv.html (accessed 30 June 2010). [1]

Domenighetti, G., A. Casabianca, F. Gutzwiller, and S. Martinoli. 1993. Revisiting the most informed consumer of surgical services: The physician-patient. *Intl. J. Technol. Assess. Health Care* **9**:505–513. [1]

Domingos, P. 1999. The role of Occam's Razor in knowledge discovery. *Data Min. Knowl. Discov.* **3**:409–425. [17]

Domingos, P., and M. Pazzani. 1997. On the optimality of the simple Bayesian classifier under zero-one loss. *Machine Learn.* **29**:103–130. [17]

Donald, A. 2005. Putting evidence into practice: What we have learnt in 10 years. Bazian. http://www.bazian.com/pdfs/Bazian_PuttingEvidenceIntoPractice.pdf (accessed 16 March 2010). [16]

Donner-Banzhoff, N., A. Schmidt, E. Baum, and M. Gulich. 2003. Der evidenzbasierte Praktiker: Ein Beitrag zum hausärztlichen Informationsmanagement. *Z. Allgemeinmed.* **79**:501–506. [13]

Donohue, J. M., M. Cevasco, and M. B. Rosenthal. 2007. A decade of direct-to-consumer advertising of prescription drugs. *N. Engl. J. Med.* **357**:673–681. [18]

Doran, E., and D. Henry. 2008. Disease mongering: Expanding the boundaries of treatable disease. *Intern. Med. J.* **38**:858–861. [13]

Dranove, D. 2001. The Economic Evolution of American Health Care: From Marcus Welby to Managed Care. Princeton: Princeton Univ. Press. [19]

Drug Safety. 2007. The Erice Manifesto: For global reform of the safety of medicines in patient care. *Drug Safety* **30**:187–190. [18]

DTC Perspectives. 2008. Spending review. *DTC Perspectives* **7(10)**. [14]

Dunwoody, S. 1999. Scientists, journalists, and the meaning of uncertainty. In: Communicating Uncertainty: Media Coverage of New and Controversial Science, ed. S. M. Friedman et al., pp. 59–79. Mahwah: Lawrence Erlbaum. [11]

Dunwoody, S., and H. P. Peters. 1992. Mass media coverage of technology and environmental risks: A survey of research in the U.S. and Germany. *Public Underst. Sci.* **1**:199–230. [11]

EC. 2008. Public Consultation: Legal Proposal on Information to Patient. Brussels: European Commission. http://ec.europa.eu/enterprise/pharmaceuticals/pharmacos/docs/doc2008/2008_02/info_to_patients_consult_200802.pdf (accessed 10 April 2010). [18]

———. 2009. Seventh framework programme (FP7): Health research. Brussels: European Commission. http://cordis.europa.eu/fp7/health/. [5]

Bibliography

ECETOC. 2010. European centre for ecotoxicology and toxicology of chemicals. http://www.ecetoc.org/overview (accessed 28 April 2010). [6]

Economist. 2009. Editorial: What a waste: American health care. *Economist* October 17. [19]

———. 2010. Editorial: Signed, sealed, delivered. *Economist* March 27. [19]

Eddy, D. M. 1982. Probabilistic reasoning in clinical medicine: Problems and opportunities. In: Judgment under Uncertainty: Heuristics and Biases, ed. D. Kahneman et al., pp. 249–267. Cambridge: Cambridge Univ. Press. [1, 9]

Eddy, D. M. 1984. Variations in physician practice: The role of uncertainty. *Health Affairs* 3:74–89. [3]

Edwards, A., and G. Elwyn, eds. 2009. Shared Decision Making in Health Care: Achieving Evidence-based Patient Choice. Oxford: Oxford Univ. Press. [4]

Edwards, A., G. Elwyn, J. Covey, E. Mathews, and R. Pill. 2001. Presenting risk information: A review of the effects of "framing" and other manipulations on patient outcomes. *J. Health Commun.* 6:61–82. [9]

Egger, M., C. Bartlett, and P. Juni. 2001. Are randomised controlled trials in the BMJ different? *BMJ* 323:1253. [1, 8]

Einhorn, H. J., and R. M. Hogarth. 1975. Unit weighting schemes for decision making. *Organ. Behav. Hum. Perform.* 13:171–192. [17]

Elmer, C., F. Badenschier, and H. Wormer. 2008. Science for everybody? How the coverage of research issues in german newspapers has increased dramatically. *Journalism Mass Comm. Q.* 85:878–893. [11]

Elwyn, G., A. Edwards, and N. Britten. 2003. "Doing prescribing": How might clinicians work differently for better, safer care. *Qual. Saf. Health Care* 12(1):33–36. [4]

Elwyn, G., A. Edwards, P. Kinnersley, and R. Grol. 2000. Shared decision making and the concept of equipoise: The competences of involving patients in healthcare choices. *Br. J. Gen. Pract.* 50(460):892–899. [4]

Elwyn, G., D. Frosch, and S. Rollnick. 2009. Dual equipoise shared decision making: Definitions for decision and behaviour support interventions. *Implement. Sci.* 4:75. [19]

Elwyn, G., A. O'Connor, D. Stacey, et al. 2006. Developing a quality criteria framework for patient decision aids: Online international Delphi consensus process. *BMJ* 333:417. [13]

Elwyn, G., A. O'Connor, C. Bennett, et al. 2009. Assessing the quality of decision support technologies using the International Patient Decision Aid Standards instrument (IPDASi). *PLoS ONE* 4(3):e4705. [13, 18]

EMA. 2006. Rules for the implementation of regulation (EC) 1049/2001 on access to EMA documents. European Medicines Agency. http://www.ema.europa.eu/pdfs/general/manage/mbar/20335906en.pdf (accessed 28 April 2010). [6]

———. 2009. Information on benefit-risk of medicines: Patients', consumers' and healthcare professionals' expectations. European Medicines Agency. http://www.ema.europa.eu/pdfs/human/pcwp/4092609en.pdf. [18]

———. 2010a. The EMA road map to 2010: Preparing the ground for the future. European Medicines Agency. http://www.ema.europa.eu/pdfs/general/direct/directory/3416303enF.pdf. [6]

———. 2010b. Human medicines. European Medicines Agency. http://www.emea.europa.eu/index/indexh1.htm (accessed 28 April 2010). [6]

Ende, J., L. Kazis, A. Ash, and M. Moskowitz. 1989. Measuring patients' desire for autonomy: Decision making and information-seeking preferences among medical patients. *J. Gen. Intern. Med.* 4:23–30. [4]

Entwistle, V., and M. Hancock-Beaulieu. 1992. Health and medical coverage in the UK national press. *Public Underst. Sci.* **1(4)**:367–382. [11]

Epstein, R. M., and R. Street. 2007. Patient-centered Communication in Cancer Care: Promoting Healing and Reducing Suffering. Bethesda: NIH/NCR. [5]

EQUATOR Network. 2010. Enhancing the quality and transparency of health research. http://www.equator-network.org (accessed 4 May 2010). [6–8]

Erin, M. W., D. F. Debra, E. B. Hanna, et al. 2005. Pulse versus continuous terbinafine for onychomycosis: A randomized, double-blind, controlled trial. *J. Am. Acad. Dermatol.* **53(4)**:578–584. [18]

ESIP. 2008. Response to the European Commission public consultation on a legal proposal on information to patients: Joint position paper of the European social insurance platform and Medicine Evaluation Committee (MEDEV) of the European Social Health Insurance Forum. Brussels: European Social Insurance Platform. http://ec.europa.eu/enterprise/sectors/pharmaceuticals/files/patients/respons_publ_consult_200805/social_insurance/medev_en.pdf (accessed 10 April 2010). [18]

Estrada, C., V. Barnes, C. Collins, and J. C. Byrd. 1999. Health literacy and numeracy. *JAMA* **282**. [9]

European Parliament. 2001. Richtlinie 2001/83/EG des Europäischen Parlaments und des Rates vom 6. November 2001 zur Schaffung eines Gemeinschaftskodexes für Humanarzneimittel. Amtsblatt der Europäischen Gemeinschaften. [18]

Evans, K., P. Hodkinson, H. Rainbird, and L. Unwin. 2006. Improving Workplace Learning. London: Rutledge. [15]

Evans, R., A. Edwards, J. Brett, et al. 2005. Reduction in uptake of PSA tests following decision aids: Systematic review of current aids and their evaluations. *Patient Educ. Couns.* **58**:13–26. [19]

Eysenbach, G., and C. Köhler. 2002. How do consumers search for and appraise health information on the world wide web? Qualitative study using focus groups, usability tests, and in-depth interviews. *BMJ* **324**:573–577. [11]

Eysenbach, G., J. Powell, O. Kuss, and E. Sa. 2002. Empirical studies assessing the quality of health information for consumers on the world wide web. *JAMA* **287**: 2691–2700. [11]

FachInfo. 2010. Ratiopharm GmbH: Fachinformation "Terbinafin-ratiopharm® 250 mg Tabletten," Juni 2008. http://www.fachinfo.de/ (accessed 21 June 2010). [18]

Fagerlin, A., P. A. Ubel, D. M. Smith, and B. J. Zikmund-Fisher. 2007. Making numbers matter: Present and future research in risk communication. *Am. J. Health Behav.* **31(1)**:S47–S56. [2]

Fagerlin, A., C. Wang, and P. A. Ubel. 2005. Reducing the influence of anecdotal reasoning on people's health care decisions: Is a picture worth a thousand statistics? *Med. Decis. Making* **25**:398–405. [19]

Fahey, T., S. Griffiths, and T. J. Peters. 1995. Evidence based purchasing: Understanding results of clinical trials and systematic reviews. *BMJ* **311**:1056–1069. [9]

Faigman, D. L. 1999. Legal Alchemy: The Use and Misuse of Science in the Law. New York: W. H. Freeman. [1]

Fanelli, D. 2009. How many scientists fabricate and falsify research? A systematic review and meta-analysis of survey data. *PLoS ONE* **4(5)**:e5738. [13]

Farmer, A. P., F. Légaré, L. Turcot, et al. 2008. Printed educational materials: Effects on professional practice and health care outcomes. *Cochrane Database Syst. Rev.* **3**:CD004398. [15]

FAZ. 2009. Bayer muß sich selbst geißeln. *Frankfurter Allgemeine Zeitung* **79**:20 (3 April 2009). [18]

FDA. 2007. Amendments Act, Public Law 110-85, 110th Congress. Washington, D.C.: GPO. [6]

————. 2009. Draft guidance for industry: Postmarketing safety reporting for human drug and biological products including vaccines. U.S. Dept. of Health and Human Services. http://www.fda.gov/BiologicsBloodVaccines/Guidance ComplianceRegulatoryInformation/Guidances/Vaccines/ucm074850.htm#WHO MUSTREPORT (accessed 28 April 2010). [6]

————. 2010a. 21 C.F.R. § 202.1: Prescription-drug advertisements. GPO. http://law. justia.com/us/cfr/title21/21-4.0.1.1.3.0.1.1.html (accessed 5 May 2010). [14]

————. 2010b. Drugs@FDA: FDA approved drug products. http://www.accessdata. fda.gov/Scripts/cder/DrugsatFDA/ (accessed 20 May 2010). [14]

FDAAA. 2007. FDA Amendments Acts. http://www.fda.gov/Regulatory Information/Legislation/FederalFoodDrugandCosmeticActFDCAct/ SignificantAmendmentstotheFDCAct/FoodandDrugAdministrationAmendments Actof2007/default.htm (accessed 5 May 2010). [14]

Feufel, M. A., G. Antes, and G. Gigerenzer. 2010. How to cope with uncertainty: Lessons learned from the pandemic influenza (H1N1) 2009. *Bundesgesundheitsblatt*, in press.

Figueras, A., and J. R. Laporte. 2003. Failures of the therapeutic chain as a cause of drug ineffectiveness. *BMJ* **326**:895–896. [18]

Finzer, B., and T. Erickson. 2006. Fathom dynamic data software. Emeryville: Key Curriculum Press. http://www.keypress.com/x5656.xml. [12]

Fisher, E. S., D. E. Wennberg, T. A. Stukel, and D. J. Gottlieb. 2004. Variations in the longitudinal efficiency of academic medical centers. *Health Affairs* **23**:19–32. [12]

Fisher, E. S., D. E. Wennberg, T. A. Stukel, et al. 2003a. The implications of regional variations in Medicare spending. Part 1: The content, quality, and accessibility of care. *Ann. Int. Med.* **138(4)**:273–287. [1, 3]

————. 2003b. The implications of regional variations in Medicare spending. Part 2: Health outcomes and satisfaction with care. *Ann. Int. Med.* **138(4)**:288–298. [1, 3]

Fixsen, D. L., K. A. Blase, S. Naoom, M. Van Dyke, and F. Wallace. 2005. Implementation research: A synthesis of the literature. FHMI Publication No. 231. Tampa: University of South Florida, National Implementation Research Network. [5]

Fleck, L. 1980. Entstehung und Entwicklung einer wissenschaftlichen Tatsache. Frankfurt am Main: Suhrkamp. [13]

Folino-Gallo, P., S. Montilla, M. Bruzzone, and N. Martini. 2008. Pricing and reimbursement of pharmaceuticals in Italy. *Eur. J. Health Econ.* **9**:305–310. [5]

Forsetlund, L., A. Bjørndal, A. Rashidian, et al. 2009. Continuing education meetings and workshops: Effects on professional practice and health care outcomes. *Cochrane Database Syst. Rev.* **15**:CD003030. [15]

Fowler, F. J., Jr, J. E. Wennebrg, R. P. Timothy, et al. 1988. Symptom status and quality of life following prostatectomy. *JAMA* **259(20)**:3018–3022. [3]

Fox, R. D., P. E. Mazmanian, and R. W. Putnam. 1989. Changing and Learning in the Lives of Physicians. New York: Praeger Publishers. [15]

Fraenkel, L., and S. McGraw. 2007. Participation in medical decision making: The patients' perspective. *Med. Decis. Making* **27**:533–538. [4]

Frauen Zimmer. 2010. Neu: Antibaby-pille ohne Chemie. http://www.frauenzimmer.de/ cms/html/de/pub/liebe-singles/video/antibaby-pille-ohne-chemie.phtml (accessed 21 June 2010). [18]

Friedman, S. M., S. Dunwoody, and S. C. L. Rogers, eds. 1999. Communicating Uncertainty: Media Coverage of New and Controversial Science. Mahwah: Lawrence Erlbaum. [11]

Fröhlich, G. 2008. Wissenschaftskommunikation und ihre dysfunktionen: Wissenschaftsjournale, peer review, impactfaktoren. In: WissensWelten: Wissenschaftsjournalismus in Theorie und Praxis, ed. H. Hettwer et al., pp. 64–80. Gütersloh: Verlag Bertelsmann Stiftung. [11]

Frosch, D. L., R. M. Kaplan, and V. Felitti. 2001. The evaluation of two methods to facilitate shared decision making for men considering the prostate-specific antigen test. *J. Gen. Intern. Med.* 16:391–398. [3, 19]

Frosch, D. L., P. M. Krueger, R. C. Hornik, P. F. Cronholm, and F. K. Barg. 2007. Creating demand for prescription drugs: A content analysis of television direct-to-consumer advertising. *Ann. Fam. Med.* 5(1):6–13. [14]

FSA. 2008. Kodex für die Zusammenarbeit zwischen der pharmazeutischen Industrie mit Ärzten, Apothekern und anderen Angehörigen medizinischer Fachberufe. http://www.fs-arzneimittelindustrie.de (accessed 31 May 2010). [18]

Gagliardi, A., and A. R. Jadad. 2002. Examination of instruments used to rate quality of health information on the internet: Chronicle of a voyage with an unclear destination. *BMJ* 324:569–573. [11, 13]

Gagnon, M. A., and J. Lexchin. 2008. The cost of pushing pills: A new estimate of pharmaceutical promotion expenditures in the United States. *PLoS Med.* 5:e1. [18]

Galbraith, R. M., R. E. Hawkins, and E. Holmboe. 2008. Making self-assessment more effective. *J. Contin. Educ. Health Prof.* 28(1):20–24. [15]

Galesic, M., and R. Garcia-Retamero. 2010. Statistical numeracy for health: A cross-cultural comparison with probabilistic national samples. *Arch. Intern. Med.* 170(5):462–468. [2]

Galesic, M., R. Garcia-Retamero, and G. Gigerenzer. 2009. Using icon arrays to communicate medical risks: Overcoming low numeracy. *Health Psychol.* 28:210–216. [2]

Galesic, M., G. Gigerenzer, and N. Straubinger. 2009. Natural frequencies help older adults and people with low numeracy to evaluate medical screening tests. *Med. Decis. Making* 29:368–371. [2]

Galtung, J., and M. H. Ruge. 1965. The structure of foreign news: The presentation of Congo, Cuba and Cyprus crisis in four Norwegian newspapers. *J. Peace Res.* 2:64–91. [11]

Gandhi, G. Y., M. H. Murad, A. Fujiyoshi, et al. 2008. Patient-important outcomes in registered diabetes trials. *JAMA* 299:2543–2549. [13]

Garattini, S. 2007. The independent clinical trials of AIFA. http://www.ambitalia.org.uk/Clinical_GL/Garattini.pdf (accessed 27 April 2010). [13]

Garfield, J., and D. Ben-Zvi. 2007. How students learn statistics revisited: A current review of research on teaching and learning statistics. *Intl. Stat. Rev.* 75:372–296. [2, 12]

Gawande, A. 2009. The cost conundrum: What a Texas town can teach us about health care. *New Yorker*, 1 June 2009. [1]

Gawande, A., D. Berwick, E. Fisher, and M. B. McClellan. 2009. 10 steps to better health care. *New York Times*, August 13. [1]

Gazmararian, J. A., J. W. Curran, R. M. Parker, J. M. Bernhardt, and B. A. DeBuono. 2005. Public health literacy in America: An ethical imperative. *Am. J. Prev. Med.* 28:317–322. [12]

General Medical Council. 1998. Seeking patients' consent: The ethical considerations. London: GMC. [2]

Geraedts, M. 2006. Versorgungsforschung in der operativen Medizin am Beispiel der Mamma-Karzinom-Chirurgie. *Gesundheitsfor. Gesundheitsschutz* 49:160–166. [1]

Bibliography

Ghosh, A. K., and K. Ghosh. 2005. Translating evidence-based information into effective risk communication: Current challenges and opportunities. *J. Lab. Clin. Med.* **145**:171–180. [1, 9]

Giacomini, K. M., R. M. Krauss, D. M. Roden, et al. 2007. When good drugs go bad. *Nature* **446**:975–977. [18]

Giersdorf, N., A. Loh, C. Bieber, et al. 2004. Entwicklung eines Fragebogens zur partizipativen Entscheidungsfindung. *Bundes. Gesundheitsfor. Gesundheitsschutz* **47**:969–976. [4]

Gigerenzer, G. 2002. Calculated Risks: How to Know When Numbers Deceive You. New York: Simon & Schuster. [Reckoning with Risk: Learning to Live with Uncertainty, Penguin.] [1, 2, 9–11]

———. 2004. Mindless statistics. *J. Socio. Econ.* **33(5)**:587–606. [10]

———. 2007. Gut Feelings: The Intelligence of the Unconscious. New York: Viking Press. [1]

———. 2008. Moral intuition = Fast and frugal heuristics? In: Moral Psychology, vol. 2., The Cognitive Science of Morality: Intuition and Diversity, ed. W. Sinnott-Armstrong, pp. 1–26. Cambridge, MA: MIT Press. [19]

Gigerenzer, G., and H. Brighton. 2009. Homo heuristicus: Why biased minds make better inferences. *Top. Cogn. Sci.* **1**:107–143. [17]

Gigerenzer, G., and A. Edwards. 2003. Simple tools for understanding risks: From innumeracy to insight. *BMJ* **327**:741–744. [12, 16]

Gigerenzer, G., W. Gaissmaier, E. Kurz-Milcke, L. M. Schwartz, and S. Woloshin. 2007. Helping doctors and patients make sense of health statistics. *Psychol. Sci. Publ. Interest* **8**:53–96. [1–3, 8–12, 16, 19]

Gigerenzer, G., and D. G. Goldstein. 1996. Reasoning the fast and frugal way: Models of bounded rationality. *Psychol. Rev.* **103**:650–669. [17]

Gigerenzer, G., and U. Hoffrage. 1995. How to improve Bayesian reasoning without instruction: Frequency formats. *Psychol. Rev.* **102**:684–704. [2, 9]

———. 1999. Helping people overcome difficulties in Bayesian reasoning: A reply to Lewis and Keren (1999) and Mellers and McGraw (1999). *Psychol. Rev.* **106**:425–430. [2, 9]

Gigerenzer, G., U. Hoffrage, and A. Ebert. 1998. AIDS counselling for low-risk clients. *AIDS Care* **10**:197–211. [1, 9]

Gigerenzer, G., J. Mata, and R. Frank. 2009. Public knowledge of benefits of breast and prostate cancer screening in Europe. *J. Natl. Cancer Inst.* **101**:1216–1220. [1, 2, 9, 11]

Gigerenzer, G., Z. Swijtink, T. Porter, L. Daston, J. Beatty, and L. Krüger. 1989. The empire of chance: How probability changed science and everyday life. Cambridge: Cambridge Univ. Press. [9, 13]

Gilbody, S., P. Wilson, and I. Watt. 2005. Benefits and harms of direct to consumer advertising: A systematic review. *Qual. Saf. Health Care* **14**:246–250. [18]

Giles, J. 2005. Internet encyclopedias go head to head. *Nature* **438**:900–901. [19]

Gillespie, R., D. Florin, and S. Gillam. 2002. Changing Relationships: Findings from the Patient Involvement Project. London: King's Fund. [4]

Glasgow, R. E., E. Fisher, D. Haire-Joshu, and M. G. Goldstein. 2007. National Institutes of Health science agenda: A public health perspective. *Am. J. Public Health* **97**:1936–1938. [5]

Glasziou, P., and B. Haynes. 2005. The paths from research to improved health outcomes. *Evid. Based Nurs.* **8**:36–38. [16]

Glickman, S. W., J. McHutchison, E. Peterson, et al. 2009. Ethical and scientific implications of the globalization of clinical research. *N. Engl. J. Med.* **360**:816–823. [5]

GLISC. 2007. Guidelines for the production of scientific and technical reports: How to write and distribute grey literature (Version 1.1.). Grey Literature International Steering Committee. http://www.glisc.info (accessed 7 June 2010). [6]

Glover, J. A. 1938. The incidence of tonsillectomy in children. *Proc. R. Soc. Med.* **31**:1219–1236. [3]

Gold, J. L. 2003. Paternalistic or protective? Freedom of expression and direct-to-consumer drug advertising policy in Canada. *Health Law Rev.* **11**:30–36. [18]

González, A. B., M. Mahesh, K.-P. Kim, et al. 2009. Projected cancer risks from computed tomographic scans performed in the United States in 2007. *Arch. Intern. Med.* **169(22)**:2071–2077. [1]

Goodman, S. N., J. Berlin, S. W. Fletcher, and R. H. Fletcher. 1994. Manuscript quality before and after peer review and editing at *Annals of Internal Medicine. Ann. Int. Med.* **121**:11–21. [7]

Gøtzsche, P. C., A. Hrobjartsson, H. K. Johansen, et al. 2006. Constraints on publication rights in industry-initiated clinical trials. *JAMA* **295(14)**:1645–1646. [7]

———. 2007. Ghost authorship in industry-initiated randomised trials. *PLoS Med.* **4(e19)**. [13]

Gøtzsche, P. C., and M. Nielsen. 2006. Screening for breast cancer with mammography. *Cochrane Database Syst. Rev.* **4**:CD001877. [2, 9]

GRADE Working Group. 2004. Grading quality of evidence and strength of recommendations. *BMJ* **328**:1490. [12]

———. 2010. http://www.gradeworkinggroup.org (accessed 30 April 2010). [6]

Gray, J. A. M. 2002. The Resourceful Patient. Oxford: eRosetta Press. [1]

Green, L. A., and D. R. Mehr. 1997. What alters physicians' decisions to admit to the coronary care unit? *J. Fam. Pract.* **45**:219–226. [17]

Green, L. W., J. Ottoson, C. Garcia, and R. Hiatt. 2009. Diffusion theory and knowledge dissemination, utilization, and integration in public health. *Annu. Rev. Public Health* **30**:151–174. [5]

Greenhalgh, T. 2006. How to Read a Paper? The Basics of Evidence-based Medicine. London: BMJ Books. [11]

Greiner, A. C., and E. Knebel, eds. 2003. Health Professions Education: A Bridge to Quality. Washington, D.C.: National Academies Press. [15]

Griffiths, K. M., and H. Christensen. 2005. Website quality indicators for consumers. *J. Med. Internet Res.* **7**:e55. [11]

Grill, M. 2007. Kranke Geschäfte: Wie die Pharmaindustrie uns manipuliert. Reinbek: Rowohlt. [12]

———. 2009. Alarm und Fehlalarm. *Der Spiegel.* http://www.spiegel.de/spiegel/print/d-65089115.html (accessed 30 June 2010). [11]

Grime, J., A. Blenkinsopp, D. K. Raynor, K. Pollock, and P. Knapp. 2007. The role and value of written information for patients about individual medicines: A systematic review. *Health Expect.* **10**:286–298. [18]

Griscti, O., and J. Jacono. 2006. Effectiveness of continuing education programs in nursing: Literature review. *J. Adv. Nurs.* **55(4)**:449–456. [15]

Grol, R. 2001. Improving the quality of medical care: Building bridges among professional pride, payer profit, and patient satisfaction. *JAMA* **186(20)**:2578–2585. [15]

Grol, R., M. Wensing, J. Mainz, et al. 2000. Patients in Europe evaluate general practice care: An international comparison. *Br. J. Gen. Pract.* **50(460)**:882–887. [13]

362 *Bibliography*

Gross, C. P., G. Anderson, and N. Powe. 1999. The relation between funding by the National Institutes of Health and the burden of disease. *N. Engl. J. Med.* **340**:1881–1887. [5]

Gross, L. 2009. A broken trust: Lessons from the vaccine-autism wars. *PLoS Biol.* 7:e1000114. [10]

Groves, T. 2008. Mandatory disclosure of trial results for drugs and devices. *BMJ* **336**:170. [6]

GU. 2010. Gesundheits-Uni Jena. http://www.gesundheitsuni.uniklinikum-jena.de/ (accessed 1 June 2010). [19]

Guadagnoli, E., and P. Ward. 1998. Patient participation in decision making. *Soc. Sci. Med.* **47**:329–339. [4]

Guyatt, G. H., A. D. Oxman, G. E. Vist, et al. 2008. GRADE: An emerging consensus on rating quality of evidence and strength of recommendations. *BMJ* **336**:924–926. [6]

Guyatt, G. H., and D. Rennie. 1993. Users' guides to the medical literature. *JAMA* **270**:2096–2097. [11]

Guyatt, G. H., D. Rennie, M. Meade, and D. Cook. 2008. Users' Guide to the Medical Literature: A Manual for Evidence-based Clinical Practice. Chicago: McGraw Hill. [6]

Guyatt, G. H., D. L. Sackett, J. C. Sinclair, et al. 1995. Users' guides to the medical literature IX: A method for grading health care recommendations. *JAMA* **274**:1800–1804. [11]

Hallowell, N., H. Statham, F. Murton, J. Green, and M. Richards. 1997. Talking about chance: The presentation of risk information during genetic counseling for breast and ovarian cancer. *J. Genet. Couns.* **6**:269–286. [2, 12]

Halstead, L. S. 1976. Team care in chronic illness: A critical review of the literature of the past 25 years. *Arch. Phys. Rehab. Med.* **57**:507–511. [15]

Ham, C. 2008. World class commissioning: A health policy chimera. *J. Health Serv. Res. Policy* **13**:116–121. [16]

Hamann, J., B. Neuner, J. Kasper, et al. 2007. Participation preferences of patients with acute and chronic conditions. *Health Expect.* **10**:358–363. [4]

Hamm, R. M., and S. L. Smith. 1998. The accuracy of patients' judgments of disease probability and test sensitivity and specificity. *J. Fam. Pract.* **47**:44–52. [2]

Hammersley, M. 2005. Is the evidence-based practice movement doing more good than harm? Reflections on Iain Chalmers' case for research-based policy making and practice. *Evid. Policy* **1**:85–100. [16]

Hammerstein, P., E. H. Hagen, A. V. M. Herz, and H. Herzel. 2006. Robustness: A key to evolutionary design. *Biol. Theory* **1**:90–93. [17]

Hand, D. J. 2006. Classifer technology and the illusion of progress. *Stat. Sci.* **21**:1–14. [17]

Hansen, R. A., J. C. Schommer, R. R. Cline, et al. 2005. The association of consumer cost-sharing and direct-to-consumer advertising with prescription drug use. *Res. Soc. Admin. Pharm.* **1**:139–157. [18]

Harrison Survey. 2008. Academic CME in North America: The 2008 AAMC/SACME Harrison Survey. AAMC. [15]

Hartz, J., and R. Chappell. 1997. Worlds Apart: How the Distance between Science and Journalism Threatens America's Future. Nashville: First Amendment Center. [2]

Hastings, G. 2007. Social Marketing: Why Should the Devil Have All the Best Tunes? Amsterdam: Elsevier Butterworth Heinemann. [13]

Hawker, G. A., J. G. Wright, P. C. Coyte, et al. 2001 Determining the need for hip and knee arthroplasty: The role of clinical severity and patients' preferences. *Med. Care* **39(3)**:206–216. [3]

Hawley, S. T., B. J. Zikmund-Fisher, P. A. Ubel, et al. 2008. The impact of the format of graphical presentation on health-related knowledge and treatment choices. *Patient Educ. Couns.* **73**:448–455. [2]

Hayek, F. A. 1945. The use of knowledge in society. *Am. Econ. Rev.* **35**:519–530. [1]

Haynes, R. B. 1993. Where's the meat in clinical journals? *ACP J. Club* **119**:A23–A24. [16]

Haynes, R. B., A. McKibbon, and R. Kanani. 1996. Systematic review of randomised trials of interventions to assist patients to follow prescriptions for medications. *Lancet* **348**:383–386. [16]

Haywood, K., S. Marshall, and R. Fitzpatrick. 2006. Patient participation in the consultation process: A structured review of intervention strategies. *Patient Educ. Couns.* **63**:12–23. [4]

Headrick, L. A. 2000. Learning to improve complex systems of care. In: Collaborative Education to Ensure Patient Safety. Washington, D.C.: HRSA/Bureau of Health Professions. [15]

Health News Review. 2010. Independent expert reviews of news stories. http://www.healthnewsreview.org/ (accessed 25 May 2010). [12]

Higgins, J. P. T., and S. Green, eds. 2009. Cochrane handbook for systematic reviews of interventions, version 5.0.2 (updated Sept 2009). http://www.cochrane-handbook.org (accessed 24 May 2010). [12]

Hill, K. P., J. S. Ross, D. S. Egilman, and H. M. Krumholz. 2008. The ADVANTAGE seeding trial: A review of internal documents. *Ann. Int. Med.* **149**:251–258. [13]

Ho, K., S. Jarvis-Selinger, F. Borduas, et al. 2008. Making interprofessional education work: The strategic roles of the Academy. *Acad. Med.* **83(10)**:934–940. [15]

Hoffrage, U., and G. Gigerenzer. 1998. Using natural frequencies to improve diagnostic inferences. *Acad. Med.* **73**:538–540. [3, 9, 16]

Hoffrage, U., G. Gigerenzer, S. Krauss, and L. Martignon. 2002. Representation facilitates reasoning: What natural frequencies are and what they are not. *Cognition* **84**:343–352. [2, 9]

Hoffrage, U., S. Lindsey, R. Hertwig, and G. Gigerenzer. 2000. Communicating statistical information. *Science* **290**:2261–2262. [1, 12]

Holte, R. C. 1993. Very simple classification rules perform well on most commonly used datasets. *Machine Learn.* **11**: 63–91. [17]

HoN. 2010. Health on the Net Foundation. http://www.hon.ch (accessed 9 June 2010). [13]

Hopewell, S., S. Dutton, L.-M. Yu, A.-W. Chan, and D. G. Altman. 2010. The quality of reports of randomised trials in 2000 and 2006: Comparative study of articles indexed in PubMed. *BMJ* **340**:c723. [8]

Hopkins Tanne, J. 2003. US guidelines say blood pressure of 120/80 mm Hg is not "normal." *BMJ* **326**:1104. [13]

Hornbostel, S. 1997. Wissenschaftsindikatoren: Bewertungen in der Wissenschaft. Opladen: Westdeutscher Verlag. [11]

Horton, R. 2004. The dawn of McScience. *New York Rev. Books* **51(4)**:7–9. [1]

House of Commons. 2005. The Influence of the Pharmaceutical Industry: Fourth Report of Session 2004–05. London: House of Commons, Health Committee. [18]

Hugman, B., and I. R. Edwards. 2006. The challenge of effectively communicating patient safety information. *Expert Opin. Drug. Saf.* **5**:495–499. [18]

HWG. 2006. Gesetz über die Werbung auf dem Gebiete des Heilwesens. Bekanntmachung vom 19 Oktober 1994 (BGBl. I S. 3068), zuletzt geändert durch Artikel 2 des Gesetzes (BGBl. I S. 984) vom 26 April 2006. Heilmittelwerbegesetz. [18]

ICMJE. 2010. Uniform requirements for manuscripts submitted to biomedical journals http://www.icmje.org/ (accessed 7 June 2010). [6]

Ikonen, T. S., H. Anttila, H. Gylling, et al. 2009. Surgical Treatment of Morbid Obesity, Report 16, pp. 22–25. Helsinki: National Institute for Health and Welfare. [8]

Impiccatore, P., C. Pandolfini, N. Casella, and M. Bonati. 1997. Reliability of health information for the public on the world wide web: Systemic survey of advice on managing fever in children at home. *BMJ* **314**:1875–1879. [2]

Information Standard. 2010. http://www.theinformationstandard.org (accessed 2 June 2010). [13]

Ioannidis, J. 2005. Why most published research findings are false. *PLoS Med.* **2**:e124. [10, 16, 19]

Ioannidis, J., S. Evans, P. Gøtzsche, et al. 2004. Better reporting of harms in randomized trials: An extension of the CONSORT statement. *Ann. Int. Med.* **141**:781–788. [12]

IOM. 2001. Crossing the Quality Chasm: A New Health System for the 21st Century. Institute of Medicine. Washington, D.C.: National Academies Press. [16]

———. 2004. Health Literacy: A Prescription to End Confusion. Institute of Medicine. Washington, D.C.: National Academies Press. [12, 16]

IQWiG. 2009. Pfizer conceals study data. Cologne: IQWiG. http://www.iqwig.de/index.868.en.html?random=405f75 (accessed 28 April 2010). [6]

ISDB. 2006. International society of drug bulletins' program for promoting independent information. http://www.icf.uab.es/informacion/boletines/bg/ISDB.pdf (accessed 1 June 2010). [18]

ISDB, MiEF, HAI, and AIM. 2008. Open letter: The European Commission's "proposal on information to patients" will boost drug sales not serve patients' interests. Response to the consultation on the legal proposal on information to patients. http://www.isdbweb.org/documents/uploads/theee.pdf (accessed 31 May 2010). [18]

Jadad, A. R., and M. Enkin. 2007. Randomized Controlled Trials: Questions, Answers and Musings. Oxford: Blackwell. [16]

Jadad, A. R., M. Moher, G. P. Browman, L. Booker, and C. Sigouin. 2000. Systematic reviews and meta-analyses on treatment of asthma: Critical evaluation. *BMJ* **320**:537–540. [7]

Jefferson, T., and F. Godlee. 1999. Peer Review in Health Sciences. London: BMJ Books. [7]

JNCI. 2010. Reporting on cancer research. http://www.oxfordjournals.org/our_journals/jnci/resource/reporting_on_cancer.html (accessed 19 May 2010). [10]

Johnson, E. J., and D. Goldstein. 2003. Do defaults save lives? *Science* **302**:1338–1339. [19]

Johnson, T. 1998. Shattuck lecture: Medicine and the media. *N. Engl. J. Med.* **339**:87–92. [11]

Jorgensen, K. J., and P. C. Gøtzsche. 2004. Presentation on websites of possible benefits and harms from screening for breast cancer: Cross sectional study. *BMJ* **328**:148. [1, 2]

———. 2006. Content of invitations for publicly funded screening mammography. *BMJ* **332**:538–541. [2]

Kahn, C. E., A. Santos, C. Thao, et al. 2007. A presentation system for just-in-time learning in radiology. *J. Digit. Imag.* **20**:6–16. [15]

Kahneman, D., P. Slovic, and A. Tversky, eds. 1982. Judgment under Uncertainty: Heuristics and Biases. New York: Cambridge Univ. Press. [2]

Kaiser Family Foundation. 2008. Prescription drug trends. http://www.kff.org/rxdrugs/upload/3057_07.pdf (accessed 31 May 2010). [18]

Kaiser, J. 2008. Making clinical data widely available. *Science* **322**:217–218. [18]

Kaiser, T., H. Ewers, A. Waltering, et al. 2004. Sind die Aussagen medizinischer werbeprospekte korrekt? *Arznei Telegramm* **35**:21–23. [1, 9, 18]

Kallen, A., S. Woloshin, J. Shu, E. Juhl, and L. Schwartz. 2007. Direct-to-consumer advertisements for HIV antiretroviral medications: A progress report. *Health Affairs* **26**:1392–1398. [14]

Kant, I. 1784. Beantwortung der Frage: Was ist Aufklärung? *Berl. Monatsschr.* **Dez.**:481–494. [9]

Kaphingst, K. A., W. DeJong, R. E. Rudd, and L. H. Daltroy. 2004. A content analysis of direct-to-consumer television prescription drug advertisements. *J. Health Commun.* **9**:515–528. [2, 18]

Kaphingst, K. A., R. E. Rudd, W. DeJong, and L. H. Daltroy. 2005. Comprehension of information in three direct-to-consumer television prescription drug advertisements among adults with limited literacy. *J. Health Commun.* **10**:609–619. [2]

Kaplan, R., and D. Frosch. 2005. Decision making in medicine and health care. *Annu. Rev. Clin. Psych.* **1**:525–556. [4]

Kasper, J. F., A. G. Mulley, Jr., and J. E. Wennberg. 1992. Developing shared decision-making programs to improve the quality of health care. *Qual. Rev. Bull.* **18(6)**:183–190. [3]

Kawachi, I., and P. Conrad. 1996. Medicalization and the pharmacological treatment of blood pressure. In: Contested Ground: Public Purpose and Private Interests in the Regulation of Prescription Drugs, ed. P. Davis. New York: Oxford Univ. Press. [18]

Kees, B. 2002. Newsroom training: Where's the investment? Miami: Knight Foundation. http://www.knightfoundation.org/research_publications/detail.dot?id=178205 (accessed 27 April 2010). [2, 10, 12]

Kell, C. M. 2007. The influence of an undergraduate curriculum on development of students' academic belief systems. *Learn. Health Soc. Care* **6(2)**:83–93. [15]

Kennedy, A. D., M. J. Sculpher, A. Coulter, et al. 2002. Effects of decision aids for menorrhagia on treatment choices, health outcomes, and costs: A randomized controlled trial. *JAMA* **288**:2701–2708. [3]

Kerner, J., B. Rimer, and K. Emmons. 2005. Dissemination research and research dissemination: How can we close the gap? *Health Psychol.* **24**:443–446. [5]

Kindel, A. 1998. Erinnern von Radio-Nachrichten: Empirische Studie über die Selektionsleistungen der Hörer von Radio-Nachrichten. Munich: Reinhard Fischer. [11]

Kirkpatrick, D. L. 1979. Techniques for evaluating training programs In: Classic Writings on Instructional Technology, ed. D. P. Ely and T. Plomp, pp. 231–241. vol. 1. Englewood: Libraries Unlimited Inc. [13]

Kitano, H. 2004. Biological robustness. *Nat. Rev. Genet.* **5**:826–837. [17]

Klemperer, D., B. Lang, K. Koch, et al. 2009. 10te Jahrestagung des Deutschen Netzwerks Evidenzbasierte Medizin: Evidenzbasierte Patienteninformationen, Vorstellung eines Standards. Berlin: Gute Praxis Gesundheitsinformation. [18]

Klemperer, D., B. Lang, K. Koch, et al. 2010. Die "Gute Praxis Gesundheitsinformation." *Z. Evid. Fortbild. Qual. Gesundhwes.* **104**:66–68. [13]

Kohn, L. T., J. M. Corrigan, and M. S. Donaldson, eds. 2000. To Err Is Human: Building a Safer Health System. Washington, D.C.: National Academy Press. [1]

Kohring, M. 1998. Der Zeitung die Gesetze der Wissenschaft vorschreiben? Wissenschaftsjournalismus und Journalismus-Wissenschaft. *Rundf. Fernsehen* **46**:175. [11]

———. 2005. Wissenschaftsjournalismus: Forschungsüberblick und Theorieentwurf. Konstanz: UVK Verlagsgesellschaft. [11]

Kommission der EU Gemeinschaftern. 2008a. Verordnung des Europäischen Parlaments und des Rates zur Änderung der Verordnung EG Nr. 726/2004 zur Festlegung von Gemeinschaftsverfahren für die Genehmigung und Überwachung von Human- und Tierarzneimitteln und zur Errichtung einer Europäischen Arzneimittel-Agentur hinsichtlich der Pharmakovigilanz von Humanarzneimitteln. http://eur-lex.europa. eu/LexUriServ/LexUriServ.do?uri=COM:2008:0664:FIN:DE:PDF (accessed 21 June 2010). [18]

————. Vorschlag für eine des Europäischen Parlaments und des Rates zur Änderung der Richtlinie 2001/83/EG zur Schaffung eines Gemeinschaftskodexes für Humanarzneimittel hinsichtlich der Pharmakovigilanz. http://eur-lex.europa.eu/ LexUriServ/LexUriServ.do?uri=COM: 2008:0665:FIN:DE:PDF (accessed 21 June 2010). [18]

Kondro, W. 2009. Exit interview with Dr. Alan Bernstein. *CMAJ* **177**:844–845. [5]

Konold, C., and C. D. Miller. 2005. TinkerPlots dynamic data exploration (Version 1.0, Computer software). Emeryville, CA: Key Curriculum Press. http://www.keypress. com/tinkerplots. [12]

Krantz, D., A. Baum, and M. von Wideman. 1980. Assessment of preferences for self-treatment and information in health care. *J. Pers. Soc. Psych.* **5**:977–990. [4]

Kravitz, R. L., R. M. Epstein, M. D. Feldman, et al. 2005. Influence of patients' requests for direct-to-consumer advertised antidepressants: A randomized controlled trial. *JAMA* **293(16)**:1995–2002. [18]

Krleza-Jeric, K., A.-W. Chan, K. Dickersin, et al. 2005. Principles for international registration of protocol information and results from human trials of health related interventions: Ottawa statement (part 1). *BMJ* **330**:956–958. [6]

Krueger, J., and R. A. Mueller. 2002. Unskilled, unaware, or both? The better-than-average heuristic and statistical regression predict errors in estimates of own performance. *J. Pers. Soc. Psych.* **82**:189–192. [16]

Kruger, J., and D. Dunning. 1999. Unskilled and unaware of it: How difficulties in recognizing one's own incompetence lead to inflated self-assessments. *J. Pers. Soc. Psychol.* **77 (6)**:1121–1134. [16]

Kuhn, T. S. 1962. The Structure of Scientific Revolutions. Chicago: Univ. Chicago Press. [19]

————. 1996. The Structure of Scientific Revolutions, 3rd ed. Chicago: Univ. Chicago Press. [5]

Kunnamo, I., and J. Jousimaa. 2004. Tietoverkot ja sähköinen maailma hoitosuositusten toteuttamisessa (in Finnish). *Duodecim* **120**:119–126. [12]

Kurz-Milcke, E., G. Gigerenzer, and L. Martignon. 2008. Transparency in risk communication: Graphical and analog tools. In: Strategies for Risk Communication: Evolution, Evidence, Experience, ed. W. T. Tucker et al., pp. 18–28. New York: Blackwell. [2, 5]

Kurzenhäuser, S. 2003. Welche Informationen vermitteln deutsche Gesundheits-broschüren über die Screening-Mammographie? [What information do German health brochures provide on mammography screening?]. *Z. Ärzt. Fortbild. Qualität.* **97**:53–57. [2]

Kurzenhäuser, S., and U. Hoffrage. 2002. Teaching Bayesian reasoning: An evaluation of a classroom tutorial for medical students. *Med. Teacher* **24(5)**:516–521. [9]

Labarge, A. S., R. J. McCaffrey, and T. A. Brown. 2003. Neuropsychologists' ability to determine the predictive value of diagnostic tests. *Arch. Clin. Neuropsychol.* **18**:165–175. [9]

Lai, W. Y. Y., and T. Lane. 2009. Characteristics of medical research news reported on front pages of newspapers. *PLoS ONE* 4:e6103. [11]

Lancet. 1937. Editorial: Mathematics and medicine. *Lancet* 1:31 [2, 12]

Langley, P., W. Iba, and K. Thompson. 1992. An analysis of Bayesian Classifiers. In: Proc. 10th Natl. Conf. on Artificial Intelligence, pp. 399–406. San Jose, CA: AAAI Press. [17]

Larsson, A., A. D. Oxman, C. Carling, and J. Herrin. 2003. Medical messages in the media: Barriers and solutions to improving medical journalism. *Health Expect.* 6:323–331. [11]

Lasser, K. E., P. D. Allen, S. J. Woolhandler, et al. 2002. Timing of new black box warnings and withdrawals for prescription medications. *JAMA* **287(17)**:2215–2220. [18]

Laurent, M. R., and T. J. Vickers. 2009. Seeking health information online: Does Wikipedia matter? *J. Am. Med. Inform. Assoc.* **16**:471–479. [19]

Law, M. R., S. R. Majumdar, and S. B. Soumerai. 2008. Effect of illicit direct to consumer advertising on use of Etanercept, Mometasone, and Tegaserod in Canada: Controlled longitudinal study. *BMJ* **337**:a1055. [18]

Lean, M. E. J., J. I. Mann, J. A. Hoek, R. M. Elliot, and G. Schofield. 2008. Translational research. *BMJ* **337**:a863. [12]

Lee, M. D., N. Loughlin, and I. B. Lundberg. 2002. Applying one reason decision-making: The prioritization of literature searches. *Aust. J. Psychol.* **54**:137–143. [17]

Légaré, F., S. Ratté, K. Gravel, and I. D. Graham. 2008. Barriers and facilitators to implementing shared decision-making in clinical practice: Update of a systematic review of health professionals' perceptions. *Patient Educ. Couns.* **73**:526–535. [19]

Légaré, F., S. Ratté, D. Stacey, et al. 2010. Interventions for improving the adoption of shared decision making by healthcare professionals. *Cochrane Database Syst. Rev.* 5:CD006732. [19]

Lenzer, J. 2009. Prominent celecoxib researcher admits fabricating data in 21 articles. *BMJ* **338**:966 [13]

Lepore, J. 2009. Editorial: It's spreading. *The New Yorker*, pp. 46–50, June 1. [10]

Levi, R. 2001. Medical Journalism: Exposing Fact, Fiction, Fraud. Oxford: Iowa State Univ. Press. [11]

Levin, L. A., and J. G. Palmer. 2007. Institutional review boards should require clinical trial registration. *Arch. Intern. Med.* **167**:1576–1580. [6]

Levinson, W., A. Kao, A. Kuby, and R. A. Thisted. 2005. Not all patients want to participate in decision making. *J. Gen. Intern. Med.* **20**:531–535. [4]

Lewenstein, B. 1995. Science and the media. In: Handbook of Science and Technology Studies, ed. G. E. Markle et al., pp. 343–360. London: Sage. [11]

Lewis, T. R., J. H. Reichman, and A. D. So. 2007. The case for public funding and public oversight of clinical trials. *Economists' Voice* **4(3)**. [13]

Lexchin, J., L. A. Bero, B. Djulbegovic, and O. Clark. 2003. Pharmaceutical industry sponsorship and research outcome and quality: Systematic review. *BMJ* **326**:1167–1170. [1, 13, 16, 18]

Lexchin, J., and B. Mintzes. 2002. Direct-to-consumer advertising of prescription drugs: The evidence says no. *J. Publ. Pol. Market.* **21**:194–201. [18]

Li, M., S. Chapman, K. Agho, and C. J. Eastman. 2008. Can even minimal news coverage influence consumer health-related behaviour? A case study of iodized salt sales, Australia. *Health Educ. Res.* **23**:543–548. [11]

Liao, L., J. G. Jollis, E. R. DeLong, et al. 1996. Impact of an interactive video on decision making of patients with ischemic heart disease. *J. Gen. Intern. Med.* **11(6)**:373–376. [3]

Lieberman, J. A., T. S. Stroup, J. P. McEvoy, et al. 2005. Effectiveness of antipsychotic drugs in patients with chronic schizophrenia. *N. Engl. J. Med.* **353**:1209–1223. [13]

Lipkus, I. M. 2007. Numeric, verbal, and visual formats of conveying health risks: Suggested best practices and future recommendations. *Med. Decis. Making* **27**:696–713. [2]

Lipkus, I. M., G. Samsa, and B. K. Rimer. 2001. General performance on a numeracy scale among highly educated samples. *Med. Decis. Making* **21**:37–44. [2]

Little, J., J. P. T. Higgins, J. P. A. Ioannidis, et al. 2009. Strengthening the reporting of genetic association studies (STREGA): An extension of the STROBE statement. *PLoS Med.* **6(2)**:e1000022. [6]

Llewellyn-Thomas, H. 2006. Measuring patients' preferences for participating in health care decisions: Avoiding invalid observations. *Health Expect.* **9**:305–306. [4]

Lo, B., and M. J. Field, eds. 2009. Committee on Conflict of Interest in Medical Research, Education, and Practice, S4–S5. Washington, D.C.: National Academies Press. [12, 13]

Loh, A., D. Simon, C. E. Wills, et al. 2007. The effects of a shared decision making intervention in primary care of depression: A cluster-randomized controlled trial. *Patient Educ. Couns.* **67**:324–332. [4]

Ludwig, W.-D., M. Hildebrandt, and G. Schott. 2009. Interessenkonflikte und Arzneimittelstudien: Einfluss der pharmazeutischen Industrie und daraus resultierende Gefahren für die Integrität der medizinischen Wissenschaft. *Z. Evid. Fortbild. Qual. Gesundhwes.* **103**:149–154. [18]

Lurie, J. D., N. J. Birkmeyer, and J. N. Weinstein. 2003. Rates of advanced spinal imaging and spine surgery. *Spine* **28(6)**:616–620. [3]

Machiavelli. 1513. Il Principe. http://www.fordham.edu/halsall/basis/machiavelli-prince.html [accessed 2 June 2010]. [19]

Macias, W., and L. S. Lewis. 2005. How well do direct-to-consumer, DTC, prescription drug web sites meet FDA guidelines and public policy concerns? *Health Mark Q.* **22**:45–71. [18]

Macias, W., K. Pashupati, and L. S. Lewis. 2007. A wonderful life or diarrhea and dry mouth? Policy issues of direct-to-consumer drug advertising on television. *Health Commun.* **22(3)**:241–252. [18]

Macintyre, S., I. Chalmers, R. Horton, and R. Smith. 2001. Using evidence to inform health policy: Case study. *BMJ* **322**:222–225. [16]

Mackenzie, F. J., C. F. C. Jordens, R. A. Ankeny, J. McPhee, and I. H. Kerridge. 2007. Direct-to-consumer advertising under the radar: The need for realistic drugs policy in Australia. *Intern. Med. J.* **37(4)**:224–228. [18]

Madore, O., and S. Norris. 2006. Federal Funding for Health Research. Ottawa: Parliamentary Information and Research Service. [5]

Maguire, P., and C. Pitceathly. 2002. Key communication skills and how to acquire them. *BMJ* **325**:697–700. [4]

Mäkelä, M., and R. Roine. 2009. Health technology assessment in Finland. *Intl. J. Technol. Assess. Health Care* **25(S1)**:102–107. [8]

Makoul, G., and M. Clayman. 2006. An integrative model of shared decision making in medical encounters. *Patient Educ. Couns.* **60**:301–312. [4]

Makridakis, S., and M. Hibon. 1979. Accuracy of forecasting: An empirical investigation (with discussion). *J. R. Stat. Soc. Ser. A* **142**:79–145. [17]

Malenka, D. J., J. A. Baron, S. Johansen, J. W. Wahrenberger, and J. M. Ross. 1993. The framing effect of relative versus absolute risk. *J. Gen. Intern. Med.* **8**:543–548. [2]

Mansfield, P. R., J. Lexchin, L. S. Wen, et al. 2006. Educating health professionals about drug and device promotion: Advocates' recommendations. *PLoS Med* **3(11)**:e451. [18]

Marinopoulous, S. S., T. Dorman, and N. Ratanawongsa. 2007. Effectiveness of Continuing Medical Education. Rockville, MD: Agency for Healthcare Research and Quality. [15]

Marsick, V. J. 1987. New paradigms for learning in the workplace. In: Learning in the Workplace, ed. V. J. Marsick, pp. 1–30, 187. London: Croom Helm. [15]

Martignon, L., and S. Krauss. 2009. Hands on activities with fourth-graders: A tool box of heuristics for decision making and reckoning with risk. *IEJME* **4(3)**:227–258. [8]

Martignon, L., and E. Kurz-Milcke. 2006. Educating children in stochastic modeling: Games with stochastic urns and colored tinkercubes. Proc. of the ICOTS 7 Conf. in Teaching Statistics. Brazil: ICOTS. [12]

Mathieu, S., I. Boutron, D. Moher, D. G. Altman, and P. Ravaud. 2009. Comparison of registered and published primary outcomes in randomized controlled trials. *JAMA* **302**:977–984. [6, 13]

Maudsley, R., D. Wilson, V. Neufeld, et al. 2000. Educating future physicians for Ontario: Phase II. *Acad. Med.* **75(2)**:113–126. [15]

McAlister, F. A., H. D. Clark, C. van Walraven, and S. E. Straus. 1999. The medical review article revisited: Has the science improved? *Ann. Int. Med.* **131**:947–951. [7]

McDonough, J. E. 2000. Experiencing Politics. Berkeley: Univ. of California Press. [5]

McGettigan, P., K. Sly, D. O'Connell, S. Hill, and D. Henry. 1999. The effects of information framing on the practices of physicians. *J. Gen. Intern. Med.* **14**:633–642. [9]

McGlynn, E. A., S. M. Asch, J. Adams, et al. 2003. The quality of health care delivered to adults in the United States. *N. Engl. J. Med.* **348(26)**:2635–2645. [15]

McGowan, J., W. Hogg, C. Campbell, and M. Rowan. 2008. Just-in-time information improved decision-making in primary care: A randomized controlled trial. *PLoS ONE* **3(11)**:e3785. [15]

McKibbon, K., N. Wilczynski, and R. Haynes. 2004. What do evidence-based secondary journals tell us about the publication of clinically important articles in primary healthcare journals? *BMC Med.* **2(1)**:33. [7]

McPherson, K., J. E. Wennberg, and C. P. Hovind. 1982. Small-area variations in the use of common surgical procedures: An international comparison of New England, England, and Norway. *N. Engl. J. Med.* **307(21)**:1310–1314. [3]

McQuail, D. 1992. Media Performance: Mass Communication and the Public Interest. London: Sage. [11]

McShane, L. M., D. G. Altman, W. Sauerbrei, et al. 2005. Reporting recommendations for tumor marker prognostic studies (REMARK). *J. Natl. Cancer Inst.* **97(16)**:1180–1184. [6]

Mechanic, D. 2001. How should hamsters run? Some observations about sufficient patient time in primary care. *BMJ* **323**:266–268. [19]

———. 2004. In my chosen doctor I trust: And that trust transfers from doctors to organizations. *BMJ* **329**:1418–1419. [12]

Mechanic, D., D. D. McAlpine, and M. Rosenthal. 2001. Are patients' office visits with physicians getting shorter? *N. Engl. J. Med.* **344**:198–204. [19]

Media Doctor Australia. 2010. Improving the accuracy of medical news reporting. http://www.mediadoctor.org.au (accessed 1 June 2010). [11]

Melander, H., J. Ahlqvist-Rastad, G. Meijer, and B. Beermann. 2003. Evidence b(i)ased medicine-selective reporting from studies sponsored by pharmaceutical industry: Review of studies in new drug applications. *BMJ* **326**:1171–1173. [13]

Mello, M. M., D. M. Studdert, and T. A. Brennan. 2009. Shifting terrain in the regulation of off-label promotion of pharmaceuticals. *N. Engl. J. Med.* **360(15)**:1557–1566. [18]

Merenstein, D. 2004. Winners and loosers. *JAMA* **291**:15–16. [1]

Merton, R. K. 1985. Entwicklung und Wandel von Forschungsinteressen. Aufsätze zur Wissenschaftssoziologie. Frankfurt am Main: Suhrkamp. [11]

MEZIS. 2010. http://www.mezis.de (accessed 1 June 2010). [8]

MHH. 2010. Patientenuniversität der MHH. http://www.mh-hannover.de/7083.html (accessed 1 June 2010). [19]

MIBBI. 2010. Minimum Information for Biological and Biomedical Investigations http://www.mibbi.org/index.php/Main_Page (accessed 28 April 2010). [6]

Miller, K. 1992. Smoking Up a Storm: Public Relations and Advertising in the Construction of the Cigarette Problem 1953–1954. Columbia, SC: AEJMC. [11]

Ministry of Health. 2006. Direct-to-Consumer Advertising of Prescription Medicines in New Zealand: Consultation Document. Wellington: Ministry of Health. [18]

Mintzes, B. 2002. For and against: Direct to consumer advertising is medicalising normal human experience. *BMJ* **324**:908–909. [18]

———. 2005. Educational initiatives for medical and pharmacy students about drug promotion: An international cross-sectional survey, WHO/PSM/PAR/2005.2. Geneva: WHO/Health Action International. [18]

———. 2006. What are the public health implications? Direct-to-consumer advertising of prescription drugs in Canada. Toronto: Health Council of Canada. [18]

Mintzes, B., M. L. Barer, R. L. Kravitz, et al. 2003. How does direct-to-consumer advertising (DTCA) affect prescribing? A survey in primary care environments with and without legal DTCA. *CMAJ* **169**:405–412. [18]

Mintzes, B., S. Morgan, and J. M. Wright. 2009. Twelve years' experience with direct-to-consumer advertising of prescription drugs in Canada: A cautionary tale. *PLoS ONE* **4(5)**:e5699. [18]

Moher, D., A. Liberati, J. Tetzlaff, and D. G. Altman. 2009. Preferred reporting items for systematic reviews and meta-analyses: The PRISMA statement. *Ann. Int. Med.* **151(4)**:264–269. [6, 7]

Moher, D., K. F. Schulz, and D. G. Altman. 2001. The CONSORT statement: Revised recommendations for improving the quality of reports of parallel-group randomised trials. *Lancet* **357**:1191–1194. [6, 7]

Moher, D., J. Tetzlaff, A. C. Tricco, M. Sampson, and D. G. Altman. 2007. Epidemiology and reporting characteristics of systematic reviews. *PLoS Med.* **4**:448. [7]

Mokdad, A. H., J. S. Marks, D. F. Stroup, and J. L. Gerbeding. 2004. Actual causes of death in the United States, 2000. *JAMA* **291**:1238–1245. [19]

Monahan, J. 2007. Statistical literacy. A prerequisite for evidence-based medicine. *Psychol. Sci. Publ. Interest* **8**:i–ii. [1]

Montori, V. M., R. Jaeschke, H. J. Schunemann, et al. 2004. Users' guide to detecting misleading claims in clinical research reports. *BMJ* **329**:1093–1096. [6]

Moore, D. E. 2008. How physicians learn and how to design learning experiences for them: An approach based on an interpretive review of evidence. In: Continuing Education in the Health Professions: Improving Healthcare through Lifelong Learning, ed. M. Hager et al., pp. 30–56. New York: Josiah Macy, Jr. Foundation. [15]

Morgan, M. W., R. B. Deber, H. A. Llewellyn-Thomas, et al. 2000 Randomized, controlled trial of an interactive videodisc decision aid for patients with ischemic heart disease. *J. Gen. Intern. Med.* **15(10)**:685–693. [3]

Moses, H., III. 2009. Researchers, funding, and priorities: The razor's edge. *JAMA* **302**:1001–1002. [5]

Moses, H., III, E. Dorsey, D. Matheson, and S. O. Thier. 2005. Financial anatomy of biomedical research. *JAMA* 294:1333–1342. [5]

Moxey, A., D. O'Connell, P. McGettigan, and D. Henry. 2003. Describing treatment effects to patients: How they are expressed makes a difference. *J. Gen. Intern. Med.* 18:948–959. [9]

Moynihan, R. 2003a. Who pays for the pizza? Redefining the relationships between doctors and drug companies. 1: Entanglement. *BMJ* 326:1189–1192. [18]

———. 2003b. Who pays for the pizza? Redefining the relationships between doctors and drug companies. 2: Disentanglement. *BMJ* 326:1193–1196. [18]

Moynihan, R., L. Bero, D. Ross-Degnan, et al. 2000. Coverage by the news media of the benefits and risks of medications. *N. Engl. J. Med.* 342(22):1645–1650. [2, 10, 11]

Moynihan, R., and A. Cassels. 2005. Selling Sickness: How Drug Companies Are Turning Us All into Patients: Allen and Unwin. [13]

Moynihan, R., I. Heath, D. Henry, and P. C. Gøtzsche. 2002. Selling sickness: The pharmaceutical industry and disease mongering. Commentary: Medicalisation of risk factors. *BMJ* 324(7342):886–891. [18]

Moynihan, R., and M. Sweet. 2000. Medicine, the media and monetary interests: The need for transparency and professionalism. *Med. J. Aust.* 173:631–634. [11]

Mühlhauser, I., and M. Berger. 2002. Patient education: Evaluation of a complex intervention. *Diabetologia* 45:1723–1733. [12]

Mühlhauser, I., J. Kasper, and G. Meyer. 2006. FEND: Understanding of diabetes prevention studies: Questionnaire survey of professionals in diabetes care. *Diabetologia* 49:1742–1746. [1, 2, 9]

Mühlhauser, I., and F. Oser. 2008. Does wikipedia provide evidence-based health care information? A content analysis. *Z. Evid. Fortbild. Qual. Gesundhwes.* 102:e1–e7. [19]

Mulley, A. G., Jr. 1989. Assessing patients' utilities: Can the ends justify the means? *Med. Care* 27:S269–S228l. [3]

———. 1990. Medical decision making and practice variation. In: The Challenges of Medical Practice Variation, ed. T. F. Anderson and G. Mooney, pp. 59–75. London: MacMillan. [3]

———. 1993a. Clinicians' Guide to the Treatment Choices for Breast Cancer Shared Decision Making Program. Boston: Foundation for Informed Medical Decision Making. [3]

———. 1993b. Clinicians' Guide to Treating Your Breast Cancer: The Surgery Decision Shared Decision Making Program. Boston: Foundation for Informed Medical Decision Making. [3]

———. 1995a. Clinicians' Guide to the Treatment Choices for Ischemic Heart Disease Shared Decision Making Program. Boston: Foundation for Informed Medical Decision Making. [3]

———. 1995b. Outcomes research: Implications for policy and practice. In: Outcomes into Clinical Practice, ed. R. Smith and T. Delamothe. London: BMJ Publ. Group. [3]

———. 2009. Inconvenient truths about supplier induced demand and unwarranted variation in medical practice. *BMJ* 339:1007–1009. [3]

Mulrow, C. W. 1987. The medical review article: State of the science. *Ann. Int. Med.* 106:485–488. [7]

Nannenga, M. R., V. M. Montori, A. J. Weymiller, et al. 2009. A treatment decision aid may increase patient trust in the diabetes specialist. The statin choice randomized trial. *Health Expect.* 12(1):38–44. [12]

National Science Board. 2008. Science and Engineering Indicators, vol. 1–2. Arlington, VA: National Science Foundation. [10]

Nature. 2006. Editorial: Britannica attacks. *Nature* **440**:582 [19]

————. 2010. Editorial: *Nature's* peer review debate. www.nature.com/nature/peerreview/debate/index.html. [11]

Nature Reviews Drug Discovery. 2008. Editorial: Advertising oversell? *Nat. Rev. Drug Discov.* **7(10)**:787. [18]

Naylor, C. D., E. Chen, and B. Strauss. 1992. Measured enthusiasm: Does the method of reporting trial results alter perceptions of therapeutic effectiveness? *Ann. Int. Med.* **117**:916–921. [2, 9]

NCI. 1998. Breast Cancer Risk Tool: An Interactive Patient Education Tool. Bethesda: National Cancer Institute. [1]

————. 2005. Fact sheet: Breast cancer prevention studies. Bethesda: National Cancer Institute. http://www.cancer.gov/cancertopics/factsheet/Prevention/breast-cancer. [1]

————. 2006. Centers of Excellence in Cancer Communication Research (CECCR) Initiative: Midcourse Update. Bethesda: NIH/Natl. Cancer Institute. [5]

Neidhardt, F. 2006. Fehlerquellen und Fehlerkontrollen in den Begutachtungssystemen der Wissenschaft. In: Wie Viel (In-)Transparenz Ist Notwendig? Peer Review Revisited, ed. S. Hornbostel and D. Simon, pp. 7–14. Bonn: IFQ. [11]

Nelson, D. E., B. Hesse, and R. Croyle. 2009. Making Data Talk. New York: Oxford Univ. Press. [5]

NHMRC. 2009. A Draft National Strategy for Medical Research and Public Health Research. Canberra: National Health and Medical Research Council. [5]

NHS. 2009. Research that is relevant to people's needs and concerns: Patient and public awareness. http://www.nihr.ac.uk/awareness/Pages/default.aspx (accessed 28 April 2010). [5]

————. 2010. UK database of uncertainties about the effects of treatments. http://www.library.nhs.uk/DUETs/Default.aspx (accessed 2 June 2010). [7, 13]

NHS Choices. 2010. Your health, your choices. http://www.nhs.uk/Pages/HomePage.aspx (accessed 2 June 2010). [7, 12]

NHS Surveys. 2010. http://www.nhssurveys.org/ (accessed 2 June 2010). [13]

Nickerson, R. S. 1998. Confirmation bias: A ubiquitous phenomenon in many guises. *Rev. Gen. Psychol.* **2**:175–220. [13]

Nicolson, D., P. Knapp, D. K. Raynor, and P. Spoor. 2009. Written information about individual medicines for consumers. *Cochrane Database Syst. Rev.* **2**:CD002104. [18]

NIH. 2009a. Glossary of clinical trials terms. http://clinicaltrials.gov/ct2/info/glossary (accessed 27 May 2010). [18]

————. 2009b. NIH Roadmap for Medical Research. Bethesda: National Institutes of Health. http://nihroadmap.nih.gov (accessed 10 April 2010). [5]

NIHR Awareness. 2010. http://www.nihr.ac.uk/awareness/Pages/default.aspx (accessed 9 June 2010). [8]

NIHR CCF. 2010. http://www.nihr-ccf.org.uk/site/default.cfm (accessed 9 June 2010). [8]

NIPH. 1996. First annual Nordic Workshop. How to critically appraise and use evidence in decisions about healthcare. Oslo: National Institute of Public Health. [16]

No Free Lunch. 2010. http://www.nofreelunch.org/aboutus.htm (accessed 11 June 2010). [8]

Nowlen, P. M. 1988. A New Approach to Continuing Education for Business and the Professions. New York: Macmillan. [15]

NTCM. 2000. Principles and Standards for School Mathematics. Reston: National Council of Teachers of Mathematics. [2]

Nuovo, J., J. Melnikow, and D. Chang. 2002. Reporting number needed to treat and absolute risk reduction in randomized controlled trials. *JAMA* **287**:2813–2814. [1, 2, 9]

Nutley, S. M., I. Walter, and H. T. O. Davies. 2007. Using Evidence: How Research Can Inform Public Services. Bristol: Policy Press. [16]

NVL. 2010. Nationale Versorgungs Leitlinien. http://www.versorgungsleitlinien.de/english (accessed 24 May 2010). [12]

Nyström, L., I. Andersson, N. Bjurstam, et al. 2002. Long-term effects of mammography screening: Updated overview of the Swedish randomised trials. *Lancet* **359**:909–919. [9]

Nyström, L., L.-G. Larsson, S. Wall, et al. 1996. An overview of the Swedish randomised mammography trials: Total mortality pattern and the representativity of the study cohorts. *J. Med. Screen.* **3**:85–87. [9]

O'Brien, M. A., N. Freemantle, and A. D. Oxman. 2001. Continuing education meetings and workshops: Effects on professional practice and health care outcomes. *Cochrane Database Syst. Rev.* **2**:CD003030. [15]

O'Connor, A. M., C. Bennett, D. Stacey, et al. 2007. Do patient decision aids meet effectiveness criteria of the international patient decision aid standards collaboration? A systematic review and meta-analysis. *Med. Decis. Making* **27**:554–574. [19]

———. 2009. Decision aids for people facing health treatment or screening decisions. *Cochrane Database Syst. Rev.* **3**:CD001431. [4, 19]

O'Connor, A. M., D. Stacey, V. Entwistle, et al. 2003. Decision aids for people facing health treatment or screening decisions. *Cochrane Database Syst. Rev.* **3**: CD001431. [3]

O'Connor, A. M., J. E. Wennberg, F. Legare, et al. 2007. Toward the "tipping point": Decision aids and informed patient choice. *Health Affairs* **26(3)**:716–725. [13]

O'Neill, O. 2002. Question of Trust: The BBC Reith Lectures. Cambridge: Cambridge Univ. Press. [12]

Ober, J. 2008. Democracy and Knowledge. Princeton, NJ: Princeton Univ. Press. [1]

OHRI. 2010. Patient decision aids. Ottawa Hospital Research Institute. http://decisionaid.ohri.ca/ (accessed 1 June 2010). [13, 19]

Oliver, R., and J. Herrington. 2003. Interactive learning environments, exploring technology-mediated learning from a pedagogical perspective. *Interact. Learn. Environ.* **11(2)**:111–126. [15]

Olsen, L., D. Aisner, and J. M. McGinnis, eds. 2008. The Learning Healthcare System: IOM Roundtable on Evidence-based Medicine Workshop Summary. Institute of Medicine of the National Academies. Washington, D.C.: National Academies Press. [3]

Oxman, A. D., and G. H. Guyatt. 1988. Guidelines for reading literature reviews. *CMAJ* **128**:697–703. [7]

Oxman, A. D., G. H. Guyatt, D. J. Cook, et al. 1993. An index of scientific quality for health reports in the lay press. *J. Clin. Epidemiol.* **46**:987–1001. [11]

Ozolins, M., E. A. Eady, A. J. Avery, et al. 2004. Comparison of five antimicrobial regimens for treatment of mild to moderate inflammatory facial acne vulgaris in the community: Randomised controlled trial. *Lancet* **364**:2188–2195. [13]

Paling, J. 2003. Strategies to help patients understand risks. *BMJ* **327**:745–748. [2]

Parnes, B., P. C. Smith, C. Gilroy, et al. 2009. Lack of impact of direct-to-consumer advertising on the physician-patient encounter in primary care: A SNOCAP report. *Ann. Fam. Med.* **7(1)**:41–46. [18]

PatientsLikeMe. 2010. Patients + data = insight. http://partners.patientslikeme.com (accessed 1 June 2010). [19]

Patsopoulos, N. A., J. P. A. Ioannidis, and A. A. Analatos. 2006. Origin and funding of the most frequently cited papers in medicine: database analysis. *BMJ* 332:1061–1064. [7]

Peters, H. P. 1994. Risikokommunikation in den Medien. In: Die Wirklichkeit der Medien. Eine Einführung in die Kommunikationswissenschaft, reprint of vol. 1, ed. K. Merten et al., pp. 329–351. Opladen: Westdeutscher Verlag. [11]

Peters, P. 2002. The role of the jury in modern malpractice law. *Iowa Law Rev.* 87:909–969. [1]

Petticrew, M. 2001. Systematic reviews from astronomy to zoology: Myths and misconceptions. *BMJ* 322:98–101. [11]

Phillips, D. P., E. J. Kanter, B. Bednarcyk, and P. L. Tastad. 1991. Importance of the lay press in the transmission of medical knowledge to the scientific community. *N. Engl. J. Med.* 325:1180–1183. [11]

PhRMA. 2008. Guiding principles: Direct to consumer advertisements about prescription medicines. Washington D.C.: Pharmaceutical Research and Manufacturers of America. http://www.phrma.org/files/attachments/PhRMA%20Guiding%20Principles_Dec%2008_FINAL.pdf. [18]

————. 2009. Pharmaceutical industry profile. Washington, D.C.: Pharmaceutical Research and Manufacturers of America. http://www.phrma.org/files/attachments/PhRMA%202009%20Profile%20FINAL.pdf (accessed 28 April 2010). [5]

PIES. 2010. Prostate interactive education system. http://www.temple.edu/imits/piesweb/ (accessed 22 May 2010). [12]

Pisano, G. 2006. Science Business. Boston: Harvard Business School Press. [5]

Pitt, M. A., I. J. Myung, and S. Zhang. 2002. Toward a method of selecting among computational models of cognition. *Psychol. Rev.* 109:472–491. [17]

Plint, A. C., D. Moher, A. Morrison, et al. 2006. Does the CONSORT checklist improve the quality of reports of randomised controlled trials? A systematic review. *Med. J. Aust.* 185 (5):263–267. [6]

Politi, M. C., P. Han, and N. Col. 2007. Communicating the uncertainty of harms and benefits of medical interventions. Eisenberg Center 2006 White Paper Series. *Med. Decis. Making* 7(5):681–695. [12]

Popper, K. R. 1963. Conjectures and Refutations: The Growth of Scientific Knowledge. London: Routledge. [11]

Pöschl, U. 2004. Interactive journal concept for improved scientific publishing and quality assurance. *Learned Publishing* 17:105–113. [11]

Postman, N. 1986. Amusing Ourselves to Death: Public Discourse in the Age of Show Business. New York: Penguin Books. [11]

Pozen, M. W., R. B. D'Agostino, H. P. Selker, P. A. Sytkowski, and W. B. Hood. 1984. A predictive instrument to improve coronary-care-unit admission practices in acute ischaemic heart disease. *N. Engl. J. Med.* 310:1273–1278. [17]

Pratt, B. M., and S. R. Woolfenden. 2002. Interventions for preventing eating disorders in children and adolescents. *Cochrane Database Syst. Rev.* 2:CD002891. [13]

Prescribing Observatory for Mental Health. 2007. Topic 4 Report: Benchmarking the Prescribing of Anti-dementia Drugs. London: Royal College of Psychiatrists. [16]

Prescrire International. 2009. Editorial: A look back at 2008: Pharmaceutical quality problems. *Prescrire Intl.* 18:84–88. [18]

Probublica. 2010. http://www.probublica.org (accessed 9 June 2010). [11]

Proctor, E. K., and A. Rosen. 2008. From knowledge production to implementation: Research challenges and imperatives. *Res. Soc. Work. Pract.* **18**:285–291. [5]

Pronovost, P., D. Needham, S. Berenholtz, et al. 2006. An intervention to decrease catheter-related bloodstream infections in the ICU. *N. Engl. J. Med.* **355**:2725–2732. [1, 8]

Psaty, B. M., C. D. Furberg, W. A. Ray, and N. S. Weiss. 2004. Potential for conflict of interest in the evaluation of suspected adverse drug reactions: Use of cerivastatin and risk of rhabdomyolysis. *JAMA* **292**:2622–2631. [13]

Psaty, B. M., and R. A. Kronmal. 2008. Reporting mortality findings in trials of rofecoxib for Alzheimer disease or cognitive impairment: A case study based on documents from rofecoxib litigation. *JAMA* **299**:1813–1817. [13]

Quam, L., and R. Smith. 2005. What can the UK and US health systems learn from each other? *BMJ* **330**:530–533. [16]

Quick, J. D., H. V. Hogerzeil, L. Rago, R. V, and K. de Joncheere. 2003. Ensuring ethical drug promotion: Whose responsibility? *Lancet* **362**:747. [18]

Rager, G. 1994. Dimensionen der Qualität. Weg aus den allseitig offenen Richter-skalen. In: Publizistik in der Gesellschaft. Festschrift für Manfred Rühl, ed. G. Bentele, pp. 189–209. Konstanz: Universitäts-Verlag. [11]

Ransohoff, D. F., and R. P. Harris. 1997. Lessons from the mammography screening controversy: Can we improve the debate? *Ann. Int. Med.* **127**:1029–1034. [2]

Rao, G. 2008. Physician numeracy: Essential skills for practicing evidence-based medicine. *Fam. Med.* **40**:354–358. [1]

Rásky, É., and S. Groth. 2004. Informationsmaterialien zum Mammographiescreening in Österreich: Unterstützen sie die informierte Entscheidung von Frauen? [Information on mammography screening in Austria: Does it facilitate women's informed decisions?]. *Sozial und Präventivmedizin* **49**:301–397. [2]

Rawlins, M. D. 2009. The decade of NICE. *Lancet* **374**:351–352. [16]

Ray, W. A., and C. M. Stein. 2006. Reform of drug regulation: Beyond an independent drug-safety board. *N. Engl. J. Med.* **354(2)**:194–201. [18]

Raynor, D. K., and D. Dickinson. 2009. Key principles to guide development of consumer medicine information: Content analysis of information design texts. *Ann. Pharmacother.* **43(4)**:700–706. [18]

Reeves, S., M. Zwarenstein, J. Goldman, et al. 2008. Interprofessional education: Effects on professional practice and health care outcomes. Cochrane Database of Systematic Reviews. *Cochrane Database Syst. Rev.* **1**:CD002213. [15]

Rennie, D. 1997. Thyroid storm. *JAMA* **277**:1238–1243. [1]

Research Australia. 2009. Trends in health and medical research funding. Sydney: Research Australia. [5]

Research!America. 2008. Rebuilding Our Economy: Investing in Research Critical to Our Nation's Health. Alexandria, VA: Research!America. [5]

Reyna, V. F., and C. J. Brainerd. 2007. The importance of mathematics in health and human judgment: Numeracy, risk communication, and medical decision making. *Learn. Individ. Differ.* **17**:147–159. [2]

Reyna, V. F., W. L. Nelson, P. K. Han, and N. F. Dieckmann. 2009. How numeracy influences risk comprehension and medical decision making. *Psychol. Bull.* **135**:943–973. [2]

Richardson, J. R., and S. Peacock. 2006. Reconsidering theories and evidence of supplier induced demand. Centre for Health Economics Research Paper 13. Victoria Monash University. [3]

Ridolfi, D. R., and J. S. Vander Wal. 2008. Eating disorders awareness week: The effectiveness of a one-time body image dissatisfaction prevention session. *Eat. Disor.* **16**:418–443. [13]

Rigby, M., J. Forsstrom, R. Roberts, and J. Wyatt. 2001. Verifying quality and safety in health informatics services. *BMJ* **323**:552–556. [2]

Ringel, J. S., F. Girosi, A. Cordova, C. C. Price, and E. A. McGlynn. 2010. Analysis of the patient protection and affordable care act (H.R. 3590): RAND Policy Brief. http://www.rand.org/pubs/research_briefs/RB9514/ (accessed 2 April 2010). [19]

Risch, N., R. Herrel, T. Lehner, et al. 2009. Interaction between the serotonin transporter gene (5-HTTLPR), stressful life events, and risk of depression. *JAMA* **301**:2462–2471. [10]

RMI. 2006. Code of Practice. Researched Medicines Industry Association of New Zealand Incorporated. http://www.rmianz.co.nz/codeofpractice.pdf (accessed 31 May 2010). [18]

Robert Koch Institute. 2009. Saisonbericht 2008. Arbeitsgemeinschaft Influenza (AGI). http://influenza.rki.de/Saisonberichte/2008.pdf (accessed 10 April 2010). [8]

Roberts, S., and H. Pashler. 2000. How persuasive is a good fit? A comment on theory testing. *Psychol. Rev.* **107**:358–367. [17]

Rochon, P. A., J. H. Gurwitz, and R. W. Simms. 1994. A study of manufacturer-supported trials of nonsteroidal anti-inflammatory drugs in the treatment of arthritis. *Arch. Intern. Med.* **154**:157–163. [7, 13]

Roland, M. 2004. Linking physician pay to quality of care: A major experiment in the United Kingdom. *N. Engl. J. Med.* **351**:1448–1454. [16]

Ross, J. S., K. P. Hill, D. S. Egilman, and H. M. Krumholz. 2008. Guest authorship and ghostwriting in publications related to rofecoxib: A case study of industry documents from rofecoxib litigation. *JAMA* **299**:1800–1812. [13]

Rothman, S. M., and D. J. Rothman. 2009. Marketing HPV vaccine: Implications for adolescent health and medical professionalism. *JAMA* **302(7)**:781–786. [18]

Royeen, C., G. M. Jensen, and R. A. Harvan, eds. 2008. Leadership in Interprofessional Health Education and Practice. Sudbury, MA: Jones and Bartlett Publishers. [15]

Rozin, P., K. Kabnick, E. Pete, C. Fischler, and C. Shields. 2003. The ecology of eating: Smaller portions sizes in France than in the United States help explain the French paradox. *Psychol. Sci.* **14**:450–454. [19]

Ruhrmann, G. 2003. Risikokommunikation. In: Öffentliche Kommunikation: Handbuch Kommunikations- und Medienwissenschaft, ed. G. Bentele, pp. 539–549. Wiesbaden: Westdeutscher Verlag. [11]

Russ-Mohl, S. 1992. Am eigenen Schopfe: Qualitätssicherung im Journalismus–Grundfragen, Ansätze, Näherungsversuche. *Publizistik* **37**:83–96. [11]

———. 2009. Kreative Zerstörung: Niedergang und Neuerfindung des Zeitungsjournalismus in den USA. Konstanz: UVK Verlagsgesellschaft. [11]

Sackett, D. L., and B. Haynes. 1995. On the need for evidence-based medicine. *EBM* **1**:5–6. [11]

Sackett, D. L., and A. D. Oxman. 2003. HARLOT plc: An amalgamation of the world's two oldest professions. *BMJ* **327**:1442–1445. [1]

Sackett, D. L., W. M. C. Rosenberg, J. A. M. Gray, R. B. Haynes, and W. S. Richardson. 1996. Evidence based medicine: What it is and what it isn't. *BMJ* **312**:71–72. [7, 11, 16]

Sackett, D. L., S. E. Straus, W. S. Richardson, W. Rosenberg, and R. B. Haynes. 2000. Evidence-based Medicine. How to Practise and Teach EBM, 2 ed. Edinburgh: Churchill Livingstone. [15]

Saelens, B. E., J. F. Sallis, J. B. Black, and D. Chen. 2003. Neighborhood-based differences in physical activity: An environment scale evaluation. *Am. J. Public Health* **93**:1552–1558. [19]

Santiago, M., H. Bucher, and A. Nordmann. 2008. Accuracy of drug advertisements in medical journals under new law regulating the marketing of pharmaceutical products in Switzerland. *BMC Med. Inform. Decis. Mak.* **8(1)**:61. [18]

Sarfati, D., P. Howden-Chapman, A. Woodward, and C. Salmond. 1998. Does the frame affect the picture? A study into how attitudes to screening for cancer are affected by the way benefits are expressed. *J. Med. Screen.* **5**:137–140. [2]

Say, R., M. Murtagh, and R. Thomson. 2006. Patients' preference for involvement in medical decision making: A narrative review. *Patient Educ. Couns.* **60**:102–114. [4]

SBU. 2009. About SBU. http://www.sbu.se/en/About-SBU/ (accessed 28 April 2010). [5]

Schatz, H., and W. Schulz. 1992. Qualität von Fernsehprogrammen: Kriterien und Methode zur Beurteilung von Programmqualität im dualen Fernsehsystem. *Media Perspektiven* **1992**:690–712. [11]

Schillinger, D., K. Grumbach, J. Piette, et al. 2002. Association of health literacy with diabetes outcomes. *JAMA* **288(4)**:475–482 [12]

Schott, G., H. Pachl, U. Limbach, et al. 2010a. The financing of drug trials by pharmaceutical companies and its consequences. Part 1: A qualitative, systematic review of the literature on possible influences on the findings, protocols, and quality of drug trials. *Dtsch. Arztebl. Int.* **107(16)**:279–285. [18]

———. 2010b. The financing of drug trials by pharmaceutical companies and its consequences. Part 2: A Qualitative, systematic review of the literature on possible influences on authorship, access to trial data, and trial registration and publication. *Dtsch. Arztebl. Int.* **107(17)**:295–301. [13, 18]

Schröder, F. H., J. Hugosson, M. J. Roobol, et al. 2009. Screening and prostate-cancer mortality in a randomized European study. *N. Engl. J. Med.* **360(13)**:1320–1328. [1, 2]

Schubert, K., and G. Glaeske. 2006. Einfluss des pharmazeutisch-industriellen Komplexes auf die Selbsthilfe. Bremen: Zentrum für Sozialpädagogik. http://www.sekis-berlin.de/uploads/media/glaeske-studie.pdf (accessed 10 April 2010). [12]

Schulz, K. F., I. Chalmers, R. J. Haynes, and D. G. Altman. 1995. Empirical evidence of bias: Dimensions of methodological quality associated with estimates of treatment effects in controlled trials. *JAMA* **273**:408–412. [7]

Schünemann, H. J., A. D. Oxman, G. E. Vist, et al. 2008. Presenting results and "summary of findings" tables. In: Cochrane Handbook for Systematic Reviews of Interventions, ed. J. P. T. Higgins and S. Green. Chichester: Wiley-Blackwell. [12]

Schüssler, B. 2005. Im Dialog: Ist Risiko überhaupt kommunizierbar, Herr Prof. Gigerenzer? *Frauenheilkunde Aktuell* **14**:25–31. [9]

Schwabe, U., and D. Paffrath, eds. 2009. Arzneiverordnungs-Report 2009. Heidelberg: Springer. [18]

Schwartz, B. 2004. The Paradox of Choice: Why More is Less. New York: Ecco. [19]

Schwartz, L. M., and S. Woloshin. 2009. Lost in transmission: FDA drug information that never reaches clinicians. *N. Engl. J. Med.* **361(18)**:1717–1720. [13, 14]

Schwartz, L. M., S. Woloshin, W. C. Black, and H. G. Welch. 1997. The role of numeracy in understanding the benefit of screening mammography. *Arch. Int. Med.* **127**:966–972. [2, 9]

Schwartz, L. M., S. Woloshin, E. L. Dvorin, and H. G. Welch. 2006. Ratio measures in leading medical journals: Structured review of accessibility of underlying absolute risks. *BMJ* **333**:1248–1252. [2, 9]

Schwartz, L. M., S. Woloshin, F. J. Fowler, and H. G. Welch. 2004. Enthusiasm for cancer screening in the United States. *JAMA* **291**:71–78. [1]

Schwartz, L. M., S. Woloshin, and H. G. Welch. 1999a. Misunderstandings about the effects of race and sex on physicians' referrals for cardiac catheterization. *N. Engl. J. Med.* **341(4)**:279–283. [2]

———. 1999b. Risk communication in clinical practice: Putting cancer in context. *Monogr. Natl. Cancer Inst.* **25**:124–133. [1]

———. 2007. The drug facts box: Providing consumers with simple tabular data on drug benefit and harm. *Med. Decis. Making* **27**:655–662. [14, 18]

———. 2009. Using a drug facts box to communicate drug benefits and harms: Two randomized trials. *Ann. Int. Med.* **150**:516–527. [14, 18]

Schwitzer, G. 2008. How do US journalists cover treatments, tests, products, and procedures? An evaluation of 500 stories. *PLoS Med.* **5**:e95. [11]

———. 2009. The state of health journalism in the US: A report to the Kaiser family foundation. Menlo Park: http://www.kff.org/entmedia/upload/7858.pdf (accessed 10 July 2010). [11]

Sedlmeier, P., and G. Gigerenzer. 2001. Teaching Bayesian reasoning in less than two hours. *J. Exp. Psychol.* **130**:380–400. [1]

Sedrakyan, A., and C. Shih. 2007. Improving depiction of benefits and harms: Analyses of studies of well-known therapeutics and review of high-impact medical journals. *Med. Care* **45**:523–528. [1, 9]

Sepkowitz, K. 2007. Under the influence? Drug companies, medical journals, and money. http://www.slate.com/id/2173652 (accessed 30 April 2010). [6]

Sepucha, K. R., F. J. Fowler, Jr, and A. G. Mulley, Jr. 2004. Policy support for patient-centered care: The need for measurable improvements in decision quality. *Health Affairs* http://content.healthaffairs.org/cgi/content/abstract/hlthaff.var.54 (accessed 10 July 2010). [3]

Sepucha, K. R., and E. Ozanne. 2010. How to define and measure concordance between patients' preferences and medical treatments: A systematic review of approaches and recommendations for standardization. *Patient Educ. Couns.* **78**:12–23. [19]

Shaughnessy, A. F., D. C. Slawson, and J. H. Bennett. 1994. Becoming an information master: A guidebook to the medical information jungle. *J. Fam. Pract.* **39**:489–499. [12]

Shaw, S. E., and T. Greenhalgh. 2008. Best research—for what? Best health—for whom? A critical exploration of primary care research using discourse analysis. *Soc. Sci. Med.* **66**:2506–2519. [5]

Sheridan, S. L., R. P. Harris, and S. H. Woolf. 2004. Shared decision making about screening and chemoprevention: A suggested approach from the U.S. Preventive Services Task Force. *Am. J. Prev. Med.* **26(1)**:56–66. [13]

Shi, L., and D. A. Singh. 2008. Delivering Health Care in America: A Systems Approach, 4th ed. Sudbury, MA: Jones and Bartlett Publishers. [8]

Shiffman, R. N., P. Shekelle, J. M. Overhage, et al. 2003. Standardized reporting of clinical practice guidelines: A proposal from the conference on guideline standardization. *Ann. Int. Med.* **139(6)**:493–498. [6]

Shuchman, M. 2007. Drug risks and free speech: Can Congress ban consumer drug ads? *N. Engl. J. Med.* **356(22)**:2236–2239. [18]

Siegfried, T. 2010. Odds are, it's wrong. *Science News* **177(26)**. [10]

SIEID. 2008. Science Statistics: Estimates of Total Spending on Research and Development in the Health Field in Canada, 1996 to 2007. Ottawa: Science, Innovation and Electronic Information Division. http://dsp-psd.pwgsc.gc.ca/collection_2008/statcan/88-001-X/88-001-XIE2008003.pdf (accessed 10 July 2010). [5]

Silver, H. J., and A. Sharpe. 2008. Behavioral and Social Science Research in the Administration's FY 2008 Budget. Washington, D.C.: AAAS. http://www.aaas.org/spp/rd/rd08main.htm (accessed 28 April 2010). [5]

Simon, D., L. Kriston, A. Loh, et al. 2010. Confirmatory factor analysis and recommendations for improvement of the Autonomy-Preference-Index (API). *Health Expect.* doi: 10.1111/j.1369-7625.2009.00584.x. [4]

Simon, D., A. Loh, and M. Härter. 2007. Measuring (shared) decision-making: A review of psychometric instruments. *Z. Ärzt. Fortbild. Qualität.* 101:259–267. [4]

Simon, H. A. 1990. Invariants of human behavior. *Annu. Rev. Psychol.* 41:1–19. [17]

———. 1992. What is an "explanation" of behavior? *Psychol. Sci.* 3:150–161. [19]

Singer, N. 2009. A push to spell out a drug's risks and benefits. *New York Times*, February 25. [14]

Sirovich, B., P. M. Gallagher, D. E. Wennberg, and E. S. Fisher. 2008 Discretionary decision making by primary care physicians and the cost of U.S. health care. *Health Affairs* **27(3)**:813–823. [3]

Sirovich, B., and H. Welch. 2004. Cervical cancer screening among women without a cervix. *JAMA* **291**:2990–2993. [1]

Slaytor, E. K., and J. E. Ward. 1998. How risks of breast cancer and benefits of screening are communicated to women: Analysis of 58 pamphlets. *BMJ* **317**:263–264. [2]

Smidt, N., J. Overbeke, H. de Vet, and P. Bossuyt. 2007. Endorsement of the STARD statement by biomedical journals: Survey of instructions for authors. *Clin. Chem.* **53(11)**:1983–1985. [6]

Smith, R. 1996. What clinical information do doctors need? *BMJ* **313**:1062–1068. [16]

———. 2005. Medical journals are an extension of the marketing arm of pharmaceutical companies. *PLoS Med.* **2(5)**:e138. [1, 8, 13]

———. 2006. Peer review: A flawed process at the heart of science and journals. *J. R. Soc. Med.* **99**:178. [16]

———. 2008. Most cases of research misconduct go undetected, conference told. *BMJ* **336(7650)**:913. [13]

———. 2009. In search of an optimal peer review system. *J. Part. Med.* **1(1)**:e13. [16]

Smith, R., and I. Roberts. 2006. Patient safety requires a new way to publish clinical trials. *PLoS Clin. Trial.* **1(1)**:e6. [6, 8]

Sox, C. M., J. N. Doctor, T. D. Koepsell, and D. A. Christakis. 2009. The influence of types of decision support on physicians' decision making. *Arch. Dis. Child.* **94**:185–190. [16]

Spiegelhalter, D. 2010. Understanding uncertainty. http://understandinguncertainty.org/ (accessed 24 May 2010). [12, 13]

Spot.Us. 2010. Nonprofit project of the Center for Media Change. http://www.spot.us (accessed 9 June 2010). [11]

Sridharan, L., and P. Greenland. 2009. Editorial policies and publication bias: The importance of negative studies. *Arch. Intern. Med.* **169**:1022–1023. [6]

Stacey, D., M. A. Murray, F. Légaré, et al. 2008. Decision coaching to support shared decision making: A framework, evidence, and implications for nursing practice, education, and policy. *Worldviews Evid. Based Nurs.* **5**:25–35. [19]

Stafford, N. 2009. German agency refuses to rule on drug's benefits until Pfizer discloses all trial results. *BMJ* **338**:b2521. [6]

Starfield, B., K. W. Lemke, R. Herbert, W. D. Pavlovich, and G. Anderson. 2005. Comorbidity and the use of primary care and specialist care in the elderly. *Ann. Fam. Med.* **3(3)**:215–222. [16]

Steckelberg, A., B. Berger, S. Köpke, C. Heesen, and I. Mühlhauser. 2005. Kriterien für evidenzbasierte Patienteninformationen [Criteria for evidence-based information for patients]. *Z. Ärzt. Fortbild. Qualität.* **99**:343–351. [2, 12, 18]

Steckelberg, A., C. Hülfenhaus, J. Kasper, and I. Mühlhauser. 2009. Ebm@school: A curriculum of critical health literacy for secondary school students: Results of a pilot study. *Intl. J. Public Health* **54**:1–8. [12, 19]

Steckelberg, A., C. Hülfenhaus, J. Kasper, J. Rost, and I. Mühlhauser. 2007. How to measure critical health competences: Development and validation of the Critical Health Competence Test (CHC Test). *Adv. Health Sci. Educ.* **14(4)**:11–22. [12]

Steinert, Y., S. Cruess, R. Cruess, and L. Snell. 2005. Faculty development for teaching and evaluating professionalism: From programme design to curriculum change. *Med. Educ.* **39(2)**:127–136. [15]

Steinert, Y., and L. S. Snell. 1999. Interactive lecturing: Strategies for increasing participation in large group presentations. *Med. Teacher* **21(1)**:37–42. [15]

Sterling, T. 1959. Publication decisions and their possible effects on inferences drawn from tests of significance or vice versa. *J. Am. Stat. Assoc.* **54**:30–34. [6]

Steurer, J., U. Held, M. Schmidt, et al. 2009. Legal concerns trigger PSA testing. *J. Eval. Clin. Pract.* **15**:390–392. [1]

Stevenson, F. A., K. Cox, N. Britten, and Y. Dundar. 2004. A systematic review of the research on communication between patients and health care professionals about medicines: The consequences for concordance. *Health Expect.* **7**:235–245. [12]

Stiftung Experimentelle Biomedizin. 2010. http://www.recherchepreis-wissenschaftsjournalismus.ch (accessed 9 June 2010). [11]

Stiftung Warentest. 2004. Urologen im Test: Welchen Nutzen hat der PSA-Test? *Stiftung Warentest* **2**:86–89. [1, 9]

Stigler, S. M. 1983. Who discovered Bayes's theorem? *Am. Stat.* **37**:290–296. [19]

———. 1986. The History of Statistics: The Measurement of Uncertainty before 1900. Cambridge, MA: Harvard Univ. Press. [17]

———. 1999. Statistics on the Table: The History of Statistical Concepts and Methods. Cambridge, MA: Harvard Univ. Press. [17]

Stine, G. J. 1999. AIDS Update 1999: An Annual Overview of Acquired Immune Deficiency Syndrome. Upper Saddle River, NJ: Prentice-Hall. [9]

Stolovitch, H. D., E. J. Keeps, and G. Finnegan. 2000. Handbook of human performance technology: Improving individual and organizational performance worldwide. *Performance Improvement* **39(5)**:38–44. [15]

Stone, M. 1974. Cross-validatory choice and assessment of statistical predictions. *J. R. Stat. Soc. Ser. B* **36**:111–147. [17]

Story, M., K. M. Kaphingst, R. Robinson-O'Brien, and K. Glanz. 2008. Creating healthy food and eating environments: Policy and environmental approaches. *Annu. Rev. Public Health* **29**:253–272. [19]

Strappato. 2009. Wenig klar mir Klära. Gesundheit Blogger. http://www.gesundheit. blogger.de/stories/1350278 (accessed 21 June 2010). [18]

Stroup, D. F., J. A. Berlin, S. C. Morton, et al. 2000. Meta-analysis of observational studies in epidemiology. *JAMA* **283(15)**:2008–2012. [6]

Strull, W., B. Lo, and G. Charles. 1984. Do patients want to participate in medical decision making? *JAMA* **252**:2990–2994. [4]

Studdert, D. M., M. M. Mello, A. A. Gawande, et al. 2006. Claims, errors, and compensation payments in medical malpractice litigation. *N. Engl. J. Med.* **354**:2024–2033. [1]

Studdert, D. M., M. M. Mello, W. M. Sage, et al. 2005. Defensive medicine among high-risk specialist physicians in a volatile malpractice environment. *JAMA* **293**: 2609–2617. [1]

Swart, E., C. Wolff, P. Klas, S. Deh, and B.-P. Robra. 2000. Häufigkeit und kleinräumige variabilität von operationen. *Chirurg* **71**:109–114. [1]

Tanenbaum, S. J. 1994. Knowing and acting in medical practice: The epistemological politics of outcomes research. *J. Health Polit. Policy Law* **19**:27–44. [13]

Tang, K. C., D. Nutbeam, C. Aldinger, et al. 2009. Schools for health, education and development: A call for action. *Health Promot. Intl.* **24**:68–77. [13]

Tetroe, J. M., I. D. Graham, R. Foy, et al. 2008. Health research funding agencies' support and promotion of knowledge translation: An international study. *Milbank Q.* **86**:125–155. [5]

Thaler, R. H., and C. R. Sunstein. 2008. Nudge: Improving Decisions about Health, Wealth, and Happiness. New Haven: Yale Univ. Press. [1, 2, 19]

Tharyan, P. 2007. Ethics committees and clinical trials registration in India: Opportunities, obligations, challenges and solutions. *Indian J. Med. Ethics* **4**. [6]

Thomaselli, R. 2004. DTC agencies, clients clash: Category spending surges, but reviews, cost pressures fray ties. *Advert. Age* **75**:1. [18]

Tinetti, M. E., S. T. Bogardus, Jr., and J. V. Agostini. 2004. Potential pitfalls of disease-specific guidelines for patients with multiple conditions. *N. Engl. J. Med.* **351**(27):2870–2874. [16]

't Jong, G. W., B. H. C. Stricker, and M. C. J. M. Sturkenboom. 2004. Marketing in the lay media and prescriptions of terbinafine in primary care: Dutch cohort study. BMJ **328**:931. [13, 18]

Tong, A., P. Sainsbury, and J. Craig. 2007. Consolidated criteria for reporting qualitative research (COREQ): A 32-item checklist for interviews and focus groups. *Intl. J. Qual. Health Care* **19**(6):349–357. [6]

Toop, L., D. Richards, T. Dowell, et al. 2003. Direct to Consumer Advertising of Prescription Drugs in New Zealand: For Health or for Profit? Dunedin: University of Otago. [18]

Towle, A. 1997. Physician and Patient Communication Skills: Competencies for Informed Shared Decision Making. Vancouver: Univ. British Columbia. [4]

Tramer, M. R., D. J. M. Reynolds, R. A. Moore, and H. J. McQuay. 1997. Impact of covert duplicate publication on meta-analysis: A case study. *BMJ* **315**:635–640. [7]

Trevena, L. J., H. M. Davey, A. Barratt, P. Butow, and P. Caldwell. 2006. A systematic review on communicating with patients about evidence. *J. Eval. Clin. Pract.* **12**:13–23. [2, 12]

Tunis, S. R., D. B. Stryer, and C. M. Clancy. 2003. Practical clinical trials: Increasing the value of clinical research for decision making in clinical and health policy. *JAMA* **290**:1624–1632. [13]

Turner, E. H., A. M. Matthews, and E. Linardatos. 2008. Selective publication of antidepressant trials and its influence on apparent efficacy. *N. Engl. J. Med.* **358**:252–260. [13]

U.S. Congress. 2010. The Patient Protection and Affordable Care Act. Public Law 111–148. [14]

U.S. GAO. 2006. Prescription Drugs: Improvements needed in FDA's oversight of direct-to-consumer advertising. Washington, D.C.: GPO. [18]

UKCRC. 2006. UK health research analysis. London: UK Clinical Research Collaboration. http://www.ukcrc.org/publications/reports/ (accessed 28 April 2010). [5]

US Preventive Services Task Force. 2002. Guide to Clinical Preventive Services: Report of the U.S. Preventive Services Task Force. Baltimore: Williams and Wilkins. [9]

USA Today. 2002. Drugmakers' gifts to doctors finally get needed scrunity. *USA Today*, October 14. [12]

van Tol-Geerdink, J. J., P. F. M. Stalmeier, E. N. van Lin, et al. 2006. Do prostate cancer patients want to choose their own radiation treatment? *Intl. J. Radiat. Oncol. Biol. Phys.* **66**:1105–1111. [12]

Vedula, S., L. Bero, S. RW, and K. Dickersin. 2008. Outcome reporting in industry-sponsored trials of gabapentin for off-label use. *N. Engl. J. Med.* **361(20)**:1963–1971. [6]

Velo, G., and U. Moretti. 2008. Direct-to-consumer information in Europe: The blurred margin between promotion and information. *Br. J. Clin. Pharmacol.* **66**:626–628. [18]

Verhoeven, P. 2008. Where has the doctor gone? The mediazation of medicine on Dutch television, 1961–2000. *Public Underst. Sci.* **17**:461–472. [11]

Villanueva, P., S. Peiró, J. Librero, and I. Peireró. 2003. Accuracy of pharmaceutical advertisements in medical journals. *Lancet* **361**:27–32. [1]

Vogel, B., R. Leonhart, and A. Helmes. 2009. Communication matters: The impact of communication and participation in decision making on breast cancer patients' depression and quality of life. *Patient Educ. Couns.* **77**:391–197. [4]

von Elm, E., D. G. Altman, M. Egger, et al. 2007. The strengthening the reporting of observational studies in epidemiology (STROBE) statement: Guidelines for reporting observational studies. *Ann. Int. Med.* **147(8)**:573–577. [6, 7]

————. 2008. The strengthening the reporting of observational studies in epidemiology (STROBE) statement: Guidelines for reporting observational studies. *J. Clin. Epidemiol.* **61(4)**:344–349. [7]

von Elm, E., G. Poglia, B. Walder, and M. R. Tramer. 2004. Different patterns of duplicate publication: An analysis of articles used in systematic reviews. *JAMA* **291**:974–980. [7]

Voss, M. 2002. Checking the pulse: Midwestern reporters' opinions on their ability to report health care news. *Am. J. Public Health* **92**:1158–1160. [1, 2, 10]

Wagner, A. 2005. Robustness and Evolvability in Living Systems. Princeton, NJ: Princeton Univ. Press. [17]

Wagner, J. T., L. M. Bachmann, C. Boult, et al. 2006. Predicting the risk of hospital admission in older persons: Validation of a brief self-administered questionnaire in three European countries. *J. Am. Geriatr. Soc.* **54**:1271–1276. [17]

Wainer, H. 1976. Estimating coefficients in linear models: It don't make no nevermind. *Psychol. Bull.* **83**:213–217. [17]

Wallsten, T. S., D. V. Budescu, R. Zwick, and S. M. Kemp. 1993. Preference and reasons for communicating probabilistic information in numerical or verbal terms. *Bull. Psych. Soc.* **31**:135–138. [2, 12]

Weber, B., and G. Rager. 1994. Zeile für Zeile Qualität: Was Journalisten über Qualität in der Zeitung denken. In: Zeile für Zeile: Qualität in der Zeitung, ed. G. Rager et al., pp. 1–15. Münster: Lit-Verlag. [11]

Webkinz. 2010. Come in and play. http://www.webkinz.com (accessed 25 May 2010). [12]

Wegwarth, O., W. Gaissmaier, and G. Gigerenzer 2009. Smart strategies for doctors and doctors-in-training: Heuristics in medicine. *Med. Educ.* **43**:721–728. [5]

Wegwarth, O., and G. Gigerenzer. 2010a. There is nothing to worry about: Gynecologists' counseling on mammography. *Patient Educ. Couns.* doi:10.1016/j.pec.2010.1007.1025. [9]

———. 2010b. Trust-your-doctor: A social heuristic in need of a proper environment. In: Simple Heuristics in a Social World, ed. R. Hertwig et al. New York: Oxford Univ. Press, in press. [19]

Weichert, S., and L. Kramp. 2009. Das verschwinden der Zeitung? Internationale Trends und medienpolitische Problemfelder. Berlin: Friedrich-Ebert-Stiftung. http://fes-stabsabteilung.de/docs/FES_Zeitungsverschwinden_2009.pdf (accessed 27 April 2010). [11]

Weinstein, J. N., T. D. Tosteson, J. D. Lurie, et al. 2006. Surgical vs. nonoperative treatment for lumbar disk herniation: The spine patient outcomes research trial (SPORT): A randomized trial. *JAMA* **296(20)**:2441–2450. [3]

Weischenberg, S. 2001. Nachrichten Journalismus: Anleitungen und Qualitäts Standards für die Medienpraxis. Wiesbaden: Westdeutscher Verlag. [11]

Weischenberg, S., W. Loosen, and M. Beuthner, eds. 2006. Medien-Qualitäten: Öffentliche Kommunikation zwischen ökonomischem Kalkül und Sozialverantwortung. Konstanz: UVK Verlagsgesellschaft. [11]

Weiss, B., ed. 2007. Removing Barriers to Better, Safer Care: Health Literacy and Patient Safety. Help Patients Understand. Manual for Clinicians, 2nd ed. Chicago: AMA Foundation. [12]

Welch, H. G., L. M. Schwartz, and S. Woloshin. 2000. Are increasing 5-year survival rates evidence of success against cancer? *JAMA* **283**:2975–2978. [1, 9]

Wennberg, D. E., M. A. Kellett, J. D. Dickens, et al. 1996. The association between local diagnostic testing intensity and invasive cardiac procedures. *JAMA* **275**:1161–1164. [3]

Wennberg, J. E. 1996. On the appropriateness of small-area analysis for cost containment. *Health Affairs* **15**:164–167. [5]

Wennberg, J. E., J. P. Bunker, and B. Barnes. 1980. The need for assessing the outcome of common medical practices. *Annu. Rev. Public Health* **1**:277–295. [3]

Wennberg, J. E., and M. M. Cooper, eds. 1999. The Quality of Medical Care in the United States: A Report on the Medicare Program. Chicago: American Health Association Press. [16]

Wennberg, J. E., E. S. Fisher, D. C. Goodman, and J. S. Skinner. 2008. Tracking the Care of Patients with Severe Chronic Illness: The Dartmouth Atlas of Health Care 2008. Lebanon, NH: Dartmouth Atlas Project. [8]

Wennberg, J. E., and A. Gittelsohn. 1973. Small area variations in health care delivery. *Science* **182**:1102–1108. [3]

Wennberg, J. E., A. G. Mulley, Jr., D. Hanley, et al. 1988. An assessment of prostatectomy for benign urinary tract obstruction: Geographic variations and the evaluation of medical care outcomes. *JAMA* **259(20)**:3027–3030. [3]

WHCA. 2010. Health literacy, Part 2: Evidence and case studies. Somerset, U.K.: World Health Communication Associates Ltd. http://www.whcaonline.org/publications.html (accessed 28 April 2010). [5]

WHO. 2009a. Patient Safety: A World Alliance for Safer Health Care. Geneva: WHO. [1]

———. 2009b. WHO strategy on research for health. http://www.who.int/rpc/research_strategy/en/ (accessed 15 March 2010). [5]

WHO. 2010. Track 2: Health literacy and health behavior. http://www.who.int/healthpromotion/conferences/7gchp/track2/en/index.html (accessed 23 May 2010). [12]

WHO/HAI. 2009. Understanding and responding to pharmaceutical promotion: A practical guide, 1st ed. Working draft for pilot field testing. World Health Organization, Health Action International Global. http://www.haiweb.org/11062009/drug-promotion-manual-CAP-3-090610.pdf (accessed 31 May 2010). [18]

Wild, C., and B. Piso, eds. 2010. Zahlenspiele in der Medizin. Vienna: Kremayr & Scheriau. [8]

Wilde, J. 2009. PSA screening cuts deaths by 20%, says world's largest prostate cancer study. ERSPC Press Office, Carver Wilde Communications. http://blog.taragana.com/pr/psa-screening-cuts-deaths-by-20-says-worlds-largest-prostate-cancer-study-601/ (accessed 27 April 2010). [2]

Wilf-Miron, R., I. Lewenhoff, Z. Benyamini, and A. Aviram. 2003. From aviation to medicine: Applying concepts of aviation safety to risk management in ambulatory care. *Qual. Saf. Health Care* **12(1)**:35–39. [8]

Wilkes, M. S., R. A. Bell, and R. L. Kravitz. 2000. Direct-to-consumer prescription drug advertising: Trends, impact, and implications. *Health Affairs* **19(2)**:110–128. [18]

Wilksch, S. M., and T. D. Wade. 2009. Reduction of shape and weight concern in young adolescents: A 30-month controlled evaluation of a media literacy program. *J. Am. Acad. Child Adolesc. Psychiatry* **48**:652–661. [13]

Wilson, A., B. Bonevski, A. Jones, and D. Henry. 2009. Media reporting of health interventions: Signs of improvement, but major problems persist. *PLoS ONE* **4**:e4831. [11]

WMA. 2009. Declaration of Helsinki: Ethical principles for medical research involving human subjects. World Medical Association. http://www.wma.net/en/30publications/10policies/b3/index.html (accessed 28 April 2010). [6]

Woloshin, S., and L. M. Schwartz. 2002. Press releases: Translating research into news. *JAMA* **287**:2856–2858. [1, 12]

———. 2009. Numbers needed to decide. *J. Natl. Cancer Inst.* **101(17)**:1163–1165. [2]

Woloshin, S., L. M. Schwartz, and B. S. Kramer. 2009. Promoting healthy skepticism in the news: Helping journalists get it right. *J. Natl. Cancer Inst.* **101**:1596 –1599. [11]

Woloshin, S., L. M. Schwartz, J. Tremmel, and H. G. Welch. 2001. Direct to consumer drug advertisements: What are Americans being sold? *Lancet* **358(9288)**:1141–1146. [14]

Woloshin, S., L. M. Schwartz, and H. G. Welch. 2004. The value of benefit data in direct-to-consumer drug ads. *Health Affairs* **W4**:234–245. [12, 14]

———. 2008. The risk of death by age, sex, and smoking status in the United States: Putting health risks in context. *J. Natl. Cancer Inst.* **100(12)**:845–853. [12]

Wong, N., and T. King. 2008. The cultural construction of risk understandings through illness narratives. *J. Consum. Res.* **34(5)**. [12]

Wormer, H. 2006. Selling science in a soap selling style? *J. Sci. Comm.* **5**:1–2. [11]

———. 2008a. Reviewer oder nur Reporter? Kritik und Kontrolle als künftige Aufgaben des Wissenschaftsjournalismus in der wissenschaftlichen Qualitätssicherung. In: WissensWelten: Wissenschaftsjournalismus in Theorie und Praxis, ed. H. Hettwer et al., pp. 219–238. Gütersloh: Verlag Bertelsmann Stiftung. [11]

———. 2008b. Wie seriös ist Dr. Boisselier? Quellen und Recherchestrategien für Themen aus Wissenschaft und Medizin. In: WissensWelten: Wissenschaftsjournalismus in Theorie und Praxis, ed. H. Hettwer et al., pp. 345–362. Gütersloh: Verlag Bertelsmann Stiftung. [11]

Wübben, M., and F. von Wangenheim. 2008. Instant customer base analysis: Managerial heuristics often "get it right." *J. Marketing* **72**:82–93. [17]

Wynder, E. L., I. T. Higgins, and R. E. Harris. 1990. The wish bias. *J. Clin. Epidemiol.* **43**:619–621. [13]

Young, J. M., P. Glasziou, and J. E. Ward. 2002. General practitioners' self rating of skills in evidence based medicine: A validation study. *BMJ* **324**:950–951. [1, 9]

Young, M. E., G. R. Norman, and K. R. Humphreys. 2008. Medicine in the popular press: The influence of the media on perceptions of disease. *PLoS ONE* **3(10)**:e3552. [13]

Young, N. S., J. P. A. Ioannidis, and O. Al-Ubaydli. 2008. Why current publication practices may distort science. *PLoS Med.* **5(10)**:e201. [16]

Zachry, W. M., III, M. Shepherd, M. Hinich, et al. 2002. Relationship between direct-to-consumer advertising and physician diagnosing and prescribing. *Am. J. Health Syst. Pharm.* **59(1)**:42–49. [18]

Zarcadoolas, C., A. F. Pleasant, and D. S. Greer. 2006. Advancing Health Literacy: A Framework for Understanding and Action. San Francisco: Jossey-Bass. [12]

Zehr, S. C. 1999. Scientists' representations of uncertainty. In: Communicating Uncertainty: Media Coverage of New and Controversial Science, ed. S. M. Friedman et al., pp. 3–21. Mahwah: Lawrence Erlbaum. [11]

Zeleny, J. 2008. Obama weighs quick undoing of Bush policy. *New York Times*, November 9. [19]

Zerhouni, E. 2007. Testimony before the House Subcommittee on Labor-HHS-Education Appropriations. Washington, D.C.: Office of Legislative Policy and Analysis. http://www.nih.gov/about/director/budgetrequest/fy2009directorssenatebudgetrequest.htm (accessed 15 March 2010). [5]

Zhu, L., and G. Gigerenzer. 2006. Children can solve Bayesian problems: The role of representation in mental computation. *Cognition* **98**:287–308. [2]

Zikmund-Fisher, B. J., A. Fagerlin, and P. A. Ubel. 2008. Improving understanding of adjuvant therapy options by using simpler risk graphics. *Cancer Nurs.* **113**:3382–3390. [2]

Zikmund-Fisher, B. J., P. A. Ubel, D. M. Smith, et al. 2008. Communicating side effect risks in a tamoxifen prophylaxis decision aid: The debiasing influence of pictographs. *Patient Educ. Couns.* **73**: 209–214. [2]

Subject Index